Doing Qualitative Research

SECOND EDITION

BENJAMIN F. CRABTREE

WILLIAM L. MILLER

EDITORS

Sage Publications, Inc.
International Educational and Professional Publisher
Thousand Oaks ▪ London ▪ New Delhi

For information:

Sage Publications, Inc.
2455 Teller Road
Thousand Oaks, California 91320
E-mail: order@sagepub.com

Sage Publications Ltd.
6 Bonhill Street
London EC2A 4PU
United Kingdom

Sage Publications India Pvt. Ltd.
M-32 Market
Greater Kailash I
New Delhi 110 048 India

Printed in the United States of America

Library of Congress Cataloging-in-Publication Data

Main entry under title:

   Doing qualitative research, 2nd edition/edited by
Benjamin F. Crabtree and William L. Miller
      p. cm.
   Includes bibliographical references (p.   ) and index.
   ISBN 0-7619-1497-8 (cloth: acid-free paper)
   ISBN 0-7619-1498-6 (pbk: acid-free paper)
      1. Primary care (Medicine)—Research—Methodology.
   2. Social medicine—Research—Methodology. 3. Social sciences—
   Research—Methodology. I. Crabtree, Benjamin F.
   II. Miller, William L. (WilliamLloyd), 1949–
      R853.S64   D65 2000
      362.1′072—dc21   99-6645

      00   01   02   03   10   9   8   7   6   5   4   3   2

Acquiring Editor:	C. Deborah Laughton
Editorial Assistant:	Eileen Carr
Production Editor:	Diana E. Axelsen
Editorial Assistant:	Nevair Kabakian
Typesetter/Designer:	Danielle Dillahunt
Cover Designer:	Ravi Balasuriya

Contents

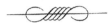

Part III Interpretation: Strategies of Analysis

Part IV Special Designs

Part V Putting It All Together

Part VI Summary

Acknowledgments

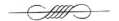

Eight years ago, we put together the first edition of this book. We were flushed with the enthusiasm of our colleagues and the new possibilities for primary care research. That book far exceeded our expectations and has opened many opportunities to meet others and to explore those possibilities. Thank you, Moira Stewart and fellow editors of the Primary Care Research Series and the publishers at Sage, for encouraging and supporting our dream. The many enriching dialogues and research adventures that were stimulated by that first edition humbly remind us that what we label as ours is only the individual voicing of a community of discourse. We express deep thanks to all the devoted and courageous kindred spirits who have participated in this community.

We especially want to use this opportunity to gratefully acknowledge several of the people who significantly influenced and supported our emotional and intellectual development at fragile moments in our growth. Dr. David Evans at Wake Forest University was a patient and creative shepherd for Will during his undergraduate and graduate school years. J. Jerome Smith of the University of South Florida and Pertti Pelto of the University of Connecticut served similar roles for Ben. Will's first adventures into family practice were nurtured by his practice partners, Mike Abgott, Dale Grove, and his dad—Warren Miller. In 1985, the late David Schmidt, MD, brought us together at the Department of Family Medicine, University of Connecticut, where, along with our remarkable colleagues and Director of Research, Patrick O'Connor, we began exploring the exciting opportunities of collaborative, multi-method primary care research. A special thanks to all of you for your friendship and support.

The authors of the chapters in this volume represent many of the core people who make up our community of discourse, support, and friendship. We are profoundly grateful for their insights and collaboration. We also thank Susie Sullivan at the University of Nebraska who worked so diligently getting the final drafts and references together for this second edition.

At the heart of creative abundance rests the mysterious and gracious nest of kith and kin. Our families are the deep wells from which we draw our water and to which our energies and love return. We offer our profound thanks to our wives, Eiko Crabtree and Deb Miller, and to our children, Martin, Mari, and Christina Crabtree and Ethan and Lindsay Miller. Being home together is the real garden of love and delight. Thanks everyone!

Introduction

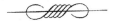

Puzzles and troubles abound. They keep disturbing the waters in which we live. These disturbances are the reason for the craft of primary health care, and the rough waters around that craft are the source of our clinical research questions. A flustered young practitioner ponders, "What is going on with the many women I see who have medically unexplained symptoms? Why do they keep coming back?" A 45-year-old woman with undiagnosed fatigue and pain stares incredulously at her younger physician and wonders, "How did this doctor learn to practice? How did he get this way?" Both patient and clinician are troubled and search for ways to discover, "What is going on here? How can I make sense of it? How could it be better?" These common primary care questions call for research approaches that preserve the complexity, storminess, and wealth of the lived experiences from which the questions arise. This book introduces strategies of inquiry using qualitative research methods that are essential for exploring these kinds of questions.

The seascape of primary care is illustrated in Figure I.1. The questions that put our research vessels into the water and the knowledges and relationships that inform and are informed by these questions are localizable on this ecological-transactional systemic map (ETS map). This map depicts a nested web of relationships where no aspect can be fully understood without accounting for the whole. Bringing qualitative methods and new paradigms of inquiry to the questions that arise from within this web greatly enhances our prospects for better, more helpful answers. The studies used to illustrate the qualitative methods described in this book touch on most of the spaces and connections on the map.

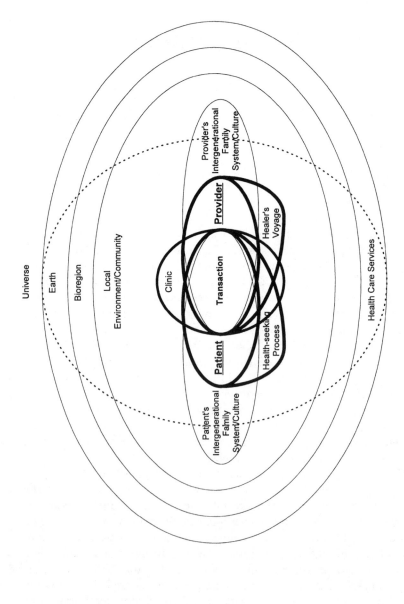

Figure I.1. The Ecological-Transactional Systemic Map of Primary Care

What goes on when primary care practitioners and patients meet in the clinical encounter or transaction? Virginia Elderkin-Thompson and Howard Waitzkin (Chapter 13) explore the use of videotapes as a means of understanding what happens when patients with somatization disorder are with their doctors. Kirsti Malterud (Chapter 17) demonstrates how to do research while seeing patients as she describes the discovery of a better way of caring with women who present with medically unexplained symptoms.

What goes on in the clinic? How does it facilitate and/or impede the process of care? How is it organized? Ben Crabtree and Will Miller (Chapter 16) present the story of answering these questions using a series of case studies that range over a 5-year period. Virginia Aita and Helen McIlvain (Chapter 14) provide more details on the case study methods used.

How do patients get to the clinic? How can health-seeking behavior be understood? Similarly, how do primary care practitioners become what they are? What goes on in the healer's voyage? Judy Brown (Chapter 6) describes the use of focus groups to help explain why patients choose to keep coming to a family practice teaching clinic. Meanwhile, Steve Bogdewic (Chapter 3) and Ritch Addison (Chapter 8) investigate the residency training experience of family physicians and illustrate, respectively, the use of participant observation and the details of interpretation with emphasis on an editing style. Jessica Muller (Chapter 12) demonstrates the use of narrative analysis to help explain how physicians in training learn to tell clinical stories through having their presentation of a patient's case restoried by their teaching attending.

What is the experience of being a primary care practitioner? How do these practitioners' lives affect their craft? How do patients' lives affect their health care decisions and experience? Will Miller and Ben Crabtree (Chapter 5) describe how to use depth interviews to explore the personal experiences and meanings of pain for family physicians and their patients. Ben and Will (Chapter 9) also discuss how Dennis Willms uses code books to help analyze his interview data about the meanings of smoking for patients in a randomized clinical trial of smoking cessation.

What are community-level health issues? What are the health care concerns at a regional level? What is going on with health care services across multiple levels and sectors of care? Valerie Gilchrist and Rob Williams (Chapter 4) give an overview of the use of key informant networks to help do time- and cost-effective community health assessment. Lynn Meadows and Diane Dodendorf (Chapter 11) walk us through the use of computer software for analyzing qualitative data about the health concerns of women 40 to 65 years old living in Alberta, Canada. The health care services question is addressed by Janecke Thesen and Anton Kuzel

(Chapter 15), who demonstrate the use of participatory research strategies for helping improve the delivery of mental health services in Norway.

The overall goals of the second edition of this book remain the same. They are to stimulate continued interest in qualitative research methods and to prepare readers for doing it. The intent is to expand existing research approaches, ways of knowing, and types of research relationships. Primary care research asks questions at multiple system levels: from global, to community, to family, to individual, to organ, to cell, to genome, to recursive interaction between and among these levels (see Figure I.1). The complex substance of primary care research is multilayered, configurational, holistic, particularistic, probabilistic, often ambiguous and complex, and wonderfully mysterious. Primary care's significance connects at the macro level with generalizations about health and healing and at the micro level with specific primary health care activities, revealing their interpretive uncertainties and value-based decisions. Given these substances and significances and the range of primary care research, a multimethod approach is called for (Brewer & Hunter, 1989; Coward, 1990; Houts, Cook, & Shadish, 1986; Light & Pillemer, 1982; McWhinney, 1991; Miller & Crabtree, 1994a; Stange, Miller, Crabtree, O'Connor, & Zyzanski, 1994; Tudiver, Cushman, & Crabtree, 1991). Primary care practitioners blend their intersubjective, longitudinal understandings of patients with their experimentally based knowledge of pathophysiology and their statistical understanding of risks and benefits. So, too, primary care researchers need to use a multimethod approach.

Multimethods aren't enough. Different ways of knowing and of relating are also needed. The ETS map in Figure I.1 is best understood in four dimensions. The flat dimensions of place are evident, but the reader should also visualize a dimension of depth where hierarchies of power are evident and then see the whole model spinning through time. These four dimensions correspond to four practical questions: (a) What are the numbers? (numeracy); (b) What do the words mean? (literacy); (c) Who benefits? (policy); and (d) What else? What are the consequences? Where do the ripples go? (ecolacy) (adapted from Hardin, 1985). Our ways of knowing must be open to all these questions. We need to view the world from many points of view.

The basic science of primary care has barely started. Most of the research knowledge in primary care is based on the assumptions and taxonomies of specialized biomedicine. For example, patients often present to primary care offices with emotional distress. There is almost no basic research on how that comes about and what happens. When do patients go to the doctor because of emotional distress? How do clinicians recognize it? What keeps emotional distress suppressed in the clinical encounter and what helps it surface? We don't know. However, there is a lot of primary care research on mental health. The problem is that it starts with *DSM-IV* diagnostic categories, derived from specialized psychiatry studies. What about all the people who don't fit the diagnostic criteria but are still quite emotionally upset? The historical reasons for this are another book, but one critical issue is the tendency for clinicians and clinical researchers to ignore culture and theory, to confuse the diagnostic category with reality.

Culture is how all humans make sense of the world. Culture is a complex set of learned categories and associated plans; it is the entire socially transmitted inheritance; it is the mental map or model of our landscape and how we understand and navigate it. Thus diagnoses are a cultural model that help us make sense of and intervene with certain experiences and observations. But there is and always will be more to reality than our constructs can account for, and there will always be alternative ways for categorizing and perceiving the same reality. What makes one cultural viewpoint preferable to another is a question of values and goals. It depends on the valued goal(s) by which the cultures are being compared. Theory is, simply, an explicit formalization of some cultural category or construct. Most of us are, usually, unaware of our culture and how it limits and directs our activities and imaginations. Clinicians have, we believe, ignored theory because they believe they are dealing directly with reality. Blood is blood and diabetes is diabetes. You don't need theory if you have Truth. Unfortunately, we don't and won't have Truth. We readily acknowledge the existence of real blood, but we can only see it, talk about it, and relate to it as we have learned from our culture. There is still more to blood than I can imagine. There will always be a cultural filter between us and reality.

The goal becomes one of ever expanding one's cultural horizons. That is the purpose of science. Science is a cultural activity, a powerful myth, that we impose on reality; it is a web for catching prejudices (Reilly, 1995). Qualitative research is a critical addition to this science, especially with the emphasis on theory development, reflexivity, and iteration. Qualitative research restores the importance of theory and culture to our work. It also reminds us of the inherent role of the observer in the observed, the impossibility of eliminating investigator bias. Qualitative traditions have devoted considerable attention to ways of incorporating and accounting for the researcher's self in the research process—an issue referred to as *reflexivity*. This may be a new, jargonesque word for primary care researchers, but it represents familiar ground for primary care clinicians. As practitioners, we have always known how to use our own feelings and reactions in clinical encounters to help us in working with patients. We have also been aware of how our own past experiences and patterns of relating can unconsciously get in the way of our clinical work with patients. This latter observation is the basis for Balint group work (Balint, 1957). These are all clinical examples of reflexivity. All of the chapters in this book

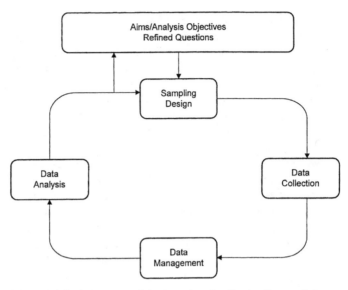

Figure I.2. Simplified Diagram of the Iterative Qualitative Research Process

address reflexivity as it relates to the topic of interest. Reflexivity is fundamental to successful qualitative research.

The simplified dynamics of the qualitative research process are illustrated in Figure I.2. Two features distinguish this process from traditional epidemiologic research design. First, no prepackaged designs exist from which to choose. Rather, multiple, specific sampling, data collection, data management, and data analysis options exist from which to select. Almost any mix and match is possible and depends on the aims, objectives, and research question. The second distinguishing feature is the iterative, cyclical nature of the process. Gathering and interpreting usually occur concurrently. Initial analysis changes sampling strategies and collection methods. Qualitative data management methods must be flexible enough to allow for these ongoing adjustments.

The organization of this book follows the structure of the above qualitative research process. This second edition represents a significant expansion from the first, covers more collection methods, and gives much more detail on the interpretive process. Chapter 1 provides an overview of how to decide what methods to use, based on aims, objectives, questions, and paradigms of knowing. Part II explores in more detail the qualitative gathering process. Chapter 2 highlights sampling issues and options. Chapters 3, 4, 5, and 6 describe the discovery strategies of participant observation, key informant interviewing, depth interviews, and focus groups. Each was chosen as a commonly used example of more general approaches. For example, key informant interviews represent one type of long-term interview relationship, whereas depth interviews and focus groups are examples, respectively, of individual and group interviews. Part III looks at interpretation and data management. Chapter 7 provides a general description of the interpretive process. This is followed in Chapters 8, 9, and 10 by detailed descriptions of actual analyses, using different analysis organizing styles. Chapter 11 gives an overview of the use of computer software for qualitative data management and demonstrates in detail the use of two particular programs, NUD*IST and Folio Views.

Part IV, represented by chapters 12 through 15, reveals the specifics of doing special qualitative designs that we believe have particular relevance to primary care research. These include the use of stories and narrative, videotape studies, case studies, and participatory research strategies. In Part V, we put the whole process together by stepping through the stories and design decisions involved in two completed qualitative investigations. Chapter 16 presents a complex, practice-based case study design requiring a large collaborative team and much money. Chapter 17 discusses a participatory, practice-based study with only one researcher and little money. Chapter 18 summarizes our present understandings concerning standards in qualitative research. Chapter 19 is more reflective and looks at the role of qualitative research in the future of primary care research.

The authors in this book effectively model the essential ingredients in writing up qualitative research (Richardson, 1990; Wolcott, 1990). These gifted researchers, many of whom are also clinicians, define their topic; reveal themselves and the context of their discussion; define the key themes and processes; provide thick, interesting, descriptive examples; explore theory; recognize the importance of culture; and share their excitement of discovery. Let's head for the sea!

Benjamin F. Crabtree
William L. Miller

PART
I

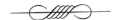

Overview of
Qualitative
Research Methods

1

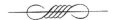

Clinical Research

A Multimethod Typology
and Qualitative Roadmap

William L. Miller
Benjamin J. Crabtree

W elcome to the excitement, diversity, and possibilities of clinical research. Welcome to a journey of adventure. This chapter presents a roadmap of research methods to facilitate the development of a multi-method approach to this adventure, with emphasis on qualitative strategies. Five styles of inquiry are briefly identified and described. Research aims and analysis goals are then matched with these styles. The research styles are also connected to three different paradigms, and this information is all used to describe the process of choosing an appropriate style of inquiry and method for a particular research interest. This chapter elaborates a typology of qualitative methods and specific strategies of inquiry and gives overviews of how to develop appropriate qualitative research designs.

A MULTIMETHOD RESEARCH TYPOLOGY

Doing research is, in many ways, like taking a descriptive and explanatory snapshot of empirical reality. For each particular photograph, the investigator must decide what kind of camera to use, what scene on which to focus, through which filter, and with what intent. At least five styles of inquiry are distinguishable, based on the primary camera, focus, filter, and

TABLE 1.1 Characteristics of Different Research Styles

	Research Styles				
Characteristics of Style	*Experiment*	*Survey*	*Documentary-Historical*	*Field*	*Philosophic*
Camera	Laboratory	Instrument	Multimethod	Researcher	Thinker
Scene of focus	Causal hypothesis	Probability sample	Artifacts	Human field	Ideal concept
Filter	Quantitative	Quantitative	Qualitative/ quantitative	Qualitative	Logic
Intent	Test causal hypothesis	Generalize to population	Description/ explanation/ prediction of nonreactive data	Holistic, realistic description/ explanation	Establish underlying principles

intent: experimental, survey, documentary-historical, field, and philosophic (see Table 1.1).

Experimental researchers create study designs that test carefully constructed causal hypotheses. The laboratory is the camera used to focus the experiment's lens on the causal hypothesis. The laboratory, whether in a building, in the field of human activity or an ecological habitat, or in a computer simulation, is where the variable of interest is *actively* and measurably *manipulated* in tightly controlled conditions. The researcher doing the experiment wears quantitative filters that selectively gaze with accurate, measurable precision. The experimental style includes the many types of experimental designs and randomized controlled trial designs.

The *survey* style of inquiry, on the other hand, focuses on a representative probability sample from a defined population by means of a research instrument, such as a structured interview, observational rating scale, or questionnaire, with the intent of generalizing the resultant descriptions and/or associations to the larger population. *Survey* is used here in the broad sense intended by the social science traditions (Babbie, 1979; Last, 1983; Lin, 1976). The epidemiologist's understanding of *survey* as cross-sectional research (Mausner & Kramer, 1985) is here understood as one example of a more encompassing survey research style. As with the experimental style, the filter and form of expression are quantitative and statistical, with emphasis on validity and reliability. Unlike the experimental style, survey research involves *passive manipulation* of the variable of interest. The observational designs of epidemiology, such as cohort, cross sectional, and case control, are examples of the survey style. Other survey designs include descriptive surveys; correlational, longitudinal, and comparative survey designs; time series designs; theory-testing correlational surveys; ex post facto designs; and quasiexperimental designs. Burkett (1990) and Marvel, Staehling, and Hendricks (1991) have presented useful typologies for organizing the survey and experimental styles of research.

The common denominator of the *documentary-historical* style is a focus on artifacts, material culture. This style is an eclectic assortment of cameras and filters. The researcher using this style gazes at an artifact through the camera and filter most appropriate for the intent. The artifacts can be archives, literature, medical records, instruments, art, clothes, or data tapes from someone else's research. Examples of documentary-historical re-search include literature review, artifact analysis, chart audits, archive analysis, historical research, secondary analysis, and meta-analysis.

The *field* researcher is personally engaged in an interpretive focus on a natural, often human, field of activity, with the goal of generating holistic and realistic descriptions and/or explanations. The field is viewed through the experientially engaged and perceptually limited lens of the researcher using a qualitative filter. *Field research is often called qualitative research.* Unlike the previously discussed research styles, field research has no prepackaged research designs. Rather, specific data collection methods, sampling procedures, and interpretive strategies are used to create unique, question-specific designs that evolve throughout the research process. These qualitative or field designs take the form of either a case study or a topical study. Case studies (Hamel, Dufour, & Fortin, 1993; Merriam, 1988; Yin, 1994) examine most or all the potential aspects of a particular distinctly bounded unit or case (or series of cases). A case can be an individual, a family, a community health center, a nursing home, a habitat or neighborhood, or an organization. Topical studies investigate only one or a few selected spheres of activity within a less distinctly bounded field, such as a study of the meaning of pain for selected persons in a community.

Lastly, there is *philosophic* inquiry, which often serves as a generator and clarifier for the other research styles. The philosophical inquirer uses analytic skills as thinker to examine an idea or concept through the filter of logic to move toward clarity and the illumination of background conditions. Philosophic inquiry often proceeds as a thought "experiment" and is frequently based on a single case or even a hypothetical case with no empirical evidence.

Research Aims

The choice of research style for a particular project depends upon the overarching aim of the research, the specific analysis goal and its associated research question, the preferred paradigm, the degree of desired research control, the level of investigator intervention, the available resources, the time frame, and aesthetics (Brewer & Hunter, 1989; Diers, 1979). There are at least five aims of scientific inquiry: identification, description, explanation-generation, explanation-testing, and control. The first three of these comprise what is often termed *exploratory research*. Qualitative methods are usually used for identification, description, and explanation-generation; quantitative methods are most commonly used for explanation-testing and control. These general guidelines have many exceptions, depending on the specific analysis goal (see Table 1.2).

The aim of *identification* is one of the most neglected aspects of scientific inquiry. All too often, investigators create concepts based on some "gut" feeling, their own reasoning, or the literature. They then produce measurement instruments that reify the concept, giving the appearance that it really exists "out there." The result may be research that is powerful (minimal Type 2 error) and minimizes false positives (Type 1 error) but may also be solving the wrong problem (Type 3 error) or solving a problem not worth solving (Type 4 error). Qualitative field research, the documentary-historical style, and philosophic inquiry are ideally suited for the essential task of identification.

At least three types of *description* are distinguishable—qualitative, quantitative, and normative. Qualitative description, using qualitative methods, explores the meanings, variations, and perceptual experiences of phenomena and will often seek to capture their holistic or interconnected nature. Quantitative description, based in descriptive statistics, refers to the distribution, frequency, prevalence, incidence, and size of one or more phenomena. Normative description seeks to establish the norms and values of phenomena (O'Connor, 1990). The choice of quantitative or qualitative methods depends on how one wishes to understand and characterize the norms of interest.

Explanation-generation/association can have at least three analytic goals—interpretive explanation-generation, statistical explanation-generation, and deductive explanation. Some research seeks to discover relationships, associations, and patterns based on personal experience of the phenomena under question. This interpretive explanation-generation is best achieved using research styles with a qualitative filter such as field and documentary-historical styles. When concepts have already been identified, described, and interpretively defined, another objective is to explore possible statistical relationships using quantitatively based styles of research. Another analytic goal is to deductively generate explanations from a set of given premises. This purpose is best met using philosophic inquiry.

Explanation-testing/prediction includes both goals or intents of confirming causality and testing theory. One form of causal confirmation is to establish predictability, and another is to definitively demonstrate causality using experimental research design. Another analysis goal is to test

TABLE 1.2 Research Aims, Analysis Objectives, Research Questions, and Appropriate Research Styles

Aim	Analysis Objective	Research Question	Research Style
Identification	Identify/name	What is this? Who is that? What is important here?	Field, doc-hist, philos
Description	Qualitative description	What is going on here? What is the nature of the phenomenon? What are the dimensions of the concept? What variations exist? What meanings/practices occur in lived experiences?	Field, doc-hist, philos
	Quantitative description	How many? How much? How often? What size? How is the phenomenon distributed over space?	Survey
	Normative description	What is the value of a phenomenon?	Field, doc-hist, survey, philos
Explanation			
Generation/ association	Interpretive, explanation, generation	What is happening here? What patterns exist? How do phenomena differ and relate to each other? How does it work? How did something occur/happen?	Field, doc-hist
	Statistical, explanation, generation	What are the measurable associations between phenomena? Does variable x relate to other variables? Why does it work? Why did something occur?	Doc-hist, survey
	Deductive, explanation	Given these premises, then _____?	Philos
Explanation			
Testing/ prediction	Causal confirmation	What will happen if ___? If ___ then ___? Does one variable cause the other?	Exper
	Theory testing	Is the original theory correct? Does the original theory fit other circumstances? Are there additional categories or relationships?	Field, doc-hist, survey, exper
Intervention/ control	Prescription testing	Is ___ more effective than ___? Does ___ have greater efficacy than ___?	Exper (RCT)
	Evaluation	How can I make "x" happen? What difference does this program/intervention make?	Field, survey

NOTE: Doc-hist = documentary-historical; exper = experiment; philos = philosophical; RCT = randomized control trial.

explanatory theory by evaluating it in different contexts. The research style used to meet this intent depends on the type of explanation being tested but may often involve field strategies, especially when the theory concerns systems and/or holistic understandings.

Intervention/control is an important aim for many clinical researchers—the testing and/or evaluation of some prescription or intervention, either intentional or natural, and associated responses. One analysis goal is to test an intervention in such a way that either its efficacy or its effectiveness can be generalized to other similar situations. This is the raison d'être for the randomized control trial (RCT). At other times, the analysis goal is to evaluate an intervention in a specific context, with no immediate expectation for generalization. Qualitative evaluation strategies are especially useful for this purpose (Chelimsky & Shadish, 1997; Patton, 1990), as well as for discovering or tracking the systemic consequences of changes or interventions. When participants are actively included in the evaluative process, field research strategies are again most helpful (Fetterman, Kaftarian, & Wandersman, 1996).

Paradigms

A paradigm represents a patterned set of assumptions concerning reality (ontology), knowledge of that reality (epistemology), and the particular ways of knowing about that reality (methodology) (Guba, 1990). These assumptions and the ways of knowing are untested givens and determine how one engages and comes to understand the world. Each investigator must decide what assumptions are acceptable and appropriate for the topic of interest and then use methods consistent with the selected paradigm. There are at least three paradigms (Habermas, 1968).

First is that knowledge that helps humans maintain physical life, our labor and technology. This is most commonly represented by positivism, the culture of biomedicine, and its associated biomedical model. Wet-lab science and quantitative methods primarily inform this knowledge, referred to here as *materialistic inquiry* (Figure 1.1). This paradigm can be metaphorically understood as "Jacob's Ladder." The materialist inquirer values progress, stresses the primacy of method, seeks an ultimate truth—a natural law—of reality, and is grounded in Western, monotheistic tradition. Materialistic inquiry is best for social engineering and its need for control and predictability. It emphasizes rationality and, within the realm of health care, strives toward the elimination of disease and the achievement of immortality (Schwartz, 1998). If one wants to understand the molecular genetics of hyperlipidemia or to develop a new drug, then this is the paradigm of choice. The materialist inquirer climbs a linear ladder to an ultimate objective truth. Most researchers using materialistic inquiry now

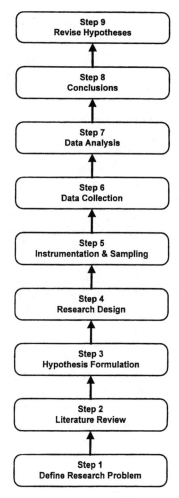

Figure 1.1. Diagram of Materialistic Inquiry

refer to their use of a postpositivist paradigm that has expanded to accept multiple constructed realities and the impact of the observer on that which is observed. The postpositivist perspective seeks successive approximations to reality but understands the unlikelihood of getting to ultimate reality.

A second paradigm is based on that knowledge that helps humans maintain cultural life, symbolic communication, and meaning, and it is referred to here as *constructivist inquiry*. This paradigm has also been called "naturalistic inquiry" (Kuzel, 1986) and "interpretivist thinking" or interpretive inquiry (Gadamer, 1976; Guba & Lincoln, 1989). We acknowledge that the choice of *constructivist* glosses over some intense debates. "Constructivists" claim that truth is the result of perspective; it is relative. There is no objective knowledge (Gergen, 1986; Goodman, 1984). "Interpretivists" trace their roots back to phenomenology (Schutz, 1967) and hermeneutics (Heidegger, 1927/1962). This tradition also recognizes the importance of the subjective human creation of meaning but doesn't reject outright some notion of objectivity. Pluralism, not relativism, is stressed, with focus on the circular dynamic tension of subject and object (Denzin, 1989b; Geertz, 1983). Although we take the more pluralistic approach, *constructivist inquiry* is the term selected because it is human constructions being studied and because it is constructions that the researcher is cocreating with the texts. This paradigm overtly acknowledges and builds upon the premise of the social construction of reality (Berger & Luckmann, 1967; Searle, 1995). We also believe the use of the word *interpretive* may be confusing, as it also refers to the methods-related task of analysis in field research. We believe it is important to keep paradigm choice and method choices separate. Qualitative methods generally inform constructivist knowledge (Figure 1.2), which can be depicted by the metaphor of "Shiva's Circle." Shiva is the Hindu Lord of the Dance and of Death. A constructivist inquirer enters an interpretive circle and must be faithful to the performance or subject, must be both apart from and part of the dance, and must always be rooted to the context. There is no ultimate truth; there are context-bound constructions that are all part of the larger universe of stories. Constructivist inquiry is best for storytelling. If one wants to understand how patients and clinicians experience pain or being informed that their cholesterol is high, then this is the paradigm of choice. The constructivist inquirer enters into Shiva's Circle, performing an ongoing iterative dance of discovery and interpretation.

A third knowledge, that which helps humans maintain social life, focuses on the reality of domination, distribution of power, associated inequalities, and ecological context and issues of sustainability (Bateson, 1979; Fay, 1987). It is referred to here as *critical/ecological inquiry*. This is the "global eye" that critically looks in at both dancers and ladder climbers and gazes at the systemic effects (Figure 1.3). The critical/ecological inquirer seeks to move from the false consciousness of present experience and ideology to a more empowered and emancipated consciousness that incorporates social justice issues and ecology by reducing the illusions through the processes of historical review and the juxtapositioning of materialistic and interpretive inquiry. Critical/ecological inquiry is best for political engagement and the study of systems. Participatory strategies of inquiry, most often using qualitative methods, are seeded and nurtured by this paradigm. Present variations on this paradigm include feminist, ethnic, and cultural studies paradigms (Denzin & Lincoln, 1994; Lather, 1991). In addition, recent

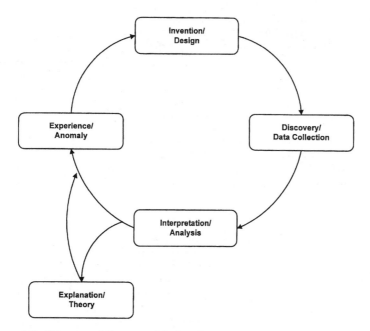

Figure 1.2. Diagram of Constructivist Inquiry

developments in the area of environmental studies and the philosophy of deep ecology (Abram, 1996; Bowers, 1997; Sessions, 1995) suggest the need to purge this paradigm of its modernist roots (i.e., individualism, anthropocentrism or humanism, belief in progress, dualism) and expand to include the larger animate and inanimate world on which human life and health depends.

It is important to remember that no particular paradigm has a final grasp on truth. The choice is most often based on the research aim and personal moral preference.

Choosing a Research Style

The determination and articulation of the research aim, analysis goal, specific research question, and appropriate mode of engagement or paradigm all shape the choice of research style. Additional factors may also influence this decision and include time frame, degree of desired researcher control, and aesthetics. For example, historical and retrospective designs are better for investigating past events. The experimental style of research is suitable if the researcher desires a high degree of control over the variables of interest. Aesthetics plays a role in the sense that each researcher

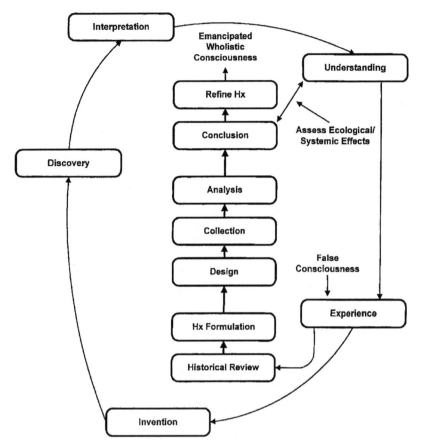

Figure 1.3. Diagram of Critical Ecological Inquiry
NOTE: Hx = history.

possesses a unique set of skills, gifts, and sensibilities that resonate better with certain styles of inquiry and/or paradigms. Research is a way to celebrate these differences. Four examples from upcoming chapters illustrate the process of choosing a research style.

The research team at McMaster University in Ontario aims to find better ways to help patients stop smoking. They specifically want to know whether the use of nicotine tobacco replacement and a simple office-based counseling strategy are efficacious interventions for this purpose. This is the analysis goal of testing an intervention, and so an experimental, randomized control design is selected. But the design does not end there.

The research team also recognizes that much is still poorly understood as to why people keep smoking or decide to stop; thus they also want to include a means for interpretive explanation-generation and include a qualitative style of inquiry as part of the larger multimethod research design. This is briefly described in Chapter 9. The field part of the study is conducted independently from the RCT because they each operate within a different paradigm. The RCT is based in classical materialistic inquiry (Wilson et al., 1988), whereas the field study of Willms uses constructivist inquiry because of his particular interest in personal meaning (Willms, Allan, et al., 1991).

Another research team, this time based in Cleveland, Ohio, aims to understand what facilitates or promotes the delivery of preventive health services in family practice offices. This is an explanation-generation aim. The specific analysis goals are to discover relationships, patterns, and statistical associations and to identify what might be happening, especially at an organizational level. These are issues of identification, interpretive explanation-generation, and statistical explanation-generation. As a result, multiple methods are selected. A survey style is used and includes chart audits and detailed observer rating scales. A field style is also selected to help with the identification and interpretive explanation-generation goals (see Chapter 9, this volume; study by Crabtree, Miller, Aita, Flocke, & Stange, 1998). The mode of engagement is essentially through materialistic inquiry, with a postpositivist slant. This choice of paradigm is based on the greater dominance of the survey methods and the long-term aim of developing interventions of control.

Crabtree and his research team in Omaha, Nebraska, also aim to better understand what is going on inside the black box of family practices relative to delivery of preventive health services. However, they are also interested in further exploring and testing a new complexity model for explaining family practices as complex systems. In other words, they seek both interpretive explanation-generation and testing theory. Because the theory being tested is systemic, a field research style based in the critical/ecological paradigm is preferred. This study is described in some detail in Chapter 16.

Kirsti Malterud is a family physician from Norway troubled by the many women patients presenting to her care with medically unexplained problems. Her research aim is to untangle this complex bundle, to help her past her feelings of helplessness, and to find new strategies for working with these patients. She is seeking emancipation; thus her mode of engagement is critical/ecological inquiry, with a participatory, feminist slant. Her specific analysis goal is to better understand the different communication styles used by the patients and herself, which is interpretive explanation-generation. A field research style of inquiry is chosen and described in Chapter 17.

The specific choice of qualitative research designs for these four multimethod and field research projects is described later in the chapter. First, we will present a typology of qualitative methods.

QUALITATIVE METHODS:
A PRIMARY CARE ROADMAP

The quest for a useful organizational map of qualitative methods is not unlike the quest for the Holy Grail. The methods derive from multiple disciplines and from at least 30 or more diverse traditions, each with its own particular language. Despite this tangled web, at least two paths to organizing qualitative methods are discernible. One approach, presented in the appendix at the end of this chapter, organizes qualitative methods on the basis of disciplinary traditions. The resulting typology enables investigators to know "who to call" at their nearby university for methods advice. The approach in the remainder of this chapter focuses on specific methods of data collection for the gathering process and on approaches to the interpretive process and offers a pragmatic perspective on how to design a qualitative or field research project.

The field research style seeks "truth from the natives in their habitat by *looking* and *listening*" (Peacock, 1986, p. 49) and by engaging. This simple statement captures the essence for a pragmatic typology of qualitative methods. Field data is collected by *observation* or *interview*. These observations or interviews usually involve the researcher being engaged with the field in some active manner. The interpretation of the resulting textual data is a subjective/objective iterative dance toward contextual truth, with three prototypical organizing styles from which to develop an analysis strategy. These organizing styles are referred to here as *template, editing,* and *immersion/crystallization*.

A field research design begins and ends with the *reflexivity process*. Reflexivity refers to self-reflection, self-criticism, and is based on the premise that the engaged field researcher is an active part of the setting, relationships, and interpretations (Altheide & Johnson, 1994). Knowing yourself and how you affect and are changed by the research enterprise are central to field research and, ideally, occur throughout the research process. Reflexivity is the first step in *describing* the research enterprise. This includes explicitly stating the research question and its aims and analysis goals, acknowledging the paradigmatic assumptions, putting together the research team and doing any necessary training, initiating the process of reflexivity, defining possible audiences for the final report, choosing and bounding the field, and selecting initial specific sampling strategies, data collection techniques, and an analytic organizing style. These latter three are chosen to maximize initial understanding of the research question and its aims and goals. Data collection and sampling are a blended activity. This is so not only because sampling determines what data is collected, but because sampling decisions frequently occur in the field as opportunities arise.

Once initial describing is done, *sampling/collecting* and *analyzing* begin almost concurrently. Analysis is a process involving the three core phases of organizing, connecting, and corroborating/legitimating. The analysis of this first phase of the research guides future decisions concerning sampling/collecting and analyzing. Analysis is actually just part of the larger five-phase iterative interpretive process, which begins its spiral with describing, includes the three phases of analysis, and ends with *representing the account* before resuming the iterative spiral again. Thus, interpretation actually begins in the beginning; when you leap into the circles of interpretation, there is no beginning. This evolving iterative process of describing-sampling/collecting-analysis-representing the account-describing-sampling/collecting is central to the field research process (see Figure 1.4). Connecting all of these phases are data management strategies, which is where the computer becomes most helpful (see Chapter 11). A basic understanding of information-rich sampling, data collection techniques, the interpretive process and organizing styles for analysis, and iterative procedures enables one to design and implement a qualitative study around a clinical research question.

Sampling/Collecting

All data collection derives from sampling decisions. Some of these are made with careful deliberation by the research team, but many others occur on the spur of the moment in the field. Anton Kuzel, in Chapter 2, reviews the many information-rich sampling strategies available and how to think about their use. Table 1.3 lists qualitative data collection techniques. *Observation* is the most available but probably the most time intensive and demanding of the collection techniques (Chapter 3). There are two continua for understanding types of observation. One refers to the degree of researcher participation in the scene being observed. The other refers to the degree of structure in the observations themselves (Patton, 1990). The observer is always a participant in the observation, but there is a great difference between being a quiet note taker staying in the *background* as much as possible (e.g., in the corner of a pharmacy), and keeping notes as a fully *participant* primary care practitioner during the course of one's duties.

The other continuum for understanding observation types refers to the *degree of structure* in the observations themselves. Any scientific observer must have a familiarity with the setting, participants, and activities, along

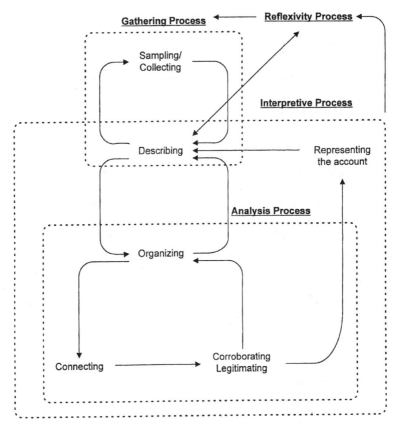

Figure 1.4. Qualitative Research Process

with a set of questions concerning these, prior to initiating observation. Contrast the situations of (a) the researcher who observes a family's first 2 days at home with a newborn to examine how the family members interact and adapt with (b) the researcher who visits the home with a checklist of mother-infant bonding behaviors. In either case, observation data are usually collected in the form of field notes but can also consist of maps and scales.

Ideally, the research question and goal determine which type of observation is most appropriate; however, this is often influenced by available funds, time, and ability and predilection of the researcher. If the goal is to understand the experience of becoming a physician (as in Chapter 8),

TABLE 1.3 Qualitative Data Gathering Techniques

Observation
    Unstructured
    Structured (direct)
        Mapping
        Category systems
        Checklists
        Rating scales
    Participant
    Recordings
        Audio
        Visual
        Audiovisual
    Self
        Diaries
        Journals
Interviewing
    Unstructured
        Everyday conversation
        Key informant
    Semistructured (Interview guide)
        Depth/focused
            Individual (depth)
            Group (focus group)
        Life history (biography)
        Oral history
        Critical incidents techniques
        Free listing
        Ethnoscience interview
        Projective techniques
        Diagram-directed techniques
            Genogram
            Ecomap
            Life space
    Structured (interview schedule)
        Pile sorts/triad comparisons (Q-sorts)
        Rank-order methods
            Paired comparisons
            Balanced incomplete block design
        Surveys/questionnaires
Material culture
    Archives/documents
    Cultural products
        Physical artifacts
        Music/art/dance
        Film/fiction/folktales/games/jokes

unstructured participant observation is highly desirable. If, on the other hand, the goal is to evaluate the hypothetical rules for being a "good intern," then *structured participant observation* facilitates the investigator's acting on the rules and observing what happens. The investigator may, however, only wish to see if residents do physical exams the way attending physicians think they should. *Structured background observation,* using a rating scale, is suitable for this question. If the goal is to understand how nurses and resident physicians communicate with each other about patients in pain, *unstructured background observation* is an acceptable initial approach because there is less known about this question and there is no preexisting "expert" consensus (see Chapters 9 and 16 for examples of some of these methods).

There are two other variations on observation. One is the use of *recordings* of conversations and events. These are becoming technically easier and more common with the advance of recording technology. The decision of whether to use an *audio* recorder or a *video* recorder depends on the question of interest and the unit of analysis (see Chapter 13). A second observation consists of those formally done by research participants through the use of *diaries, journals,* and *autobiographies.* These, too, can range from structured food-intake diaries to highly unstructured journals of dreams.

Types of *interviewing* are distinguished by exploring four dimensions that answer the questions "who," "how," "what," and "when." "Who" refers both to whether one interviews an *individual* or a *group* and to the *role context of the interviewer.* The difference between interviewing an individual or a group appears obvious, but it is often ignored in ways similar to the ecological fallacy in statistics. When a group of family practice residents is informally interviewed, as a group, in an on-call room, or when a group of caregivers is sampled for a focus group interview, the unit of analysis is the group (see chapter 6). This data is not equivalent to individual interviews with the same residents or the same caregivers. Who one decides to interview, an individual or a group, is a complex question. It partially depends on the answer to the question, "Who do I want to make inferences about, individuals or groups?" In addition, individual interviews often provide more depth about a topic, whereas group interviews frequently generate greater breadth of information (see Chapters 5 and 6; Crabtree, Yanoshik, Miller, & O'Connor, 1993).

The role context of the interviewer is an often neglected consideration. As a physician, I am identified primarily according to the clinical role; my research interests are viewed as subsidiary to my biomedical professional relationships. On the other hand, I might be identified primarily as a department chair with a vested interest in the economic success of the hospital network. Finally, I might be hired as a consultant to do research, and that role would condition my relationship with research participants. Gender, ethnic, and social class issues also factor into this dimension of interviewing.

The second dimension, "how," refers to the *degree of structure* in the interview process (see Table 1.3). As with observation, no interview is completely unstructured, but three levels of structure can be usefully delineated (Bernard, 1988). *Unstructured interviewing* is equivalent to guided everyday conversation and is often part of participant observation, particularly in the form of key informant interviews (see Chapter 4). Key informants provide expert, inside information. The researcher has one or more topic areas that are probed whenever the opportunity arises during a given period of observation. *Semistructured interviews* are guided, concentrated, focused, and open-ended communication events that are cocreated by the investigator and interviewee(s) and occur outside the stream of everyday life. The questions, probes, and prompts are written in the form of a flexible interview guide (Chapters 5 and 6). *Structured interviews,* on the other hand, are more like spoken questionnaires, with a rigidly structured interview schedule directing the interview, and may often be conducted over a telephone. Structured interviews are best when sufficient trustworthy information already exists on which to develop the interview schedule.

Which type of structured or semistructured interview is selected for a particular project depends on *"what" information* is sought. *Depth interviews* intensively plumb a particular topic (McCracken, 1988) (Chapter 5). *Life histories* reveal personal biography (Denzin, 1989b; Watson & Watson-Franke, 1985), *oral histories* get in touch with personal experience of some event, and *projective techniques* expose the shadows of personality (Pelto & Pelto, 1978). *Critical incidents technique* focuses on a semistructured exploration of defining moments. The terms and meanings of words and actions and the rules governing them are elicited through *free listings* and an *"ethnoscience interview"* (Spradley, 1979). *Pile sorts* and *rank-order methods* are structured techniques for further clarifying cognitive and decision-making activity underlying human choices (Weller & Romney, 1988). The *semistructured diagram-directed techniques* are goal specific and include some primary care examples such as the genogram (McGoldrick & Gerson, 1985; McIlvain, Crabtree, Medder, Stange, & Miller, 1998), life-space drawings (Blake & Bertuso, 1988), timelines, and family circles (Thrower, Bruce, & Walton, 1982).

"When" refers to the time factor in the interview relationship. Some interview relationships, such as key informant interviews (Chapter 4), involve a long-term relationship; others, such as most focus groups (Chapter 6) and most depth interviews (Chapter 5), consist of a one-time meeting. All of the interview methods could potentially be used in *long-term, repeated,* or *single*-time relationships.

The decision to observe, record, and/or interview is often more complex than is usually recognized. Behavior and conversations are best recorded, activities of daily living are better observed, and stories and cognitive maps are best obtained through interview. A useful maxim is *look at behavior; listen to perceptions.* A corollary of this is that if you only interview and don't do observations, you are faced with knowing only beliefs and not behavior. Thus you are at risk for the self-report fallacy. After these basic generalizations, the decision-making process becomes less obvious. A critical question guiding one to the most appropriate selection is, *How is the topic in question usually shared in the culture or group of interest?* (Briggs, 1986). For example, what if our topic of research interest concerns how particular health care practitioners learn the identity characteristics and style of their particular specialty? Surgeons often share this information in the operating room or in the trauma room in an apprentice-type interaction, therefore participant observation as an apprentice is a preferred data collection technique. Obstetricians frequently share information in the form of "near disaster" and "dramatic save" stories while sitting and waiting in the delivery room lounge. Recordings of these stories, if possible, is optimal. Many nurses and family physicians eagerly share information in the form of explanatory talk. Whenever two or more gather, they usually seize the opportunity to share experiences, puzzlements, insights, and frustrations. Interviewing works well with family doctors and nurses.

The Interpretive Process

Although there are nearly as many approaches to interpretation as there are qualitative researchers, these strategies all encompass five core phases of activities (Chapter 7). The interpretive process starts with *describing,* which is a time for reflecting on what is happening to the research team and within the research process and how all of it is influencing and shaping the interpretive process (reflexivity) and what the next steps should be. The next three phases encompass the actual analysis process and include *organizing, connecting,* and *corroborating/legitimating.* Organizing refers to how one enters the data and reorganizes it in a way that helps answer the research question. Connecting is the operation whereby one connects various segments and emerging interpretations within the data to identify and/or discover connections, patterns, themes, and new meanings. This is the heart of the analysis and interpretive process. Corroborating/legitimating concerns the issues of standards, credibility, trustworthiness, and interpretive validity (see Chapter 18) (Altheide & Johnson, 1994). These three analysis phases have their own iterative cycle, which connects and reconnects over time with describing and the sampling/collecting cycle. The analysis cycle also connects with the fifth phase of interpretation, *representing the account*. This is the process of telling the story, of writing it up, of creating some means for presenting the results of the research. Representing the account often begins early in the research process.

An important and recurrent decision point in the interpretive process comes at the organizing phase, whenever the investigative team or interpreter reenter the data. We have identified three idealized organizing styles for helping to conceptualize this phase and the necessary decision making. These three organizing styles are *template, editing,* and *immersion/crystallization*. All three styles are illustrated in Figure 1.5.

The organizing styles inherent in most of the traditional strategies of qualitative inquiry can be lumped into one of our three prototypical styles. Table 1.4 lists the three organizing styles with their associated research traditions and/or specific analytic techniques.

The *template organizing style* makes use of a template or organizing codebook that is applied to the text being analyzed. The template can be detailed or more open ended and usually undergoes revision after encountering the text. The template derives from theory, research tradition, preexisting knowledge, and/or a summary reading of the text. Templates can be codebooks developed prior to data collection, such as in the approach of Miles and Huberman (1994), or created after data collection has begun, as in ethnographic content analysis (Altheide, 1987) (see Chapter 9). Templates can also be a theoretical, behavioral, or linguistic structure. The structure-based approaches apply either interactional structures (e.g., sociolinguistics) (McLaughlin, 1984) or logical, semantic, or sequential structures (e.g., ethnoscience, ethology) to the identified units (see appendix). For example, Spradley (1979), an ethnoscientist, would read text looking for how "term X is like term Y." "Is like" is the semantic structure applied to the identified terms. Whatever the template, it is applied to the text with the intent of identifying the meaningful units or parts. The units are behavioral, as in ethology and ecological psychology studies, or language units such as words, phrases, utterances, folk terms. If the text reveals inadequacies in the template, modifications and revisions are made and the text is reexamined. The interaction of text and template may involve several iterations and include the collection of more data until no new revisions are identified. The analysis then proceeds to the connecting phase, where the units are connected into an explanatory framework consistent with the text.

The *editing organizing style* is termed "editing" because the interpreter enters the text much like an editor searching for meaningful segments,

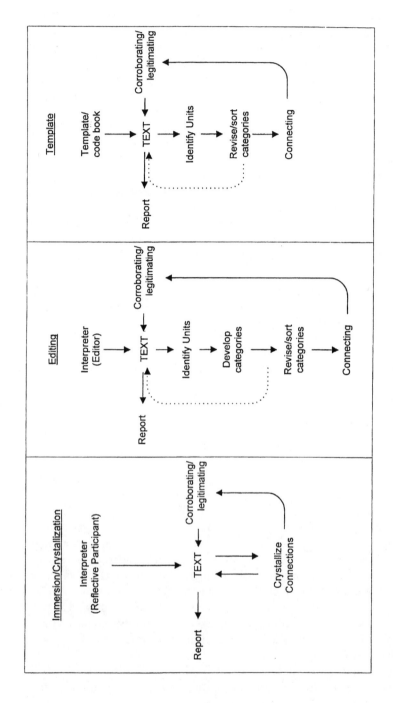

Figure 1.5. Diagrammatic Representation of Different Organizing Styles of Analysis

TABLE 1.4 Qualitative Analysis Styles, With Associated Research Traditions and Techniques

Templates (Chapter 9)
  Codebook based
    A priori
      Qualitative positivism
    A posteriori
      Ethnographic content analysis
  Structure based
    Basic content analysis
    Ethology
    Kinesics/proxemics
    Disclosure analysis
    Ethnography of communication
    Ethnoscience
Editing (Chapter 8)
  Phenomenology
  Hermeneutics
  Ethnomethodology
  Symbolic interactionism
  Grounded theory
  Ecological psychology
  Concept book approach
Immersion/crystallization (Chapter 10)
  Heuristic research
  Ethnography

cutting, pasting, and rearranging until the reduced summary reveals a helpful interpretation. The interpreter engages the text naively, without a template. The researcher attempts to identify and separate from preconceptions prior to reading the data. The interpreter searches for meaningful units or segments of text that both stand on their own and relate to the purpose of the study. Once identified, these units are sorted and organized into categories or codes. It is these categories that are explored for patterns and themes in the connecting phase of analysis. The grounded theory approach of Glaser and Strauss (1967), popular with qualitative nurse researchers (Chenitz & Swanson, 1986), and McCracken's (1988) Long Interview analysis use variations on the editing organizing style. Addison (Chapter 8) illustrates the editing style in more detail.

Immersion/crystallization consists of the analyst's prolonged immersion into and experience of the text and then emergence, after concerned reflection, with an intuitive crystallization of the data. This cycle of immersion and crystallization is repeated until the reported interpretation is reached. Note that the organizing and connecting phases are collapsed into one. The heuristic research of Moustakas (1990) and Kotarba's (1983) existential truth analysis are examples. The penetrating and revealing insights of Howard Stein (1990), well known to family physicians, are also examples of the use of this organizing style. The stories and case report insights of patients, nurses, and practicing primary care physicians are a variation of the use of this organizing style and often serve as starting points for new directions in research or further enlightening of previous studies (Miller & Crabtree, 1990).

The initial and later choices of an organizing style depend on at least five situations within the research process. These include self-analysis, the research question and aims, prior or emerging knowledge about the topic of interest, and the potential audiences for the research. Template style is especially helpful when there is good prior knowledge of the topic, a clinical audience is anticipated, a research aim is theory testing, or it is one's aesthetic preference. Editing and immersion/crystallization styles are useful when the research aim is one of exploration and/or discovery, when scant knowledge already exists, the research is participatory, or these styles have more personal aesthetic appeal to the research team. It is important to remember that multiple styles can be used during the course of the research. Chapters 8 through 10 give examples of this mixed use of organizing styles. These choices and the interpretive process as a whole are examined in more detail in Chapter 7.

It is essential, in concluding this section on interpretation, to reiterate the iterative process of qualitative research design. Interpretation begins when the research is first conceptualized and reflexivity is initiated, and analysis begins shortly after or when the first data are collected. This analysis and interpretation create new understandings, generate changes in the research question, and uncover new anomalies. The result is often a change in the sampling strategy, new collection tools, and thus changes in the analysis process, including the use of a different organizing style. This recursive cycle continues until understanding is complete enough and/or no disconfirming data are discovered.

SUMMARY

The introduction in this book opened with four primary health care puzzles—cigarette smoking, preventive health services delivery, family practices as organizational systems, and women with medically unexplained symptoms. This chapter's journey toward puzzle-solving began by constructing a roadmap or typology of research styles based on aims, goals, questions, and paradigms. At this first fork in the road, field research, usually as part of a multimethod strategy, was selected as the preferred strategy for investigating these particular puzzles. Then we explored the maze of qualitative methods used in field research by viewing them through our eyes as doers of clinical qualitative research. The design options for data collection and interpretation were identified. The remainder of this book describes these options in more detail, and each author explains his or her design decisions. Four of these decision pathways are now briefly described to illustrate how the qualitative methods typology is implemented.

Dennis Willms and his colleagues (see Chapter 9) want to understand how people enrolled in a randomized controlled trial (RCT) for smoking cessation perceive the use and meaning of cigarettes within the context of their everyday lives. Willms et al. recognize the need to gather intimate information about perceptions and meanings from individuals over time. Thus, they choose an amalgam of key informant/depth interviews at repeated intervals over the course of the RCT, with collection and interpretation going on iteratively. As what is known about smoking behavior has not been as helpful as was hoped, they decide to start fresh and initially enter their interview transcript texts using an immersion/crystallization organizing style. The results from this initial analysis are used to create a detailed codebook as a means of facilitating the identification of potentially meaningful text segments for later in the interpretive process. This is particularly important, given the need at the end of the study for relating the findings back to the RCT. Within this format, Willm's particular choice of *ethnographic analysis* is primarily an aesthetic one derived from his training as an anthropologist.

Kurt Stange and his team at Case Western Reserve (see Chapter 9) seek to discover what goes on in primary care practices relative to preventive health services delivery. The field research part of this multimethod project hopes to gain an understanding of the behaviors, moods, and activities that constitute everyday life in the sampled offices. To do so, the research nurses enter the world of primary care as participant observers. They and the other investigators want to reveal possible new patterns of behavior and explanations for the larger survey-style study of which this field research is a part. Thus, they also choose immersion/crystallization as an initial organizing style. In this case, a template is not developed until near the end as part of the corroborating/legitimating phase of analysis. The goal is to stay open to new possibilities as long as possible. The later template is also helpful in relating the qualitative findings to the quantitative ones.

Ben Crabtree and his research team (Chapter 16) want to know what goes on inside the "black box" of family practices as organizations. They hope to understand the practice as a whole. Almost no research currently exists in this area. Crabtree wants to reveal the subjective complexity, interrelatedness, and richness of life inside a family practice. There is a clearly bounded unit, so a case study strategy is used with participant observation and key informant interviews as primary collection methods supplemented with chart audits, depth interviews, and observation rating scales. The interpretive process is unusually complex, as there are multiple types of text that need to be compared both within cases and between cases. The decision making for this study is explained in Chapter 16.

Kirsti Malterud wants both to understand her experience with women patients who present with medically unexplained symptoms and to change her communication strategy in some way to improve care. Thus, she uses a participatory action research strategy in which she acts as a participant observer within her own practice. This approach enables her and her patients to iteratively explore and change their communication behavior. Her initial interpretive process is guided by speech act theory from the discipline of linguistics. The specifics of her interpretive process are detailed in Chapter 17.

The road traveled in this chapter has prepared the reader for the research adventures ahead. For pedagogical purposes, this chapter's discussion has separated the different research methods, including dividing qualitative from quantitative. In practice, we believe the various methods complement each other, and their integration is encouraged. Expand your research perspectives and join the search. Welcome to the exhilarating adventure of doing qualitative clinical research.

Appendix:
From Whence It Came—
Qualitative Research Traditions

Each of the human science disciplines has several qualitative research traditions, which have developed over the past century. For example, anthropology has ethnoscience and ethnography; sociology has symbolic interactionism, grounded theory, and ethnomethodology; and psychology has hermeneutics and ecological psychology. Other disciplines, particularly education, nursing, and marketing, have borrowed liberally from these traditions and developed their own. One unfortunate consequence has been a proliferation of conceptual jargon and difficult reading for those outside the particular tradition. This appendix serves as a brief summary reference for many of these qualitative traditions. The goal is to help the reader identify which tradition(s) and possible consultant(s) are pertinent to their research.

Table 1.4 identifies the major research traditions as they relate to the organizing styles discussed earlier in this chapter. Also included in this table are specific techniques such as *basic content analysis* (e.g., Berelson, 1971; Weber, 1985), a very structured template-style technique shared by many traditions; *ethnographic content analysis* (Altheide,

TABLE 1.5 Domains of Study and Qualitative Research Traditions

Domain	*Research Tradition*
Lived experience ("lifeworld")	**Psychology**
Intention of actor as individual	Phenomenology
Actors as access to social context	Hermeneutics (interpretive interactionism)
Individual	**Psychology and anthropology**
As person with biography	Life history (interpretive biography)
Behavior/events	Psychology
Over time and in context	Ethology
Related to environment	Ecological psychology
Social world	**Sociology**
How individuals achieve shared agreement	Ethnomethodology
How humans create and interact in a symbolic environment	Symbolic interactions (semiotics)
General relations among social categories and properties	Grounded theory
Culture	**Anthropology**
As holistic whole	Ethnography
As symbolic world	Symbolic anthropology
As cognitive map of social organizations	Ethnoscience (Cognitive anthropology)
Communication/talk	**Sociolinguistics**
Forms and mechanisms of actual conversation	Conversation analysis (Discourse analysis)
Forms and mechanisms of nonverbal communication	Kinesics/proxemics
Patterns and rules of communication	Ethnography of communication
Practice and process	**Applied professions**
Caring	Nursing research
Teaching and learning	Educational research
Managing/consuming	Organizational/market research
Evaluation	Evaluation research

1987), derived from the qualitative tradition in sociology; and the *concept book approach* to content analysis (Mostyn, 1985), emerging from psychology and more like the editing style described by Addison in Chapter 8. The a priori codebook analysis techniques elaborately presented by educational researchers Miles and Huberman (1984) are labeled *qualitative positivism* by us but are referred to by Tesch (1990) as transcendental realism.

Once an investigator decides that field research and qualitative methods are best suited for the question of interest, the next step is to decide what aspect of human life is of primary concern. The focus can be the individual as a person with a biography created over time, or behavior and events, or social life, or culture, or communication, or intentionally lived experience, or it can be specific processes and practices such as caring, consuming, managing, teaching, and evaluating. Table 1.5 outlines how these units or domains of human life relate to the different traditions of qualitative research. The boundaries between these traditions are often quite blurred. For example, symbolic anthropology borrows heavily from phenomenology, hermeneutics, and symbolic interactionism. A brief overview of each of the qualitative research traditions is now possible.

Phenomenology seeks to understand the lived experience of individuals and their intentions within their "lifeworld." It is the search for essences. It answers the questions, "What is it like to have a certain experience?" "What is the essence of this particular experience?" To accomplish this, investigators must "bracket" their own preconceptions, enter into the individual's lifeworld, and use the self as an experiencing interpreter. Paradigm cases and theories are frequently identified, and the experience is presented as descriptive narrative. Exemplars of this approach, begun by Edmund Husserl (1931), include Giorgi (1970), Colaizzi (1978), and Van Kaam (1969). Phenomenology has gained popularity among a number of nursing researchers (Bargagliotti, 1983; Oiler, 1982).

Hermeneutics is a movement beyond phenomenology in that the goal of hermeneutic research is to use the interpretation of lived experience to better understand the political, historical, and sociocultural context in which it occurs. Hermeneutics (see Chapter 6) also requires the investigator to enter an interpretive circle of intentional action (Allen & Jenson, 1990). Originating in the interpretation of Biblical text and developed for social science by philosophers such as Heidegger (1927/1962), Gadamer (1976), and Ricoeur (1981), hermeneutics as a methodology is well described by Packer and Addison (1989) and also by Denzin (1989b), who refers to it as *interpretive interactionism*.

The *life history* tradition borrows from both of the above and from ethnography with its use of key informant interviewing. Life histories provide rich narratives and portraits of an individual's life story, including its turning points and core themes. Watson and Watson-Franke (1985) and Denzin (1989a) explicate the process of doing a life history, also called *interpretive biography*.

Human ethology purports to be the biology of human behavior. Methodologically, ethology is the direct observational study of human or animal behavior over time in its natural context. Building from the work of animal ethologists Lorenz (1966) and Tinbergen (1951), human ethologists now attempt to discover the universal grammar structuring human behavior and interactions. They use video recordings to categorize form-constant behavioral sequences called "fixed action patterns" and to decipher learned behavior patterns. The goal is a theory of human behavior constructed from the rules governing the organization of the behavior patterns, often conceptually mapped as an ethogram. Eibl-Eibesfeldt (1989) has written a superb text describing the methodology, theory, and findings of human ethology research. *Proxemics,* the study of the symbolic use of space, including the concept of personal space (Hall, 1974), and *kinesics,* the study of body movement (Birdwhistell, 1970), are branches of ethology that overlap with sociolinquistics and anthropology.

Ecological psychology also focuses on behavior, but here the purpose is to discover the influence of environment on behavior. Whereas ethologists focus on the behavior itself, ecological psychologists, following the work of Barker (1968), focus and record both the "behavioral episode" and the surroundings in which the stream of behavior occurs. The goal is to develop principles and laws that explain the interdependence of the two. Descriptive statistics are frequently used along with text (field notes and/or videotapes) analysis.

Heuristic research, as defined by Clark Moustakas (1990), derives from the phenomenological tradition in psychology and places a special emphasis on self-reflection in the research experience. The heuristic inquirer uses intensive inner searching and empathic immersion in others' experiences to reach a narrative portrayal of the phenomena in question.

Garfinkel (1967) presented *ethnomethodology* in 1967. He and subsequent ethnomethodologists, such as Mehan and Wood (1975), seek to understand how people make sense of the most common everyday occurrences. They wonder, "How is it that people all know and come to agree that the act of holding a hand means one thing in the doctor's office and something else in the park?" A common methodologic technique, the "incongruity procedure," consists of "breaking the rules" and then observing how people attempt to correct the damage done. The ethics of such research remains controversial.

Symbolic interactionists owe their ancestry to Weber (1968) and Mead (1934) and their contemporary tradition to the "Chicago School" of sociology (Thomas, 1983). This tradition is also concerned with how people make sense of social interactions, but the emphasis is on how the interactions are interpreted as symbols by the participants. The goal is to explicate the meaning of a word, action, or sign and develop principles of symbolic interaction. *Semiotics,* the study of signs and their significations, and *conversation analysis* are tools commonly used by symbolic interactionists (Goodwin, 1981; Manning, 1987). The study by Becker, Geer, Hughes, and Strauss (1961) of medical students is an early example of the symbolic interactionist approach. Blumer (1969) provides an excellent source on symbolic interaction theory.

Grounded theory, a research tradition worked out by Glaser and Strauss (1967), has made major contributions to both the medical sociology and the nursing literature. One key to its popularity is the detailed descriptions of the methodology provided by Glaser and Strauss and their students. With philosophical roots in phenomenology, grounded theory searches to identify the core social psychological and/or social structural process within a given social scene. The goal is to develop classifications and theory grounded in the particular social scene investigated. "Grounded" means based on and connected to the context-dependent observations and perceptions of the social scene. The researcher constantly and recursively compares research interpretations, in the form of "memos," against the data, a process termed the "constant comparative method."

Ethnography is one of the oldest field research traditions and the cornerstone of anthropology. The goal is to tell the whole story of a defined group's daily life, to identify the meanings, patterns, and passions of a bounded cultural group. Given such a holistic task, ethnographers use multiple methods over an extended period of time while immersed in the everyday life of the culture being studied. Murdock, Ford, Hudson, et al.'s (1950) "Outline of Cultural Materials" is a commonly used guide and codebook for this research. Goetz and LeCompte (1984) describe the use of ethnography in education. Helpful general references include Pelto and Pelto (1978), Hammersley and Atkinson (1983), and Fetterman (1989). All ethnographers work from the same tool kit, but their interpretive foci often differ substantially. Some ethnographers see the culture through materialistic eyes (positivism), wearing the glasses of neoevolutionism (White, 1959) or cultural ecology (Harris, 1966). Others see through glasses of neofunctionalism (Gluckman, 1963) or neo-Marxism (Singer, 1989) and perceive culture as a source of conflict and power struggles. A third group of ethnographers emphasize the ideological aspects of culture rather than the materialistic and conflict-based perspectives. This group includes structuralism (Levi-Strauss, 1963), ethnoscience (following), and symbolic anthropology (described later) and views culture as a system of shared symbols and meanings (much like the symbolic interactionists in sociology).

Ethnoscience, also called *cognitive anthropology,* represents a blending of the ethnographic and linguistic traditions within the discipline of anthropology. The original goal was to learn a culture's "emic" constructs, or the meaning of things and events as understood by the members of the culture. This goal has translated into methods and studies that seek to map the cognitive world of a culture, the semantic rules and shared meanings governing conduct. The results are classifications and rules, often presented in the form of taxonomic trees or semantic network diagrams. The methods of ethnoscience, such as componential analysis, pile sorts, and multidimensional scaling, are especially suited for term identification and for decision modeling. Detailed descriptions of these techniques are found in Spradley (1979), Werner and Schoepfle (1987b), Weller and Romney (1988), and Gladwin (1989).

Whereas ethnoscientists rely primarily on participants' statements about symbolic meaning, *symbolic anthropologists* go beyond the statements to examine how myths, rituals, and other cultural events are actually used in the everyday context of social and cultural life. The goal is to reveal the shared cultural categories and plans that enable people to communicate and meet their needs. The outcomes are "thick descriptions" of cultural events (Geertz, 1973) and paradigm cases and/or the important cultural themes underlying and revealed by the event or ritual (Turner, 1969). These themes are often depicted in taxonomic grids (Douglas, 1982).

Sociolinguistics is home for both *discourse analysis* and the *ethnography of communication.* Both seek to understand the rules or structure of communication. Discourse analysts focus directly on conversation itself, using transcripts of naturally occurring conversations, such as those between doctor and patient (see Cassell, 1985; Mishler, 1984), to uncover a portrait of the forms, mechanisms, and rules guiding the conversation. Stubbs (1983), Van Dijk (1985), and Moerman (1988) provide good descriptions of the technique.

Ethnographers of communication, led by Hymes (Gumperz & Hymes, 1972), focus as much on the context of the conversation as on the conversation itself. They want to know not only the rules of communication but the larger cultural patterns of communication, which are often depicted graphically.

PART II

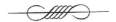

Discovery

Data Collection Strategies

2

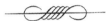

Sampling in
Qualitative Inquiry

Anton J. Kuzel

The validity, meaningfulness, and insights generated from
qualitative inquiry have more to do with the
information-richness of the cases selected and the
observational/analytical capabilities of the researcher than
with sample size.

M. Q. Patton, 1990, p. 185

Researchers are people who want to answer their questions in a careful,
systematic way, and they face a practical challenge with every inquiry:
There are more sources of data available to them for study than they can
possibly examine and understand. How do researchers select a sample from
this larger pool for closer scrutiny? How can they feel confident that the
sample they have chosen is appropriate and adequate? In particular, how
do researchers doing qualitative research answer these questions?

Patton (1990) suggests that qualitative researchers "typically focus in
depth on relatively small samples, even single cases (*n* = 1), selected
purposefully." He contrasts this with quantitative research designs, which

AUTHOR'S NOTE: I want to thank my colleagues in the Department of Family Practice at
Virginia Commonwealth University and the editors of this book for their insightful comments
and suggestions.

"typically depend on larger samples selected randomly" (p. 169). These tendencies result from the underlying purpose of sampling in traditions of inquiry that rely primarily on quantitative methods. In these research traditions, which typically employ *experimental* or *survey* styles of inquiry (Chapter 1), one's sample should be representative of some larger population to which one hopes to generalize the research findings. In qualitative research, which typically uses *field* or *documentary/historical* research styles, sampling is driven not by a need to generalize or predict, but rather by a need to create and test new interpretations. Typically, the investigator wants to increase the scope or range of data exposed to uncover multiple realities and/or to create a deeper understanding—what McWhinney (1989) calls "an acquaintance with particulars." It allows for development of theory that takes into account local conditions (Bogdan & Biklen, 1982; Glaser & Strauss, 1967; Guba & Lincoln, 1989; Lincoln & Guba, 1985; Patton, 1980, 1990). In experimental and survey research, sampling strategies focus on *representativeness*. In field or documentary/historical research, sampling strategies strive for *information-richness* (Patton, 1990).

The basic assumptions behind most qualitative research, and the usual purposes of this kind of work, make random sampling inappropriate in most cases. First, the sample size in a qualitative study is typically small—often between five to 20 units of analysis. This small size would introduce a large sampling error if one's purpose were to select a group that was representative of a larger population. Second, true random sampling assumes knowledge sufficient to define the larger population from which the random sample is drawn, and qualitative studies usually make no such claim. Third, true random sampling assumes that the characteristics of interest are normally distributed in the population. This is also not assumed or not known by investigators doing qualitative research. Fourth, some data sources are "richer" than others, and a random sampling strategy could cause the investigator to miss the best opportunities for gaining information (Marshall, 1996).

Theory development and verification in the different research paradigms also shape the process of sampling. In materialistic inquiry, one begins with a priori theory which is relatively fixed, that is, one has an explanation for something that is to be tested. This explanation is purported to hold in some universe that must be clearly defined. Theory is tested quantitatively in the context of a random sample (to avoid investigator bias), using large enough numbers of subjects to demonstrate statistical significance (Guba & Lincoln, 1989). Constructivist inquiry, on the other hand, starts with a priori theory or understanding which is flexible (Creswell, 1998; Glaser & Strauss, 1967; Lincoln & Guba, 1985). The initial question or problem allows for preliminary decisions about the boundary of the investigation. The investigator concerns him- or herself with questions such as Which data sources are information rich? Who should I talk to or what should I look at first? As interpretation develops, additional questions arise: Which data sources may confirm my understanding? challenge my understanding? enrich my understanding? (Glaser & Strauss, 1967; Guba & Lincoln, 1989; Lincoln & Guba, 1985; Marshall & Rossman, 1989, 1995, 1998; Patton, 1990). All forms of inquiry begin with some sort of prior understanding or theory about the subject of study—no investigator is a blank slate (Kuzel, 1986). They differ in that materialistic inquiry usually starts with a theory that is closed and either proven or disproven. Constructivist inquiry generally begins with a theory or understanding that is expanded, modified, and confirmed in the context of the study.

WHAT TO SAMPLE

Two studies by contibutors to this volume illustrate the practical implications of these ideas. In the first example, Miller, Yanoshik, Crabtree, and Reymond (1994) wondered why family physicians underestimate their patients' pain severity. Their question suggests inquiries that focus on personal pain experience and on the way that experience is shared with and understood by another. Miller's group, with limited resources, elected to start by exploring patients' and family physicians' personal experiences with pain through interviews with six patient-physician pairs. Their own personal experiences, prior understandings, and their reading of the literature led them to

> control for cultural factors, minimize patient-physician conflict, and control for pain context. As the number of physician-patient pairs would be small, we chose to interview a sample that was culturally homogeneous to minimize the effects of culture, ethnicity, and social class within each respondent group. All physicians and patients were selected from a nonurban area in north central Connecticut. Physicians were limited to residency-trained, board-certified family physicians of European descent, and the patients had to be of European descent, over 45 years of age, and working class (blue-collar job and no college education).
>
> The six family physicians were randomly selected from a list of physicians practicing in the target area. These six physicians each provided the name of one patient who recently experienced pain but who was not perceived by the physician as having a chronic pain syndrome. (p. 180)

The physicians and patients were separately interviewed and the interviews fully transcribed. Each respondent was asked questions that dealt with pain socialization, types of pain, personal pain management, types of pain patients, and physician pain management. The team analyzed the first four pairs using an editing organizing style (see Chapter 7). A template organizing style, based on the emerging understanding and possible alternate hypotheses, was then used to analyze the last two pairs and "identified no new categories or themes, thus providing assurances regarding adequacy of sample size" (Miller, Yanoshik, et al., 1994, p. 180).

The second example is Addison's study of the training experiences of nine family practice residents (Chapter 8). He saw the residency's "intense, stressful process as a problem for the trainees, their families, and their patients. I wanted to better understand what becoming a physician was like for the individuals involved, how the practices of resident physicians became problematic, and whether positive alternatives were possible" (Chapter 8, p. 151). Furthermore, Addison states that he "wanted to understand what they actually did as they began their residency, not just what they thought they were doing, believed they were doing, intended to do, or said they did" (p. 151).

After talking with experts in medical education and visiting a variety of residency programs in several specialties, Addison chose a university-affiliated family practice program in a semiurban county setting. He states, "I decided to focus on the first year of residency, long recognized as most stressful in terms of its encompassing demands and most significant in terms of inculcating attitudes, beliefs, values, and practices" (Chapter 8, p. 152). This inquiry was the basis of Addison's doctoral dissertation, and he invested an enormous amount of personal time and effort. He used participant observation (Chapter 3) for a full year with an incoming class of residents in both inpatient and outpatient settings. He took call with them, interviewed their peers, supervisors, and significant others, and pored over charts, memos, and schedules. After this first intensive year, he continued to selectively spend time with the residents for the final 2 years of their residency. "I followed some more closely than others, as I found some residents more welcoming of my presence, some more verbal, and some more critically reflective" (Chapter 8, p. 152).

Compared to the simpler research design of Miller, Yanoshik, et al. (1994), who only did one iterative cycle between gathering and interpretation prior to seeking disconfirming/confirming cases, Addison (1992) made innumerable loops. He speaks of the hermeneutic (interpretive), circular process of his inquiry:

> I moved from immersing myself in the residents' everyday existence wherein I developed an experiential understanding of their practices. I then made this understanding explicit in the form of an interpretation of the meaning of their practices. I then incorporated this fuller interpretation into my further observations and immersion to understand more or different aspects of their

TABLE 2.1 What to Sample: Two Case Examples

"What"	*Miller, Yanoshik, et al. (1994)*	*Addison (Chapter 8)*
Events	Stories of personal pain experiences	Morning report, grand rounds
Persons	Physicians, patients	Residents, faculty, family, friends
Artifacts	None—interviews only	Evaluations, schedules, memos
Activity	Stories of personal and professional pain	Work rounds, ambulatory patient care, taking call
Time	Retrospective recall	Residency training experience from 1st, 2nd, and 3rd years

existence . . . to flesh out underdeveloped portions of the account and to correct aspects that were not yet coherent or cohesive. (1992, pp. 116, 121)

These published studies illustrate the two key sampling concepts of *appropriateness* and *adequacy*. Issues of appropriateness begin with a consideration of whether the investigator is using a suitable paradigm or model of research (Guba & Lincoln, 1989; Kuzel, 1986; Lincoln & Guba, 1985; Patton, 1980, 1990; Chapter 1). Miller, Yanoshik, et al. (1994) were interested in how family physicians understand and treat pain; Addison wanted to uncover and help to fix problems in the training of family physicians. Clearly, both questions deal with personal and social constructs that are better addressed through qualitative methods. The *choice* of the subject of interest also sets limits on the scope of the investigation (Lincoln & Guba, 1985). Boundaries are shaped by determining "what it is you want to be able to say something about at the end of the study" (Patton, 1980, p. 100), and clarity on this issue is critical to appropriate sampling. This boundary is a sampling frame, and it may be further defined by considering what to sample.

The "what" may include events, places, persons, artifacts, activity, and time (Spradley, 1980). Choosing among these possibilities is challenging, but it helps to consider "what is the phenomenon of interest, and how is it usually represented?" (Briggs, 1986; Chapter 1). Miller, Yanoshik, et al. (1994) wanted to understand physicians' and patients' personal pain experiences, that is, "what's the meaning of this?" Addison wanted to understand the process of resident training, that is, "what's going on here (and what's wrong with that, and how might it be improved)?" These questions (and the resources available to the investigators) guided their choices of what to sample, as illustrated in Table 2.1.

Miller, Yanoshik, et al.'s work is an example of the kind of sampling typically done in studies employing depth interviews (Chapter 5) to get at the meaning of experiences. They used specific criteria to determine a homogeneous sample of individual physicians (and paired patients) who were invited to participate. Addison's study relied heavily on participant observation (Chapter 3), an approach that is suited to his general question of "what's going on here (and what's problematic about that)?" As we see in his work, this kind of research typically derives data from all six categories—events, places, persons, artifacts, activity, and time—of "what to sample." Particularly characteristic in Addison's study is sampling over time—what Guba and Lincoln refer to as "prolonged engagement" in the field (1985).

The optimal sampling strategy in case study research is more complicated. Case study research (Chapter 14) may concern a single person engaged in a particular activity at a particular place and time, a group of people engaged in several activities, or multiple cases of either type. As Aita and McIlvain point out in that chapter, the choice of the "unit of analysis" and the overall purpose of the case study project will guide sampling decisions. Focus group research (Chapter 6) has roots in market analysis and brings together people with experience and interest in the topic of study to talk about their personal stories and opinions. Membership in a given focus group may be homogeneous or heterogeneous, depending on the purpose of the investigation and the available resources. (See the later discussion on sampling strategies and Chapter 6 for more on this decision).

HOW TO SAMPLE

Specific Strategies

There are other issues besides "fit with question" and "fit with phenomenon" that determine the appropriateness of qualitative sampling. While contemplating all the options of *what* to sample, the qualitative researcher must also decide *how* to sample. This includes considering whether to observe (settings, events, or activities), examine (artifacts) or interview (individuals or groups). The researcher must consider how to record what he or she sees, hears, and thinks (i.e., videotaping or audiotaping vs. notes, memos, or diaries). She must choose which of many information-rich qualitative sampling strategies to employ. This is yet another way of asking the appropriateness question: "Is the sampling strategy consistent with the purpose of the inquiry?" Patton (1990) suggests 16 kinds of purposeful qualitative sampling, shown in Table 2.2. Several of these categories deserve emphasis because they are typical of qualitative inquiry in clinical research or thought by many authors to be desirable strategies.

TABLE 2.2 Typology of Sampling Strategies in Qualitative Inquiry (After Patton, 1990)

Type of Sampling	*Purpose*
Maximum variation	Documents diverse variations and identifies important common patterns
Homogeneous	Focuses, reduces, simplifies; facilitates group interviewing
Critical case	Permits logical generalization and maximum application of information to other cases
✓Theoretical	Finding examples of a theoretical construct and thereby elaborating and examining it
Confirming/ disconfirming	Elaborating initial analysis, seeking exceptions, looking for variation
Snowball or chain	Identifies cases of interest from people who know people who know what cases are information rich
Extreme or deviant case	Learning from highly unusual manifestations of the phenomenon of interest
Typical case	Highlights what is normal or average
Intensity	Information-rich cases that manifest the phenomenon intensely but not extremely
Politically important cases	Attracts desired attention or avoids attracting undesired attention
Random purposeful	Adds credibility to sample when potential purposeful is too large
Stratified purposeful	Illustrates subgroups; facilitates comparisons
Criterion	All cases meet some criterion; useful for quality assurance
✓Opportunistic	Follow new leads; taking advantage of unexpected
Combination or mixed	Triangulation, flexibility, meets multiple interests/needs
Convenience	Saves time, money, and effort but at expense of information and credibility ,

Maximum variation sampling occurs when one seeks to obtain the broadest range of information and perspectives on the subject of study. Guba and Lincoln (1989) claim this is the preferred strategy for constructivist inquiry. By looking for this broad range of perspective, the investigator is purposefully challenging his or her own preconceived (and developing) understandings of the phenomenon under study. This also mitigates against the tendency to make the "messiness" of reality appear unduly "neat and tidy." Maximum variation sampling appeals particularly to the investigator who values critical/ecological inquiry (Fay, 1987), for the views of the powerful as well as the disenfranchised are represented. If practical constraints preclude the use of this strategy, the investigator might defend the use of a more *homogeneous* sample on the basis of seeking to understand a particular group of individuals particularly well and/or control for context, with some appreciation of the unarticulated diversity yet to be explored and some suggestions or plans for further study. Miller, Yanoshik, et al.'s (1994) example above is a good illustration of this choice.

Patton (1990) points out that maximum variation sampling "documents unique or diverse variations that have emerged in adapting to different conditions" and "identifies important common patterns that cut across variations" (p. 182). In practice, the investigator might ask a respondent, "Who do you know who thinks very differently about this topic?" as a way of getting a wide range of opinion. Another way to seek diversity is to use specific selection criteria that seem theoretically important and choose data sources to represent the range of those criteria. For example, Crabtree and Miller describe in Chapter 16 how they chose "both urban and rural practices and practices with different intensity of preventive services delivery" (p. 299) in their Prevention and Competing Demands study. Thesen and Kuzel (Chapter 15) tell of a government-sponsored project to gather "user" perceptions of mental health services. The agency that designed the study recruited project leaders "from different sectors of the services and in different parts of the country—in psychiatric specialist services as well as in primary care, in rural and urban, southern and northern parts of the country" (p. 277).

Typical case sampling focuses directly on the ordinary and usual. It is sometimes paired with *deviant case sampling* that focuses on examples at the ends of the spectrum of a phenomenon. These extremes often help bring to the surface and challenge the "taken for granted" assumptions that guide normal behavior in typical cases.

Critical case sampling is where one looks for sources of data that are particularly information rich or enlightening. This sampling strategy "permits logical generalization and maximum application of information to other cases because if it's true of this one case it's likely to be true of all other ['similar'] cases" (Patton, 1990, p. 182). In other words, the researcher is looking for the particularly good story that illuminates the questions under study.

Theory-based sampling occurs when one samples for information in a focused manner, based on an a priori theory that is being evaluated and/or modeled. This is different from the more commonly used *theoretical sampling* of Glaser and Strauss (1967). They state, "Theoretical sampling is the process of data collection for generating theory whereby the analyst jointly collects, codes, and analyzes his data and decides what data to collect next and where to find them, in order to develop his theory as it emerges. The process of data collection is controlled by the emerging theory" (p. 44). This is clearly evident in Addison's study, in which he kept circling through the iterative cycles of gathering, including new theoretical sampling decisions and interpretation as described in his quote from earlier in this chapter.

It is important to recognize the implication of theoretical and other iterative kinds of purposeful sampling: The sample is selected serially and contingently (Guba & Lincoln, 1989). In other words, the processes of framing and reframing the research question, sample selection, data gathering, data analysis, and theory construction usually occur concurrently in constructivist inquiry. This *flexibility* of theory is a typical and important feature of constructivist research. Merriam (1988) suggests that "purposive and criterion-based sampling occur before the data are gathered, whereas theoretical sampling is done in conjunction with data collection" (p. 51).

Fixed sampling strategies, such as the *criterion-based* approach taken by Miller, Yanoshik, and colleagues (1994), are particularly helpful when doing small, exploratory studies. These can be homogeneous samples, as in the example, or a few cases that represent a range or extremes, so that one can learn from the comparisons and contrasts. This latter approach may not allow one to consider sampling to the point of "saturation" of data categories, but the next sampling strategy focuses precisely on that goal.

Confirming and disconfirming cases are sampling strategies in which one looks for data that will support or challenge the investigator's understanding of the topic of study. Patton (1990) calls this a process of "elaborating and deepening initial analysis, seeking exceptions, testing variation" (p. 183). A related concept is that of "theoretical saturation" (Glaser & Strauss, 1967), or sampling to the point of redundancy (Lincoln & Guba, 1985; Morse, 1995). Not only does this technique provide more convincing evidence of the credibility of developed theory, but it also allows one to answer the question, "When can I stop sampling?" Miller, Yanoshik, and colleagues (1994) describe how they saw the same perspectives in their last two interviews as they did in the first four and state that this enhances the validity of their analysis.

Sampling to the point of saturation is also seen in the commonly used technique of *snowball sampling* (Bogdan & Biklen, 1982; Patton, 1990).

> In this form of sampling one identifies, in whatever way one can, a few members of the phenomenal group one wishes to study. These members are used to identify others, and they in turn others. Unless the group is very large, one soon comes to a point at which efforts to net additional members cannot be justified in terms of the additional outlay of energy and resources; this point may be thought of as a point of redundancy. (Lincoln & Guba, 1985, p. 233)

As sampling to the point of saturation yields a more convincing explanation of events, so does searching for disconfirming evidence—

purposefully looking for negative cases (Lincoln & Guba, 1985). If some are found, the investigator must modify previous understanding to account for the new information. If none are found, both the investigator and the audience for the final report are still more convinced of the credibility and completeness of the espoused interpretation.

The strategies of sampling to the point of redundancy or theoretical saturation, of searching for disconfirming evidence, and of maximum variation sampling have implications for sample size. Although there are no hard and fast rules, experience has shown that five to eight data sources or sampling units will often suffice for a homogeneous sample (as in the Miller example), and 12 to 20 or more are commonly needed when looking for disconfirming evidence or trying to achieve maximum variation (Lincoln & Guba, 1985; Marshall & Rossman, 1989, 1995, 1998; McCracken, 1988; Patton, 1990). When there are subgroups, the "five to eight" rule applies to each group. Malterud (Chapter 17), for example, chose to explore a clinical problem—women's medically unexplained health problems—that was heterogeneous at many levels. She chose to focus on their responses to a key question designed to elicit patient expectations of the physician and derived seven basic categories of expectations from 35 consecutive interviews—an average of five interviews per category.

Suggested Guidelines

Several experts in qualitative research make a case for preferred sampling strategies. Morse (1995) emphasizes the importance of theoretical sampling, negative case sampling, and data saturation in her principles of saturation, which are repeated here in a condensed form:

1. Begin with a cohesive [homogeneous] sample. This reduces generalizability but makes it easier to achieve saturation.
2. Theoretical sampling also speeds the process of saturation.
3. Sampling for and saturation of negative cases promotes validity. ⅄
4. "The more complete the saturation, the easier it is to develop a comprehensive theoretical model" (Morse, 1995, p. 149).

Creswell (1998) suggests that certain kinds of qualitative research tend to favor certain kinds of sampling. These tendencies are summarized in Table 2.3.

Maxwell (1996) also sees preferences for sampling strategies but organizes these according to the purpose of the inquiry. If the purpose is to represent typicality, then a relatively homogeneous sample of typical cases is appropriate. If one wishes to portray a range of possibilities, then maximum variation sampling is clearly in order. If the purpose is to

TABLE 2.3 Sampling Tendencies in Five Qualitative Traditions (After Creswell, 1998)

Tradition	Commonly Used Sampling Strategies
Biographical	Convenience Politically important case Critical case Typical case
Phenomenological	Criterion
Grounded theory	Theoretical
Ethnography	Comprehensive Typical case Criterion

Case study	If single, same as biographical
	If multiple, then
	  Maximum variation
	  Extreme case
	  Typical case
	  Confirming/disconfirming case
	  Critical case

illuminate theory through well-chosen examples, then critical case sampling is appropriate. Finally, if one wishes to explore the reasons for differences among subgroups by contrasting and comparing them, then one should choose stratified purposeful sampling.

The theoretical sampling advocated by Glaser and Strauss (1967) and further developed by Strauss and Corbin (1990) has gained widespread use because of the enormous popularity of grounded theory research. These researchers describe subprocesses of theoretical sampling that are related to coding and data analysis using an editing organizing style. The first is "open sampling," which happens in the early, discovery phases of inquiry. Strauss and Corbin's description of this kind of sampling seems most closely related to Patton's maximum variation or opportunistic strategies. "Relational and variational" sampling occurs during "axial coding"—the process of looking for relationships between categories of data (connecting phase of analysis). Again, using Patton's terminology, this kind of sampling employs strategies of maximum variation, negative case, and extreme case. The final phase of sampling in grounded theory development is called "discriminate sampling." Here the focus is on "maximizing opportunities for verifying the story line, relationships between categories, and for filling in poorly developed categories" (Strauss & Corbin, 1990, p. 187). This seems to be another way of describing theoretical saturation (corroborating/legitimating phase of analysis).

Miles and Huberman (1994) also suggest preferred strategies when they state that three kinds of qualitative sampling are particularly likely to have a big "payoff" for the researcher: typical case, negative case, and exceptional case. They also have important advice for investigators who are dealing with complex studies. In these instances, "you are sampling people to get at characteristics of settings, events, and processes. Conceptually, the people themselves are secondary" (p. 33). In particular, Miles and Huberman warn against overreliance on the talk and behaviors of "key informants" (Chapter 4). They point out that the field researcher's drive for information-rich sources can lead to premature closure on a theory. The investigator, they say, should look at the periphery for surprises and for confirming or disconfirming evidence.

Final Thoughts

Professionals more familiar with quantitative research may have persistent misgivings about the small sample size in most qualitative studies. It is important to understand that a desirable qualitative report presents a convincing argument and allows for vicarious experience and learning. Desirable qualitative reports are useful (Elder & Miller, 1995; Inui & Frankel, 1991; Kuzel, Engel, Addison, & Bogdewic, 1994; Lincoln & Guba, 1985; Mays & Pope, 1995b; also see Chapter 18) . Skillful field or documentary/historical research can achieve this with relatively few well-chosen cases—sometimes as few as one! As Patton (1990) suggests, one only has to consider the impact of the work of Piaget or Freud to realize that sample size is not the determinant of either clinical or research significance.

All investigators work within the limitations of time and funding available for their efforts. In quantitative research, the investigator endeavors to make "N" only as big as it has to be for statistical significance. Similarly, the qualitative researcher generally samples new sources up to, but not beyond, the point of saturation. Furthermore, by using pragmatic strategies such as maximum variation or critical case sampling, investigators focus the majority of effort on information-rich cases and derive more return from effort. They may find that after the first three interviews, they are getting the same kind of information on a given topic, and they will choose, therefore, to devote relatively less time to that area in the fourth and fifth interviews in favor of exploring new, related topics or looking for information that will challenge their understanding.

In summary, researchers using constructivist or critical/ecological paradigms and employing field or documentary/historical styles of investigation must attend to two quality issues when making sampling decisions: appropriateness and adequacy. To ensure appropriateness, researchers should (a) consider how the sample fits the research purpose and the phenomenon of interest and (b) employ a sampling strategy that is consistent with the style of inquiry. To ensure adequacy, researchers should (a) select sample units serially—"who and what comes next" depends on who and what came before; (b) continuously adjust the sample in response to developing interpretations and theories; (c) sample to the point of saturation of categories and interpretations; and (d) actively search for negative cases or alternative explanations to give developing theory greater breadth and strength (Lincoln & Guba, 1985; Kuzel, 1990; Kuzel et al., 1994).

Although these guidelines are common to many of the qualitative methods texts now in use, there is no single generally agreed-on set of rules for sampling. It is better to remember that

> all descriptions purporting to be true carry with them their own interpretive standards. Here, of course, is where qualitative research becomes a craft very much dependent on the public and private standards (aesthetic, moral, and professional) held by the researchers. (Van Mannen, 1979, p. 257)

It is the investigator's responsibility to make explicit the ethical, practical, and logical rationales for the sampling strategy employed so the audience for the work can judge its quality.

3

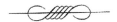

Participant Observation

Stephen P. Bogdewic

If you are a successful participant observer you will know
when to laugh at what your informants think is funny; and
when informants laugh at what you say it will be because
you meant it to be a joke.

H. R. Bernard, 1988, p. 148

Participant observation has been described as an oxymoron (Ellen,
1984). How is it possible to stand back and observe that of which you
are also an integral part? Although on initial reflection this may seem
difficult, it is in fact a process that we use in everything we do. As a result,
it can appear too simple to be considered a method. On the other hand, as
this method is the province of a range of different social scientists, it can
also be made to seem mystical, an art form that defies description.
Somewhere between these two extremes lies a method that is of use to
researchers in primary care settings. This chapter provides an introduction
to the techniques, common practices, and procedures of this method, using
examples from an investigation of the socialization of family medicine
residents to illustrate major points.

Participant observation has its roots in social and cultural anthropology.
The origin of this unique way of collecting data is generally attributed to
Malinowski's (1961) fieldwork among the Trobriand Islanders. Malinowski

is credited as being the first to use participant observation to generate specific anthropological knowledge (Ellen, 1984). The term "participant observation" can be traced to Lindemann (1924), who distinguished between "objective observers" who, primarily through the use of interviewing, approach a culture from the outside, and "participant observers" who use observation to research a culture from within (Friedrichs & Ludtke, 1974).

Hammersley and Atkinson (1983) argue that regardless of the distinct purposes of social science, the methods it employs are simply refinements of processes we use in everyday life. It is no surprise, then, that participant observation has been defined in many, albeit similar, ways. Goetz and LeCompte (1984) see it as a means for eliciting from people the ways in which they construct their definitions of reality and the manner in which they organize their world. Bogdan (1972) provides an operational definition that attempts to more completely encompass the method: "research characterized by a prolonged period of intense social interaction between the researcher and the subjects, in the milieu of the latter, during which time data, in the form of field notes, are unobtrusively and systematically collected" (p. 3).

Jorgensen (1989) offers perhaps the most detailed definition. He defines the method in terms of seven distinct features: the insiders' viewpoint, the here and now of everyday life, the development of interpretive theories, an open-ended process of inquiry, an in-depth case study approach, the researcher's direct involvement in informants' lives, and direct observation as a primary data gathering device. For Jorgensen, the ultimate aim of participant observation is to "generate practical and theoretical truths about human life grounded in the realities of daily existence" (p. 14). It is this definition of participant observation that guided the study reported in this chapter.

WHY PARTICIPANT OBSERVATION?

Most aspects of human existence can be studied using the method of participant observation. The fundamental reason to select participant observation over other research techniques relates to the significance of the cultural context and observing behaviors in answering the research question. If the focus of interest is how the activities and interactions of a setting give meaning to certain behaviors or beliefs, participant observation is the method of choice. The inhabitants of any organization or group are influenced by assumptions that they take for granted. These "assumptions" reflect the unique culture of a given organization. Rather than relying on the perceptions of inhabitants, participant observation affords the researcher direct access to these assumptions. There are several advantages to this method when it is used to investigate cultural groups:

- As time in the field passes, the inhabitants are less likely to alter their behavior due to your presence; you are accommodated rather than reacted to. As a result, your chances of witnessing the phenomenon as it actually occurs are greatly enhanced.
- Differences between real and verbal behavior are made apparent. Information obtained from interviews and questionnaires may not reflect actual behavior.
- Questions can be formed in the language of the inhabitants. Rather than constructing questions a priori, questions can be constructed using terms and colloquialisms characteristic of the people you are studying.
- The sequence and connectedness of events that contribute to the meaning of a phenomenon can be identified. Rather than attempting to piece an understanding together from various clues or repeated interviews, the context can be observed as it unfolds in everyday life.
- The richness and complexity of the human condition can be more fully appreciated and understood. There are times when discreet aspects of human interaction will be singled out for study, but there are, likewise, many times when there is no substitute for generating a holistic description of a naturally occurring phenomenon.

It is apparent from the preceding list of advantages that participant observation would not be appropriate for all types of studies. Jorgensen (1989) and Bernard (1988) suggest that it would, however, be a likely choice when

- it would be considered an intrusion to have a complete stranger present to witness and record the situation of interest,
- the situation of interest is obscured or completely hidden from the public, and/or
- the inhabitants appear to have significantly different views than do outsiders.

Given these criteria, there are many situations in primary care where participant observation could prove useful. The various organizations in which the business of primary care takes place all have their own unique cultures. How many variations of primary care organizations are there? How will these organizations respond to environmental factors such as the economic strains on society and the growing, unmet health care needs of a large number of citizens? As these organizations respond, how can the processes by which they change be understood? Likewise, the various occupational groups that are involved in the delivery of primary care each function in accordance with particular norms, language, customs, and rituals. How do these occupations interpret and carry out what they each define as primary care? How do their definitions differ? To what values are the members of these occupations socialized during their training? In summary, any research question that requires an understanding of the processes, events, and relationships, the context of a social situation, is appropriate for the method of participant observation.

There are costs associated with using participant observation. It can be very time consuming. The field work portion of a study can, and often does, take a year or even more to complete. However, it is possible to conduct applied research in as short a time as 1 to 3 months (Bernard, 1988) or even several days or weeks when part of a larger study design (see examples in Chapters 9, 14, and 16). The time required to conduct the study reported in this chapter was slightly less than 1 year. Whether participant observation is a suitable method depends entirely on the research question being asked and the overall design of the study.

A PRIMER ON PARTICIPANT OBSERVATION

In this section, I describe the various steps in participant observation, using examples from a study of residency training in family medicine. Two interests prompted this investigation (Bogdewic, 1987). My primary interest was in knowing how residents in family medicine developed their professional identity. Through what stages did they pass en route to claiming the identity of "family doctor"? What factors or forces influenced how their identity was shaped? In addition, I was interested in knowing how this identity formation process differed in the two major types of settings in which it occurred—university-based programs and community-based programs.

Overview of the Project

The selection of methods for this investigation was guided by the question, What does it mean for family medicine residents to one day call themselves family doctors? I was less interested in residents' perceptions of their identity and more interested in those behaviors and other factors within the training setting that gave meaning to this unique professional identity. Because this meaning is culturally derived, I felt it was necessary to observe the residents in the context that formed their identity. Furthermore, the resources required to conduct a time-intensive investigation were available. Two colleagues helped with data collection. Each of them observed at only one site, while I divided my time equally between the two sites. In addition to being participant observers, we each conducted key informant interviews (see Chapter 4).

Observations were limited to the outpatient care facility (Family Practice Center [FPC]) and those educational spaces that were located in or adjacent to it, for three reasons. First, the FPC is a social scene that closely approximates the type of setting in which most residents will ultimately practice. Second, the FPC is the residents' home base. It is where they routinely interact, both formally and informally, with those who share a similar commitment to their discipline. A final factor was one of practical consideration. Family medicine residents rotate through numerous other teaching services, many of which are located at other hospitals. The logistics of arranging to be with the residents while they were on these other rotations was not feasible. In summary, the FPC was selected as the primary site for observations because it was the setting most relevant to the phenomenon being studied (Mays & Pope, 1995a). A more complete discussion of the issues related to selecting a sample in qualitative investigations can be found in Chapter 2.

Interactions and activities that were observed included routine patient care activities (including interactions with support staff, preceptors, peers, and, to a lesser extent, patients), educational conferences, one-on-one and small group teaching encounters, and informal interactions with staff, faculty, and fellow residents. Although observations occurred throughout an 11-month period, the bulk of the observations took place during the first 6 months of the study. Observation days were randomly selected, and observation periods occurred throughout each part of the day.

The majority of family medicine residency programs are located in community hospitals that have some university affiliation (American Academy of Family Physicians, 1991). The second largest category of programs is those based in university hospitals. This was one reason why both types of programs were included in this study. A second reason was that it had been my observation over the prior 10 years that, within academic family medicine, there was some general level of agreement that the two types of programs were significantly different. I had always been curious about these perceived differences and thought it would be fascinating to conduct my own comparison. Finally, it was a manageable task to include both programs in this study, as they are within one hour's driving time from each other.

Gaining Entry

Once a site has been selected that you believe provides access to the data in which you are interested, you need to gain permission to conduct the study. Several things bear keeping in mind. First, rehearse in advance the way you will answer the many questions you think you may be asked.

Remember, no matter how well you frame your interest, and no matter how credible you appear, you are asking permission to partake in private matters. Along those lines, take full advantage of anyone who can help you gain entry. Finally, the process of gaining entry is when data collection begins and data analysis starts.

In the resident socialization study, I had to gain entry into two settings. In the community setting, this was accomplished by sending one letter to the residency director and then attending one faculty meeting. The primary concern expressed by the faculty in this meeting was a practical one—what's in it for us? How will we benefit from participating in this study? Once I adequately addressed this, I was given the go-ahead to conduct the study. When I asked about how I should present my proposal to the residents, I was informed that would not be necessary. I was told that the residents trusted that the faculty had their best interests in mind and that they (the residents) would support the faculty decision.

I sent the same letter to the residency director of the university program and was similarly invited to attend a faculty meeting to discuss my proposal. This is where the similarity ended. After considerable discussion, the faculty referred me to the group responsible for the management of the clinic where I would be spending the bulk of my time. The primary concern of this group was patient confidentiality. Once they were reassured that this would not be a problem, the management group decided that the residents needed to be involved in the decision-making process. Rather than letting me make initial contact with the residents, the chief resident first wrote the residents a memo, briefly explaining what I wanted to do. I then wrote each resident, providing greater detail about the design and purpose of my study. Over the course of the next 3 to 4 weeks, each resident responded to the chief resident regarding his or her willingness to participate. They all had agreed. All that was left was another meeting with the clinic management group and then the residency faculty, and I was in. This process took about 2 months.

In addition to gaining permission to conduct the study from each of the residency programs, I also had to contact the Human Subjects Committee in both institutions. Much to my surprise, formal approval was not required. More recently, Institutional Review Boards have increasingly been asking for a formal review and requiring informed consent procedures from study participants, as can be seen in the examples from other chapters in this volume.

Initial Contact

Entry has been negotiated. Now what? How do you, a stranger, walk in the door without causing everyone's head to turn? The fact is, you can't avoid it. People know you are not one of them and are curious to learn who you are and what you are doing there. Therefore, what you need, for your own comfort level as well as that of the inhabitants, is a succinct way of introducing yourself and explaining why you are there. Even if someone else has told them the purpose of your study, they will want to hear it from you. The best rule to follow is to *tell them the truth* (Bogdan, 1972). This does not mean you have to go into great detail; in fact, too much detail can alarm people. An honest, jargon-free, down-to-earth explanation will suffice. Among other things, such an explanation is much easier for someone to pass on to the other members of the organization.

One lesson I learned from my first few contacts in the field is the importance of being vague. My initial explanations to some of the staff about wanting to understand how the residency training program influenced identity formation were interpreted as my wanting to evaluate their organization. I quickly learned I was better off giving a much broader description of my purpose. Rather than putting any focus on their organization, I explained that I was primarily interested in what it meant to people to become family doctors. This statement was essentially true, and it was considered less threatening because it required no apparent judgments about the organization.

Establishing Rapport

Beyond initial introductions, it is recommended that the researcher approach the early days in the field with caution. At this point, you do not know the routines and rituals of the situation. You cannot determine yet what is considered offensive nor what roles are appropriate for you to play. Additionally, you have not yet established trust with the "natives." Behavior during this phase is guided as much by commonsense knowledge about considerate social interaction as it is by anything else (Bogdan, 1972). The goal at this stage is to develop trusting and cooperative relationships with the insiders in the field setting. Such relationships are necessary to gain access to important aspects of daily existence and to be trusted with dependable, pertinent information (Jorgensen, 1989).

Although there are no hard and fast rules for establishing and maintaining rapport, the following tips are worth considering:

Be unobtrusive. At the outset you should be more observer than participant. This phase of participant observation has been referred to as "learning the ropes" (Geer et al., 1968; Shaffir, Stebbins, & Turowetz, 1980). Your behavior and attire should not draw attention to you. Your goal is to learn what it takes to fit in. There is no precise formula to follow; however, normal social cues such as body language and obvious shifts in feeling states or interactions are to be trusted.

Be honest. People in the setting you are studying will have a limited understanding of why you are there. Questions about your interests and what you hope to find should be dealt with in an open and direct fashion. You may need, at this time, to assure people that their participation is voluntary, identities will remain anonymous, and all information will be treated confidentially (Jorgensen, 1989).

Be unassuming. It is conceivable that you have some degree of technical or professional knowledge regarding the situation you are studying. Not only could this present a bias, it also runs the risk of threatening the subjects. If anything, play down your expertise. You already know what you know. That's not why you are in the field.

Be a reflective listener. This fundamental communication skill not only helps build rapport but is also an excellent way to learn the language of the inhabitants. The particular words used in a given social situation have a certain significance or meaning to the insiders. By reflecting back what you are hearing, you can better understand how the language in this setting differs from what you know, and, simultaneously, you can move the relationship to a deeper level.

Be self-revealing. Subjects have some degree of curiosity about you, particularly as time passes. A willingness to discuss common interests and life experiences can open the door to a more trusting relationship. You have to decide just how intimate your relations with subjects can become. Avoiding intimacy, however, and opting for a more aloof stance can limit your being accepted.

As rapport is developed, you are able to begin participating in the activities in the setting. These joint activities or shared experiences with the inside members mark the boundary between outsiders and insiders. Participating in them means that you have "joined," even if yours is a special type of membership.

The Mechanics of Observation

Just what does "participation in the activities of the setting" mean? What do participant observers routinely do? One way to think about participant observation is to think of all the elements needed to tell a story—who, what, when, where, why, and how. To organize my fieldwork, I adapted the following framework from Goetz and LeCompte (1984):

Who is present? How would you characterize them? What role are they playing in the group? How did they enter the group? On what is their membership in this group based? Who did the organizing or directing of the group?

What is happening? What are people doing and saying, and how are they behaving? How did this activity/interaction begin? What things appear to be routine? To what extent are the various participants involved? What is the tone of their communication? What body language is being used?

When does this activity occur? What is its relationship to other activities or events? How long does it last? What makes it the right time (wrong time) for this to occur?

Where is this happening? What part do the physical surroundings contribute to what is happening? Can and does this happen elsewhere? Do participants use or relate to the space or physical objects differently?

Why is this happening? What precipitated this event/interaction? Are different perspectives on what is occurring evident? What contributes to things happening in this manner?

How is this activity organized? How are the elements of what is happening related? What rules or norms are evident? How does this activity or group relate to other aspects of the setting?

Obviously, not all of these categories will be recorded in a single observation. They provide one way of thinking about the range of possible ways to begin the adventure of learning about a social situation. Most of the above questions are ones that we unconsciously process as we encounter social scenes on a routine basis. Of course, we also unconsciously apply our own biases and interpretations to these scenes, often without giving them any additional thought. The difference for the participant observer is that consciously recording the specific details of that which we might normally take for granted begins to show how meanings are constructed in this particular organization or setting. To the novice field worker, it may at first seem like busywork to pay attention to details such as how people are physically located within a room. These details can, however, open doors to realizations that can contribute in ways previously unimagined to the story that is unfolding.

In the study of family medicine residents, one routine location for my observations was the preceptor room. This is the place in the outpatient clinic where individual faculty members and community practitioners (preceptors) are available to provide consultation and supervision to the residents. Residents usually come to this room with some question they would like answered or to ask the preceptor to see the patient with them.

For the first few weeks, my observations were not guided by any framework. I was simply "learning the ropes." Soon afterward, I began applying some structure to my observations. One of the first things I noticed that I had not noted previously was the difference between residents' presentation styles in the two settings. In the community program, when residents presented a patient to the preceptor, they almost always remained standing; residents in the university program, more often than not, sat down. This one difference colored the ensuing interaction with the preceptor. It also led to the development of a new category that served as a filter for screening other observations. One final comment about the above framework—it only specifies the various elements of an observation. It does not indicate the possible "types" of observations. Spradley (1980) distinguishes between three types or levels of observation: descriptive, focused, and selective. *Descriptive observations* occur early in the study and are the least systematic. They are guided by the general question, "What's going on here?" Werner and Schoepfle (1987b) have described this level of observation as the "shotgun approach." Every attempt is made to observe as much as possible. *Focused observations,* which are more selective than descriptive observations, represent choices the researcher has made based on both areas of interest and on what has been learned from being in the setting. The product of such observations may be categories or taxonomies that begin to provide initial structure to one's understanding. *Selective observations* are highly focused and enable the researcher to compare the attributes of various categories or activities. Spradley (1980) suggests that the three levels of observation be thought of as a funnel. Each level has a narrower focus.

Before beginning your fieldwork, or during your first few days in the field, *map the territory.* This means literally diagramming the physical spaces in which you are spending time. This map provides one context for the interactions you observe. It enables you to consider differences, such as the difference between group space and personal space, from a more global perspective than may be available in any other manner. It helps you see where you are spending your time and where you are not. Lastly, the exploration required to draw the map is one way of becoming familiar with the setting.

The Participation Continuum

Observation is the more passive dimension of the participant observer role. By definition, participation connotes some form of active involvement. Before considering the factors that influence the extent to which one can participate, it is useful to consider ways of conceptualizing the participant observer role.

Jaeger (1988) distinguishes between three different stances participant observers can take—the active participant, the privileged observer, and the limited observer. Jaeger's characterization depicts participation as an all or none situation. By contrast, Junker (1960) poses four theoretical social roles for conducting fieldwork—complete participant, participant as observer, observer as participant, and complete observer. This characterization depicts participation as a function of degree.

The identity of the "complete participant" is completely concealed. This person joins a group ostensibly as a regular member but with the sole purpose of conducting research. A variation of this role is seen in the work of Konner (1987). Having achieved considerable success as an anthropologist, Konner decided, in his mid-30s, to attend medical school. His training in anthropology provided an excellent foundation for providing a thorough account of his journey through medical school.

At the other end of the continuum is the "complete observer." Hammersley and Atkinson (1983) point out that complete observation has advantages and disadvantages similar to complete participation. In both situations, the researcher does not interact as a researcher with those being studied. This minimizes the problem of reactivity. However, both of these roles make it difficult, if not impossible, to question and interview subjects. Likewise, both of these roles may limit just what can be observed. Most fieldwork lies somewhere between these two extremes.

The distinction between participant as observer and observer as participant is blurred. Junker (1960) characterizes the former as marked by "subjectivity and sympathy" and the latter as a somewhat more detached role characterized by "objectivity and sympathy." Obviously, there is a significant overlap between these two roles. Distinguishing them as separate is one way of encouraging the researcher to move about the continuum and adopt the posture best suited to the situation.

The extent to which the researcher both chooses to participate and is allowed to participate depends on several factors. The purpose of the study and the particular nature of the setting are the foremost factors. My primary interest in the resident socialization study was to see the training program through the eyes of the residents. Because the setting was not highly structured, I was able to participate in a range of resident activities. I attended lectures with them, ate meals with them, sat in on their small group and one-on-one teaching encounters, and served as a sounding board to them just as their peers often did.

It is important to keep in mind that the goal of participation is not to see how many different ways the researcher can become involved in the activities of the organization. You are primarily concerned with collecting data. Participation is a way of establishing rapport. It is also how you find ways to fit into the organization that do not disturb the setting or interfere with your function as an observer (Bogdan, 1972).

Informants

Researchers who attempt to learn the insiders' view of a particular social and cultural scene do not do so alone. They are aided by knowledgeable individuals from within the culture—informants. Informants are defined as "native speakers," engaged by the participant observer to "speak in their own language" (Spradley, 1979). Informants teach the researcher through modeling and interpreting and by supplying information. Together with the researcher, informants help edit the story as it is being discovered.

Every member of a cultural group is a potential informant. Each has commonsense knowledge of his or her social world and can teach you something. However, it is usually impossible to cultivate relationships with every member, so researchers select informants, and vice versa. Selection is based on several factors. In general, you want someone who has been in the culture long enough such that they no longer think about it. Informants who fit this description are more inclined to provide an insider's account or analysis. By contrast, anyone who steps beyond the insider role and offers an analysis based on specific frameworks, such as those of social science, should be avoided (Spradley, 1979). Informants might also be selected because they represent a particular category of actor. In studying the developmental process of identity formation among residents, for example, it was essential to locate informants within each of the 3-year groups.

Informants who have special knowledge, status, or access to observations denied the researcher are referred to as "key informants" (Goetz & LeCompte, 1984). Perhaps the best advice for selecting key informants comes from Bernard (1988). He suggests you seek informants who are observant, reflective, and articulate and who also know how to tell good stories. These are the people with whom to develop and maintain relationships throughout your time in the field. A more thorough consideration of the use of informants is provided in Chapter 4.

FIELD NOTES: A DIALOGUE WITH SELF

Once a level of comfort and trust is established, the adventure of being in the field blossoms. What may amount to routine activities for the inhabitants become pieces of an intricate puzzle to the participant observer. The temptation to continue observing and participating rather than stopping to record the experience is strong. *Field notes cannot, however, be trusted to memory.* The richness and detail of an experience will be lost as a new and unexpected phenomenon occurs. The habit of regularly recording experiences as soon as possible after they occur is essential.

Field notes represent an attempt to provide a literal account of what happened in the field setting—the social processes and their contexts. Obviously, it is not possible to record everything that transpires. What eventually gets recorded depends on the style and preference of the researcher, the research questions being asked, the particulars of the setting, and the methods used to record data. There are three fundamental questions to be considered with regard to field notes (Hammersley & Atkinson, 1983): what to record, how to record it, and when to record it.

What: The Content of Field Notes

The general rule of thumb for what to record, especially during the early stages of fieldwork, is *"If in doubt, write it down."* Even with a particular research question in mind, one cannot be certain of what will eventually contribute to an understanding of the phenomenon of interest. Descriptions must include enough of the context surrounding the activity so that meaningful comparisons and contrasts can be made during analysis. Until the habits and skills of accurate recording of observations are fully developed, it is very helpful to use a framework or checklist for constructing the context. Spradley proposes one such framework:

1. Space: the physical place or places
2. Actor: the people involved
3. Activity: a set of related acts people do
4. Object: the physical things that are present
5. Act: single actions that people do
6. Event: a set of related activities that people carry out
7. Time: the sequencing that takes place over time
8. Goal: the things people are trying to accomplish
9. Feeling: the emotions felt and expressed. (Spradley, 1980, p. 78)

A framework such as this encourages thick description, and "rich field notes" are those endowed with quality descriptions (Bogdan & Biklen, 1982). Beyond the descriptive part of field notes, however, there is a reflective part. The researcher is the primary research tool in a participant observation study, so it is essential that the researcher's personal journey be included in the field notes. Before even entering the field, it is important to record your feelings, hunches, known biases, assumptions, and even expected outcomes. Doing so provides a baseline against which you can compare what actually emerges as the study develops. Once the study is under way, the reflective dimension of field notes falls into several categories (Bogdan & Biklen, 1982):

1. *Reflections on Analysis.* Throughout the investigation, themes will emerge, new hunches or possibilities will surface, patterns will develop, connections will be made, and you will experience confusion over what you are seeing. Reflecting on these dimensions of the fieldwork experience is the beginning of the dialogue you have with yourself throughout the study and from which your analysis takes form.

2. *Reflections on Method.* As a participant observation study develops, the strategies and processes used to explore various aspects of the setting change. This happens as a result of learning more about the environment and also being afforded new opportunities for observation and/or participation. In addition, not everything you attempt will work. Reflecting on how and why you select new strategies or on how you deal with difficult situations provides, in the end, an accurate record of what the study actually entailed.

3. *Reflections on Ethical Dilemmas and Conflicts.* By its very nature, fieldwork places the researcher in intimate contact with the lives of the observed. Decisions such as what to record, how to handle privileged information, what types of relationships are appropriate, and how to handle value conflicts are common occurrences. Reflecting on these issues is both an important part of the "story" and a way of working out concerns.

4. *Points of Clarification.* Not all reflections require in-depth thought. Without having to go into any detail, it is useful to include sentences in your notes that point out errors or that clarify something about which you were previously confused.

5. *Reflections on the Observer's Frame of Mind.* Every attempt should be made to explore one's preconceptions prior to entering the field, and it is inevitable that field experiences will challenge many of the researcher's assumptions. Patients, for instance, actually play more of an educational role with residents than I imagined. By reflecting on this process of discovery, the researcher not only moves from the imagined world to the empirical world but also documents important analytic constructs.

6. *Reflections on Feelings.* A critical aspect of the observer's frame of mind involves feelings. When our thoughts, assumptions, values, and reflections are challenged, we respond emotionally as well as intellectually.

The experiences we have in the field are not merely observed and recorded, they are also felt. Reflecting on feelings is essential. Only through such reflection can the researcher determine how he or she is influencing the field experience.

At one point in working with residents who were feeling significant stress from their training experience, I realized that I enjoyed the fact they seemed to feel good when they were interacting with me. Upon reflection, I realized I enjoyed it so much that I sometimes shied away from discussing certain things with them that might shift the feeling state. I learned from this that I was less secure than I thought about being in this particular setting. Once I realized this, I chose to change my behavior. I did not want to deny the residents and myself an opportunity to learn from all of their feeling states, including those of frustration, sadness, and anger. I did two things differently. First, I made a conscious effort not to send cues that would shift the feeling state, cues such as tone of voice, eye contact, and only permitting brief pauses between comments. Then, I asked a few key informants who were seniors what I might do to make it easier for the other residents to explore the total range of their feelings. These informants not only suggested certain questions I might ask based on their understanding of some of the stresses and challenges of residency training, they also launched into a more serious level of discussion regarding some of their own concerns. In essence, they were modeling for me what they thought might work.

How: The Form of Field Notes

Most field notes are not written in the field. The "field notes" that are most often referred to represent an expanded account of a variety of information obtained in the field during a given observation session and then later assembled. There are various technologies that can be used to obtain this information. These will be discussed later in this section. For now, the focus will be on the various types of "notes" that are generated during a participant observation study. Although the term *field notes* is often used interchangeably for these various notes, each serves a distinct purpose.

Jottings. The participant observer must be sensitive to what is considered normal and appropriate behavior while in the field if he or she is to be granted access to the range of possible observations. For this reason, it is unlikely that the researcher will have the opportunity to write any extensive notes during observation sessions, as this behavior is likely to be conspicuous. Situations such as lectures, where note taking is normal, are an exception. For the most part, the initial notes the researcher takes can best be described as jottings.

The word *jottings* is an accurate description of what the researcher is usually able to do in the field—jot down phrases, or even just a key word, that capture some aspect of the observation. Later, when the expanded account of the observation session is being developed, jottings serve as memory triggers. Traditionally, a small notebook, one that might fit in a pocket, was the accepted standard for recording these abbreviated notes. However, the advent of palm-top computers has introduced an effective tool that not only simplifies the ability to collect jottings but also facilitates their incorporation into field notes. No particular format is suggested for jottings; the primary objective is simply to capture some key phrase or descriptor without drawing attention to the process of doing so. What actually gets written is a matter of style or preference. Discovering the best way to write brief notes, or a condensed account, in a particular setting usually requires some experimentation. The ploy of "frequent trips to the bathroom" is one method that has been the brunt of much humor among experienced field workers.

Log or Field Diary. It is valuable in doing fieldwork to have a record of how you spend your time. Such a log has many benefits. It can be used for planning future sessions, for recording the amount of time spent in the field as well as for any associated expenses, for easy reference in reviewing who has been interviewed and where the most frequent observations have occurred, and as an appointments calendar. By providing a historical record of the entire fieldwork experience, analysis of the log can generate additional insights to the study.

Field Notes. The term *field notes* is used here to describe the expanded account, or permanent notes, that is the core of a participant observation study and the foundation for eventual analysis. It is, therefore, essential that they are as complete and accurate as possible. Field notes are written as soon as possible after an observation period and are an expression of the jottings (this is covered in greater detail in the following section). In no time at all, the number of actual pages can swell to unimagined proportions. Therefore, to manage the data, it is important that field notes be well constructed. This requirement entails several issues.

First, if relying on written field notes, each page must be properly labeled. For example, a space could be reserved in the upper right hand corner of the page for noting name of the observer, date, location, time of the observation period, and page number. The cover page on a set of notes for a given observation session could also include a title that might prove useful in recalling that particular session (e.g., "The Stormy Seminar on

Liability," "The New Preceptor"). If using a computer program (refer to Chapter 11), provide these details in the computer file.

In addition, on printed field notes, each page should have a wide margin down one side. This margin enables you and others to make comments on the notes, comments that can then be used to reflect on feeling states, possible meanings, or even theoretical hunches about what may be happening. This margin is also useful in coding the notes. Coding is a fundamental analytic process (it is more fully described in Chapters 7 and 9). Basically, coding addresses the issue that facts do not speak for themselves (Jorgensen, 1989). Therefore, as field notes are written and reviewed, it is important to make side notes that identify and label issues that seem relevant to what is being studied. This might include themes, relationships, key words or questions, patterns, sequences, and so forth (e.g., ways of being esteemed, how to look responsible, etc.). Computer programs now allow this to be done directly in the program (refer to Chapter 11).

Another consideration in writing field notes is how to accurately record dialogue. The actual words that participants use are important. Each culture has its own language, which means the language has a particular meaning for the inhabitants of the culture. The word(s) that the researcher might select for describing a phenomenon could easily have a completely different meaning from what was intended by the subject. It is essential, then, that dialogue be recorded accurately.

Unless dialogue is mechanically recorded, which is not always possible or desirable, the researcher must depend on jottings and memory to reconstruct dialogue. A consistent method for distinguishing the accuracy of dialogue is essential. The following is one suggested method:

Verbatims: If you are certain you have the actual words used in a sentence or phrase, or a key word that was expressed, place it in double quotes (" . . . ").

Paraphrase: Citations in which you have a lesser degree of certainty but are reasonably sure of what was said can be placed in single quotes (' . . . ').

Observer's comment: Words themselves can be misleading. Someone can say "yes" when, in fact, it is clear they mean "no." Often the context of an exchange is better understood by inserting an explanatory comment or description. This interjection can be separated from the rest of the text by the use of brackets ([. . .]).

Finally, be liberal in starting new paragraphs. Any event or circumstance that is new to the scene being observed merits a new paragraph. If someone new enters the room or if the mood or topic changes, start a new paragraph. By doing so, you will make your notes much easier to both read and code.

Location: Preceptor Room

Observer: SP
Date: 2/2/87
Time: 1:30-5:30 pm
Page: 3

follow up →

Upon returning from the noon conference, I made my usual pass through the staff lounge, only to find no coffee or people. I then headed for the clinic. As I approached the nursing station en route to the preceptor room, I was asked by one of the nurses if 'I could be helped.' I briefly explained my presence. She had no questions, thanked me and went about her business. She did not indicate in any fashion that she knew about my study and appeared too busy to talk at the moment. . . . [I am surprised. I thought I had become a pretty common fixture in this setting by now. Maybe she knew about the study but simply did not connect it to me personally. I need to follow up on this.]

Key informant problem ??

I entered the preceptor room and found it vacant. From the stack of charts sitting on the lone table it is apparent that a preceptor is close by. . . . [The preceptors often try to catch up on completing their patient charts while they are precepting.] . . . Before I even sit down, Dr. H. enters. He shakes my hand and says, "How's the study going? I don't mean here [this setting], just in general." I make a few vague general comments about what a challenging experience this has turned out to be. [I am reluctant to discuss "the study." I would rather discuss what is happening around us. Dr. H. has been a key informant for me. I am concerned that what this may mean to him is that we (he and I) will usually be engaged in editorial/analytical comments about the study rather than in discussing the activities that are occurring in the setting. I need to give some thought to how this happened and what I can do to change it.]

We are interrupted by a call that Dr. H. receives from a patient. As he chatted in an animated fashion with the patient, he turned to me with a big smile on his face and whispered, "This is a great couple." Several times during the conversation he called the patient "sir." Two more times he covered the receiver and commented on 'what a great couple they were.' He closed the conversation by saying that he would have 'my nurse call you back to let you know if the hospital could do a chest X ray on Saturday.' I was curious to see what Dr. H. would have to say about this "great couple," but just as he finished the call a resident came into the room and asked Dr. H. to see a patient with him. JR (second-year resident): "I've got a kid with a rash that won't go away, could you take a look at it?" Without asking any questions, Dr. H. stood up and said "Sure, let's go," and departed the preceptor room with the resident.

resolution: my way

While they were gone, one of the senior residents (BL) came in, sat down, and we exchanged greetings. I had spent quite a bit of time with this resident a few days ago, during which we were talking about her father, who was a surgeon. Within moments, we were interrupted by another senior student (WD), who came into the preceptor room ostensibly to ask the other senior what type of medication she preferred for a particular condition. They discussed the options and then disagreed about the medication, despite what the literature had to say. When WD left, I asked the remaining resident if she was comfortable with the disagreement. She replied, "Sure, there really isn't a right answer."

Figure 3.1. Sample Page of Field Notes—Expanded Account

Another way of indicating a shift or break in the observation, or in a subset of observations, is simply to insert a break line in the text (see Figure 3.1).

Journals, Memos, or Notes on Notes

The "field notes" that have just been described represent the descriptive part of the written record. Although it might be possible to include the reflective part of the fieldwork experience in these field notes, the preferred way to proceed is to keep a separate or parallel set of notes for this purpose. Reflective notes are literally the notes you write to yourself about the descriptive accounts that you have developed—notes on notes. Included in them are your thoughts, confusions, and understandings of personal, methodological, and analytic aspects of the fieldwork experience. Such notes enable the researcher to gain analytical distance from the data (Strauss & Corbin, 1990). They are the sine qua non of a participant observation study. Throughout the time in the field—the data collection stage—numerous themes, hypotheses, insights, and theoretical ideas emerge. These are recorded at the time they occur. The understandings that surface from them provide the direction for the next steps in the study. In this sense, the final analysis that is eventually achieved reflects a cumulative learning experience. The journal or "notes on notes" tracks the intellectual and emotional journey of the researcher. These notes explain how the learning and discovery process evolved. The file management capability of computer text management programs such as Folio Views and NUD*IST (Chapter 11) enables these to be incorporated directly into the field notes so that the two files may be viewed and worked on simultaneously, a feature that greatly enhances the ability to generate reflective notes while reviewing field notes.

When: The Process of Writing Field Notes

Participant observation studies can continue for extended periods of time. During that time, both the researcher's focus of interest for the study and the understanding of what the data mean take several turns before the investigation is complete. It is, therefore, essential that the researcher develop and use effective habits for writing field notes. Otherwise, invaluable data that is left to memory is lost. Following are hints for writing field notes that can help the researcher develop these habits:

1. Record your notes as soon as possible after the observation. There is no substitute for a fresh impression. The longer you wait before writing notes, the greater the risk of losing data. You may forget details or uncouple what you observed from what you felt. If enough time passes, you may even fail to record anything. This means you must schedule your activities in the field so that you have ample to write your notes immediately following observation sessions. *The discipline of daily writing is a must in a participant observation study.*

2. *Don't discuss your observation with anyone until you have it recorded.* It can be tempting to talk with others about what you have observed. Events in the field can be exciting, particularly when you begin to see connections that you believe are significant. Doing so, however, easily alters what you eventually record. There will be plenty of time later to share your thoughts and excitement.

3. *Find a private place that has the equipment you need to do your work.* Ideally, being able to use the same location each day can contribute to your sense of purpose and minimize distractions. In any event, find a convenient, quiet location where you can work undisturbed for several hours.

4. *Plan sufficient time for recording.* Estimating the time required to properly record a given observation session takes some amount of practice. Until you have gained this type of experience, it is best to give yourself more time than you think it will take. One hour of observation easily takes from 3 to 6 hours to record. With this in mind, it is a good idea to limit initial observations to 1 hour and plan recording time accordingly. Gathering large amounts of data without sufficient time for recording usually produces poor notes.

5. *Don't edit as you write or dictate.* It is possible to record notes according to topics or themes; however, the natural, chronological flow of the session usually provides the best organizing framework. Therefore, wait until you have completed your notes before you go back over them and edit or add as necessary. Along those same lines, if days later you recall something from an observation that you failed to record, go back and add it to your notes. There is one exception to this rule of thumb. If a particular observation session was lengthy, or the course of events was complex, or a given conversation was involved, consider making a brief outline of the major topics before starting to write. Doing so can reduce the tendency to reread notes as they are being written.

Recording notes is a laborious task. Observation sessions can leave you feeling drained or can leave you feeling exhilarated. In either case, the last thing you feel like doing at the end of a session is sitting down and concentrating on writing a detailed account of what transpired. This is something you must discipline yourself to overcome. Otherwise, when you are in the advanced stages of analysis and realize your data are thin, there is nothing you will be able to do except, perhaps, gather additional data.

Rich data cannot be generated retrospectively. Writing expanded accounts of your notes in a timely fashion is, therefore, the most essential habit you will need to develop to conduct a participant observation study. Such discipline also helps refine your ability to write well, a skill that is an essential component of all fieldwork (Wolcott, 1995).

TECHNOLOGIES FOR RECORDING AND MANAGING FIELD NOTES

Paper and Pencil. The mental image that first comes to mind when thinking about doing field notes is usually the indispensable paper and pencil. Although limited in their use, paper and pencil notes are often the only alternative. Tape recorders and portable computers would be conspicuous in many settings where paper and pencil seem natural. For instance, in both educational and clinical settings, there is usually a fair amount of writing activity. In such settings, a researcher who is jotting brief notes that will later serve as cues would hardly be noticed. Beyond "jottings," paper and pencil notes are of questionable value. Given the technology that currently exists, it makes little sense to hand write expanded accounts.

Audio Recording. Tape recorders are an excellent tool for making notes. They can be used to record both jottings and more expanded accounts. In the resident socialization study, my assistants and I used a minicassette recorder to record brief reminders, cues we later used in writing more complete notes. This recorder was the same type that many of the physicians were using to dictate notes for patients' charts. Its presence was seen as "normal." This same recorder was then used to develop one version of an expanded account. My home was approximately 1 hour away from the study location, and, because of both the privacy it offered and the availability of a computer, was an excellent location for writing field notes. On the drive home I dictated an account of the observation session. "Talking through" the day's activities was excellent preparation for sitting down at the word processor and letting the day's events flow onto paper. Once the typed version of the notes was completed, the recording that was made on the drive home was listened to for any additional data. In Chapter 16, Crabtree and Miller describe having field workers dictate their observations, which are then transcribed as field notes.

Tape recorders are also the optimal way to record both dialogue and interviews. In some instances, such as lectures or certain meetings, tape recorders are not uncommon and usually go unnoticed. Likewise, many people, once an interview gets under way, forget that a recorder is in use.

Like written notes, tape recordings must be transformed before they can be subjected to complex analysis. Transcribing tapes is both time consuming and expensive—factors that must be weighed in deciding how much recording will be feasible.

Computers. Personal computers have many advantages for recording and managing field notes and for conducting a thorough analysis of the data. With the advent of portable computers and palm-top computers, most of these functions can easily be performed in the field. With nothing more than a basic word processing package, it is possible to record, file, and perform various basic analyses of your recorded data. However, software advances have been dramatic over the past few years, and the ability to manage and analyze qualitative data has flourished. Chapter 11 provides a thorough account of the advantages and possibilities of using computers in conducting qualitative research.

Photography and Videotaping. Both photography and videotaping provide unique visual records of observations. Still photographs capture details as well as more global perspectives of a setting. Videotaping has the advantage of showing how scenes develop and how the movements and actions of the actors are related. Both of these technologies are, in most situations, obtrusive. The opportunity to use them depends on the unique characteristics of the setting. For instance, Family Medicine residents are routinely videotaped or observed during their patient encounters. Without having to impose any equipment in the setting, I was able to watch residents perform the core act for which they had been training.

It is important to remember that permission to use audio and visual recording devices must be obtained in each instance where they are to be used. Under no circumstances should you take for granted that permission to conduct the investigation also includes permission to take still or motion pictures or to tape-record conversations.

INDIVIDUAL VERSUS TEAM RESEARCH

To illustrate the basic elements of participant observation, the focus in this chapter was on having the investigator conduct the fieldwork and complete the study on his or her own. There are some primary care physicians who will manage to accomplish this, but a more realistic model would require a collaborative approach, one in which hired research field workers do the majority of the data collection. The use of such field workers, including how they can be properly trained, is described in the case studies reported in Chapters 9, 14 and 16. However, a few important points merit emphasis.

In a participant observation study, it is generally understood that the researcher is the *primary instrument* for both data collection and analysis. Because field workers become an extension of the primary investigator, the preceding statement attests to how important it is to have field workers be adequately trained and fully cognizant of the purposes and goals of the project. They become the eyes and ears of the primary investigator, and together, they must be able to think as one.

SUMMARY

Much that we are routinely aware of is guided by what we have come to expect, the norms to which we are accustomed. Therefore, the details of a scene, as well as the difference between the figure and the ground, often do not capture our conscious attention. In a participant observation study, until our focus becomes refined, there is no telling which details matter. It is, therefore, essential that the researcher be capable of *seeing what is before him* rather than what he is accustomed to seeing. This does not require genius; *it requires practice.* It is a skill that can be developed. For example, one way of developing the skill of observation is to practice writing descriptions of events that have become an ordinary part of your life from as many perspectives as you can imagine. Regularly scheduled meetings that you attend might be an excellent place to start. This skill is further developed by inviting a colleague to write descriptions of the same event and then comparing them. Of course, it could be argued that the best way to develop the skills of the participant observer is in the field. Certainly it is true that to become adept at these skills there is no substitute for the actual experience of participant observation. However, each of the needed skills can be developed and strengthened before the research ever enters the field.

The method of participant observation is not for everyone, but as demonstrated by Malterud in Chapter 17, even an individual physician working in his or her own practice can successfully complete a study using participant observation. It is a method that asks a great deal of the researcher and offers no promise in return. Such research can consume a great deal of time and energy. And in the end, all the data in the world won't necessarily lead to a useful interpretation. However, the best way to ensure that the data is rich and has captured some essence of the scene being studied is to be armed with the necessary skills, to be open to possibilities you have not yet imagined, and to be willing to look at yourself as intensely as you look at the events you are studying. In participant observation, who you are and what you see cannot be separated, only understood.

4

Key Informant Interviews

Valerie J. Gilchrist
Robert L. Williams

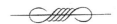

The purpose of this chapter is to familiarize the reader with key informant interviewing, a type of individual interview that involves forming a relationship over time and that is commonly used by ethnographers. Its use in clinical research represents what Arthur Kleinman (1983) has called "the translation of concepts from other fields into new ways of conceptualizing and analyzing health care problems" (p. 540).

Ethnography is what those of us who are not anthropologists think anthropologists do. The popular image is captured by the vision of Margaret Mead in her tent, taking notes while listening to the natives. The reality is more complex. The ethnographer learns about culture in basically three ways: (1) observation—what people actually do, as well as examination of artifacts of any sort; (2) discussion—what people say they think, believe, or do, and why; and (3) reflection—what the ethnographer infers or interprets (Helman, 1991). The researcher becomes an essential component of the research process. "Ethnography is neither subjective nor objective. It is interpretive, mediating two worlds through a third" (Agar, 1986, p. 19).

Ethnographers try to understand another's culture. A culture is the assumed beliefs and norms of a group, its shared sense of reality. All perceptions are "filtered, selected, and interpreted" by our culture (Burkett,

AUTHORS' NOTE: We wish to acknowledge the skills of Joanne Fabick and Susan Labuda Schrop, M.A., in organizing and editing the numerous drafts of this chapter. This chapter also benefited from the excellent direction of William Miller, M.D., and Benjamin Crabtree, Ph.D.

1991). We attribute meaning according to our culture. Although ethnography has traditionally entailed prolonged engagement studying cultures to which the researcher is a stranger, this has changed (Patton, 1990). Mishler (1984), in his book *The Discourse of Medicine,* describes the contrast and conflict between the patient's world, which he labels the "voice of the lifeworld," and the technical-scientific assumptions of medicine, labeled the "voice of medicine." These two worlds represent different cultures. Denzin (1997) describes eight features that challenge traditional ethnography and are especially pertinent for clinicians as they use a traditional technique such as key informant interviews and apply it in new ways. These eight features portray ethnography as (a) inseparable from writing or representing the account, (b) embedded in culture, (c) postcolonial and therefore multicultural, (d) necessarily self-reflexive, (e) gendered, (f) moral, (g) discontinuous, and (h) in evolution. These features need to be considered when interpreting key informant interviews.

To understand how key informant interviewing might be useful in primary care research, we will begin by defining terms and explaining the particular value of this approach, then discuss the selection of key informants for interview. The process of conducting the interview, methods of assessing the validity of the data obtained, and limitations of the approach will all be covered. Finally, specific application in primary care and clinical research will be discussed.

WHAT ARE KEY INFORMANT INTERVIEWS?

Key informant interviewing can aid in understanding cultural differences in health and disease concepts, in planning for delivery of health care, and in identifying community health resources. This chapter is titled "Key Informant Interviews"; all three of these terms require clarification.

Informant is viewed by some social science researchers as both pejorative and inadequate to capture the relationship between the researcher and the individual sharing information. Michael Agar, in a telephone interview, described the term in the following manner:

> I called the independent truckers I worked with in the last ethnography I wrote, "teachers." I decided that was really the proper term. It showed the kind of respect I feel for their knowledge. It showed the kind of role that they were really in, with reference to me, in terms of teaching me about independent trucking. But there's a lot of choices available. (Gilchrist 1992, p. 71)

Other terms that have been used are *consultant, friend, respondent, actor, participant, interviewee,* and *source.* We will use the term *informant* to mean "the individual who shares information," simply because it still seems to be the most commonly used term in the literature. We recognize that information is, however, multisensorial, contextual, emotional, social, spiritual, and, always, cultural.

Key informants are *key* to the researcher's understanding of that culture. They differ from other informants by the nature of their position in a culture, their information-rich connection to the research topic, and by their relationship to the researcher. Key informants are individuals who possess special knowledge, status, or communication skills, who are willing to share their knowledge and skills with the researcher, and who have access to perspectives or observations denied the researcher through other means (Goetz & LeCompte, 1984). Although, historically, key informants have an ongoing relationship with the researcher, they may also be individuals who bring specific information to inform a study in a more limited manner, such as aiding in questionnaire design (Lieberman, Meana, & Stewart, 1998) or as a member of the key informant tree described later in this chapter (Williams, Snider, Ryan, & the Cleveland COPC Group, 1994). Key informant interviews rarely, if ever, stand alone as a means to understand and interpret culture. Rather, their perspective is combined with observational field notes, in-depth interviews, and/or quantitative data.

An *interview* usually means some sort of formal communication. However, in this setting or context, it describes the relationship between the ethnographic researcher and the key informant from whom is negotiated an understanding of the culture or domain of interest. "Rather than studying people, ethnography means learning from people" (Spradley, 1979, p. 3). A key informant provides information through formal interviews and informal verbal interchanges or conversations. Other types of information obtained from a key informant may cover a wide range and include manuscripts, pictures, artifacts, and so on. However, it is the informant's interpretation of information that is critical. In an investigation of how experienced clinicians efficiently assessed their patients, the interpretations of their patients' presentations was clear to them but had to be explained to the physician researcher (Miller, 1992). Finally, informants communicate with the researcher in nonverbal ways—how they dress, when and how they speak, and the influence of context on their actions. This is all part of the information imparted by the key informant to the researcher and captured as part of the field notes.

WHY USE KEY INFORMANTS?

One might appropriately ask, Why use key informants? Why not just interview everyone you possibly can and get different perspectives without relying on the interpretations of just a few select individuals? There are three main reasons for using key informants: (a) to gather information efficiently, (b) to gain access to information otherwise unavailable to the researcher, and (c) to gain a particular understanding or interpretation of cultural information.

Pragmatically, one cannot interview everyone or observe everything. One cannot be in all places at all times. If one is going to use only a few key individuals, it is better to understand the limits of their information based on who they are and to develop a relationship with them to ensure the richness of that information. Efficiency also plays a role in the choice of key informants, especially in the face of limited resources. Gregor and Galazka (1990) describe how they used key informants to investigate the need for geriatric services in their community. Key informants provided them with the needed information in a cost-effective manner.

Key informants can also provide the researcher with both *access and sponsorship.* This may mean access to information that is unavailable except from the key informant. For example, knowledge about the beginning years of the Family Practice Center is available only from a senior faculty member. In addition, access based on sponsorship may be afforded to certain individuals because of the key informant's status or relationships within a community. Access may also be limited by certain personal characteristics of the key informant, such as gender and ethnicity. An example of sponsorship issues in a medical setting is described by Bosk (1979) in his study of medical mistakes. When Bosk approached a senior surgeon, asking for his cooperation, the surgeon replied that his sponsorship would be "the kiss of death" and that Bosk had best obtain entree through the house staff.

Finally, significant information available in a culture might not be appreciated by the researcher. As discussed earlier, the key informant may become a *research collaborator.* The key informant first answers questions and provides the explanations—what, when, who, why, and how (Schatzman & Strauss, 1973). As the researcher begins to formulate interpretations, it is the key informant who helps expand, modify, and clarify these interpretations. The key informant(s) will help transform the researcher's limited understanding of the culture into something with meaning for the researcher's own culture. A key informant is a *translator,* both literally and figuratively.

WHO IS A KEY INFORMANT?

Although almost anyone can become an informant, not everyone makes a good informant" (Spradley, 1979, p. 45). The informant may vary according to the topic and the relationship between the individuals. There may be several key informants or there could be one special individual. The ideal key informant is described as "articulate and culturally sensitive" (Fetterman, 1998, p. 47). This cultural sensitivity may or may not be analytic.

> Some informants use their language to describe events and actions with almost no analysis of their meaning or significance. Other informants offer insightful analysis and interpretation of events from the perspective of the native or folk theory. Both can make excellent informants. (Spradley, 1979, p. 52)

The informant needs to be thoroughly enculturated and currently active within his or her own culture, as well as reflective about that culture, to represent that culture accurately to the researcher. The researcher also needs to consider that an informant, by his or her very ability and willingness to straddle two cultures, may not represent the native culture (Lofland & Lofland, 1984; Patton, 1990; Pelto & Pelto, 1978; Spradley, 1979).

This relationship between the researcher and informant(s) is fluid and varies in intensity. The key informants may be individuals who supply information because of their position in a community (Williams et al., 1994) but have no other ongoing relationship to the research study or the researcher. The informant may start as a respondent, answering questions, and then may become an interpreter, explaining observations and expanding on questions. Later, he or she may become more of a teacher, asking questions, and, finally, the informant may become a collaborator. Researchers often share their accounts with key informants, "which serves both an ethical and a methodological function" (Michael Agar in Gilchrist, 1992, p. 77). Eventually, key informants may share authorship (Reason, 1994).

HOW TO SELECT KEY INFORMANTS

In the past, little was written about how the researcher went about finding key informants, although anthropology is full of stories about how this relationship went awry (Behar, 1996). Good luck or personal contacts somehow magically lead to the perfect key informant who is "trustworthy, observant, reflective, articulate and a good storyteller" (Johnson, 1990, p. 30).

Key informants are not selected randomly. Random sampling, as one type of probability sampling, assumes that the characteristic under study is represented equally in a study group. The knowledge or perspective being

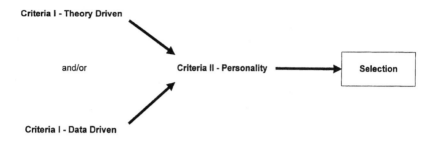

Figure 4.1. Selection Criteria for Finding Key Informants
SOURCE: Adapted from Johnson, 1990.

sought by the researcher, as well as the inclination and ability to share that with the researcher, is not equally distributed within a study group. The selection of key informants represents nonprobability sampling, referred to as purposeful, strategic, or information-rich sampling (also see Chapter 2). The selection attempts to yield a small number of informants who provide information-rich pictures of aspects of information or knowledge distributed within the study population.

Johnson describes two sets of selection criteria to be used sequentially in finding key informants (see Figure 4.1): (a) the type of information being sought, and (b) compatibility for an ongoing relationship (Johnson, 1990). In the first criterion, selection is either based on a theoretical perspective or is data driven. For example, Gregor and Galazka (1990) used a snowball method for identifying key informants from the researchers' initial contact with an individual known to staff members (emergent or data driven). Later, they specifically sought representation of the Black community (theory driven).

Another example of using data-driven criteria for determining who might be a knowledgeable key informant is described by Bernard (1995). His cultural consensus model of informant competence is based on the tendency of informants' agreement about cultural information to reflect the extent of their cultural knowledge. By quantitatively analyzing the amount of agreement between informants, one can then apply a factor analysis to identify the individuals with the most cultural information. Thus, those individuals who most often agree with the group about "the way it is" are those individuals most knowledgeable about their culture. If willing, they would make good key informants.

This first set of selection criteria, driven by theory or data, results in a pool of potential key informants. Within that pool, the researcher seeks out those who are willing and able to work with the researcher—selection criteria II. This factor is often determined by the characteristics of the researcher and key informant, such as gender, ethnicity, age, and personality. As articulated by Noblit, "a key informant for me may not be a key informant for you" (Gilchrist, 1992, p. 74).

Sometimes, good key informants are acquired serendipitously, and thus only selection II criteria are considered. For example, through friends of friends, church or community contacts, or chance acquaintance, relationships with key informants may develop. This method, or lack thereof, may yield an excellent key informant, but there is the risk of an informant discovered in this manner revealing only limited information about his or her culture. If this key informant is similar to the researcher in important ways, cultural information may be unavailable to the key informant for the same reason that it is unavailable to the researcher. Both people could be blinded by the distinct perspectives of social class, age, religion, and ethnicity. In addition, this person may be more likely to shield some aspects of culture from the researcher, thinking it is unimportant, possibly injurious to the relationship, or particularly unattractive.

LEARNING FROM KEY INFORMANTS

There are two types of discourse through which researchers learn about a culture from informants: (a) informal listening, discussing, and observing, and (b) more formal interviews or questioning. It is important to remember, however, that both are interpretive. "The manner in which an informant discusses an issue, thus revealing patterns of personal choosing, is, for the ethnographer, just as important as the revelation of social patterns themselves" (Dobbert, 1982, p. 114). The key informant interprets his or her own culture, and the researcher interprets the information the key informant reveals. "Conversations and interactions in the field can never be exactly reproduced" (Behar, 1996, p. 7).

Clinicians are most familiar with medical history taking as a type of interview. The more formal ethnographic interview differs from this medical interview, especially in regard to the greater openness of the research interview.

> Because the researcher's aim in using informants is to uncover patterns and not to get questions answered, the researcher cannot, like the interviewer, direct the conversation. Indeed, by directing the conversation, the researcher can only uncover patterns predicted in advance. . . . [With] an informant, the basic aim is to determine what patterns the informant sees and considers important enough to bring up. (Dobbert, 1982, p. 114)

Clinicians have been taught to narrow the inquiry and focus. Ethnographic questioning does just the opposite. The emphasis is on listening. "The question is not, how do you talk to an informant? But, how do you listen to an informant?" (Dobbert, 1982, p. 118). The astute clinician will recognize that these two features, following the direction of the informant and intense listening, characterize the "patient-centered clinical method" (Stewart, Brown, et al., 1995) and support the application of ethnographic tools and skills in areas of primary care, as called for by Stein (1990).

Questioning

Just as in medicine we ask certain types of questions (Can you describe the pain? Where does it hurt? What makes the pain better? What makes the pain worse?) to better understand and develop a picture of a patient's pain, so does the ethnographer ask certain types of questions to help develop an understanding of that person's culture. Spradley (1979) identifies three different types of questions: (a) *descriptive questions:* Tell me about the community health center; (b) *questions of inclusion or exclusion:* Which of these services can I get at the community health center—parenting classes, immunization. . . ? What does the community health center not provide—food stamps, legal counseling. . . ? and (c) *questions of verification:* So if I needed my prescription renewed, could I go to the community health center? Other, more specific types of informative questions include *substitution frame questions* and *card-sorting questions.* In substitution frame questions, the researcher removes one term and the informant is asked to replace it with another. For example, "If I wanted to get medication, I'd go to the community health center," is replaced with, "If I wanted to get _____, I'd go to the community health center." *Card-sorting questions* are a type of pile-sort exercise. The researcher lists terms, each on separate cards, and asks the informant to separate them according to a category.

Clinicians will be able to imagine an abundance of questions to use in their research. The function of these ethnographic questions is to expand and then to enrich the researcher's understanding of what the informant is describing. This requires, above all, *constant vigilance.* Not only can one not assume, without verification from the informant, that one's understandings and assumptions are the same as the informant's; the very framing of questions limits responses. This has a familiar clinical equivalent. As described by Mishler (1984), the physician's effort to control the medical interview "has the effect of absorbing and dissolving the patient's self-understanding of her problems into a system of purposive-rational action, namely, the framework of technical medicine" (p. 260). The way in which we question informants may, itself, limit and distort the information they give. This is especially important for most clinician-researchers who will work within their own culture where the temptation to assume shared meaning is great.

Language

"The language and other symbols in a culture do not simply refer to objects but are constitutive of them" (Schwandt, 1994, p. 123). A discussion of how the researcher tries to understand a culture by means of a verbal interchange with another individual is not complete without at least a brief examination of language. "Language is a way of organizing the world" (Patton, 1990, p. 227). "It is through discourse that material power is exercised and power relations are established and perpetuated" (Gavey, as quoted by Widdicombe, 1995, p. 107). The key informant may not only literally translate for the researcher but may also provide information about the nuances of the language and the cultural mores (i.e., what not to say). The language of clinical professionals is often very different from that of clients/patients. The same word can carry markedly different meanings (e.g., "critically ill"). The use of language will open or close relationships with a key informant and others.

Texts and Sources

Multiple interview formats are used with key informants. These may be formal, one-on-one interviews that are audiotaped and transcribed; however, much information is often revealed in casual conversation and needs to be recorded in the form of field notes. As the researcher's relationship with a key informant becomes more comfortable for both, the information transmission is likely to become less formal. The researcher needs to remain aware of that subtle transition and not lose "conversational" information. Researchers may write brief field notes during the course of the day and then, later, dictate summaries, expanding on those jottings. Field notes should be as complete as possible and include not only verbal information but nonverbal communication and descriptions of the context of the conversations. Some investigators separate descriptive notes and methodological notes. These notes must be distinguished from a diary that contains the researcher's questions, thoughts, interpretations, considerations, and reflections.

REPRESENTING THE ACCOUNT

Spradley (1979) states, "every ethnographic description is a translation" (p. 22). Geertz (1988) goes on to describe all of anthropology as "interpretations of interpretations." These quotes reflect the fact that the researcher must translate from the native culture to the researcher's culture but that the information is also filtered by both the informant and the researcher. What each one of us sees and remembers from any setting depends very much on who we are. Agar (1980) describes the understanding that evolves out of the relationship between the informant and the researcher as a "joint construction of reality." Each person contributes a perspective. The description should use "native language" and describe not only the final analysis of the study but how that analysis was obtained. Also needed is "an accounting of the relationship between field notes and the ethnography based upon them" (Sanjek, 1990, p. 401). How did the account evolve?

In addition, each person's understanding is not static. The iterative cycle of reflecting about self, reviewing and analyzing both old and new data, gathering more information, and then performing further interpretation highlights misconceptions and clarifies understandings (See Chapter 7). A research account starts with recognizing one's initial suppositions and assumptions. This full description allows the text (field notes and transcriptions) to be "deconstructed." The text created by the rendition of events by the researcher is deconstructed as his or her biases and taken-for-granted notions are exposed, and, at times, alternative ways to look at the data are introduced (Fontana & Frey, 1994).

The process of reflection and iteration is difficult to describe clearly in an ethnographic account. These accounts can be neither what Geertz (1988) calls "author-saturated" texts such as novels nor "author-evacuated" texts such as the description of a biochemical cascade. The former obscures the reality of the observations and the participants; the latter implies reproducible objectivity (p. 141). Lather uses concurrent text from interviews and her own reflections in her description of a study of women with AIDS (Lather & Smithies, 1997). Video and other media may also be used (Reason, 1994). Separate documentation, as much as is possible, of personal observation, interview information, and the constructed and co-constructed understanding by the researcher and the key informants is essential. This is all a way of saying that telling the research story is as important as the conclusion of that story.

CORROBORATING/ LEGITIMATING

What is a valid or truthful account? Because qualitative research is as much a reflection of the researcher as of the research instrument, validity has been difficult to define. Noblit defines a valid ethnographic account as one in which

> the second person finds the same story. My belief is that if I'm good enough, other people would find a story that resonates with mine. Not that it would necessarily be the same, but we would be able to understand the other person's story from our own. And that is as close as you get. (Gilchrist, 1992, p. 74)

There is full description of standards in Chapter 18, but a review of those directly pertaining to key informants is warranted.

Member Checks. This refers to the process of recycling interpretation back to key informants. This recycling should be documented in the study account, preferably with mention of the informants' comments. The research relationship may also change the key informant. Rather than ignoring this possibility, Lather (1986) describes including an assessment of what has changed, called *catalytic validity.*

> My argument is premised not only on a recognition of the reality-altering impact of the research process itself, but also on the need to consciously channel this impact so that respondents gain self-understanding and, ideally, self-determination through the research participation. (p. 68)

Searching for Disconfirming Evidence. "The job of validation is not to support an interpretation, but to find out what might be wrong with it. A proposition deserves some degree of trust only when it has survived serious attempts to falsify it" (Cronbach, as quoted in Lather, 1986, p. 65). Searching for disconfirming evidence involves both purposive sampling and prolonged engagement. Documentation of the selection process leading to the identification of key informants allows the researcher to seek accounts from other informants who may differ from the key informant in critical ways (see Chapter 2). This purposeful sampling of individuals and the inclusion of conflicting as well as complementary accounts strengthens description. The sampling and inclusion also allow consideration of potential biases due to informants' stakes in specific outcomes or due to their position in an organization. Prolonged engagement in the field of research and the "safety" of an established relationship are other ways for the researcher to confront any conflicts or apparent biases in the informants' revelations. Do they do what they say they do? Informants will report more accurately on events that are usual, frequent, or patterned and less accurately on things that are not readily observed or are inferential (Johnson,

1990). Prolonged engagement also allows the less readily observable aspects of a setting to become visible.

Triangulation. This is an essential check for the researcher. Triangulation refers to the use of both multiple data sources (for example, multiple informants) and multiple methods (such as participant observation, key informant interviewing, focus groups, and record reviews). One informant may give highly reliable but invalid information. The researcher also needs to go beyond data and methods triangulation and include multiple theoretical perspectives. "The attempt to produce value-neutral social science is increasingly being abandoned as at best unrealizable, and at worst self deceptive, and is being replaced by social sciences based on explicit ideologies" (Hess, as quoted in Lather, 1986, p. 50).

Thick Description. This is "a thorough description of the context or setting within which the inquiry took place and with which the inquiry was concerned" (Guba & Lincoln, as quoted in Kuzel & Like, 1991, p. 153). The following five aspects of key informants should be described: (a) how they were identified; (b) their initial relationship to the researcher; (c) how that relationship changed over time; (d) their physical characteristics, if important for the study (e.g., age, gender); and (e) prior experience, if important for the study (e.g., length of time living in the neighborhood).

Reflexivity. This refers to consideration of the observer as part of the setting context and culture that he or she is studying.

> What happens within the observer must be made known if the nature of what has been observed is to be understood. The subjectivity of the observer influences the course of the observed event radically as inspection influences (disturbs) the behavior of an electron. (Behar, 1996, p. 6)

The recognition that one's perspective is always partial and limited is referred to as "critical subjectivity" (Lather & Smithies, 1997). A research account is not only the presentation of data but the explanation of how the researchers defined what would be their data. What did they consider important and why? How did their considerations change? How did their presence in the setting change that setting? Lather (1986) calls for a "systematized reflexivity which gives some indication of how *a priori* theory has been changed by the logic of the data" (p. 67). Altheide and Johnson (1994) summarize reflexive accounting as including the relationship between what is observed and the larger context, the relationships among the observer and others, the issue of perspective, the role of the reader in the final product, and the issue of representational style.

ETHICAL
CONSIDERATIONS

Ethical concerns, in traditional medical research, have focused on harm, informed consent, and confidentiality. In social science research, there is also a focus around issues of deception and privacy. Working with a key informant often involves an extended, intimate, and evolving relationship built on trust. Such relationships raise questions about the researcher's stance vis-à-vis those whom he or she studies. Increasingly, researchers are calling for nonexploitive research relationships and the consideration of research subjects as partners. The involvement of subjects as participants is fundamental to participatory research (Heron, 1996; Reason, 1994; see also Chapter 15); however, the degree to which individual researchers share their research questions, assumptions, and findings may vary.

The primary task of such participatory research, and some feminist research, is empowerment and liberation through the joint construction of knowledge (Oakley, 1981; Punch, 1994; Reason, 1994). Participatory researchers, for example, view any techniques of interviewing as ways of manipulating respondents (Fontana & Frey, 1994). "The desire to create change, to lessen oppression, or to assist in the development of a more equitable world sets up a different research dynamic from that of the disengaged academic" (Tiereny & Lincoln, 1997, p. viii). It behooves researchers to consider beforehand how their relationship with a key informant may change that informant as well as themselves and their research philosophy.

All informants should be encouraged to guard information that they feel uncomfortable revealing, but they should also be reassured that the information that can be shared is valuable. All transcripts of interviews, diagrams, and notes can be shared with informants to seek their verification of the materials and allay any concern about the contents of notes or materials used in research studies. Some researchers will feel comfortable sharing their field notes and emerging understandings of a process or community with key informants, but others will not. It is important to remember that if researchers share their hypothesis with key informants, it is likely to change the way informants think about their setting. The evolving perspective of a key informant may or may not be helpful to the developing research study. A specific problem for researchers is the experience of their relationship with a key informant bridging another relationship. An example in health care when a key informant is a patient, coworker, or employee. Less than full disclosure about a study's purpose and developing assumptions can be even more disruptive in such a situation.

LIMITATIONS

It is important to recognize potential problems using key informants, especially in a clinical setting. Although it should be possible to follow rigorous approaches to sampling, interviewing, and interpretation in studies using key informants to investigate clinical care, compromises often need to be made in the practice setting. Resources are more limited, and a balance has to be struck between rigor and feasibility. These compromises do not necessarily invalidate the data, but they do emphasize the need to be aware of sources of bias and their likely effect on the data.

Most informants usually do not spontaneously describe what happens in their culture but are guided by the researcher's questions. An interviewer's questions, as well as subsequent interpretations, are driven by his or her own cultural assumptions or traditions. The questions dictate the answers. "Having been socialized into culture means that the sensory clues we perceive from the external world and from within ourselves are filtered, selected, and interpreted according to meaningful patterns we have learned" (Burkett, 1991, p. 287). This is especially problematic for clinical researchers. Rather than questioning some aspect of a culture, biomedicine for example, an assumption is made that may not be correct. It is often only through intense reflection that an assumption is even recognized as such. In Chapter 17, Malterud cautions clinician/researchers not to deny their roles as participants but rather consider their impact, find collaborators for analysis, follow sampling guides, and exercise intense reflection.

Particular care must be taken in the way that key informants are identified. Communities are usually heterogeneous groupings; key informants drawn from one grouping may not accurately represent another grouping. Key informant networks are prone to this problem, as the process of identifying new informants by using previous informants is inherently limited. Gregor and Galazka (1990), in their use of key informants to identify geriatric needs, ran into this problem when their informants were not adequately representing the views of African Americans in the community. By closely monitoring their data, however, they were able to identify the problem. By setting up a second network within the African American portion of the community, they illustrated an appropriate response to this problem. Information needed about a particular segment of the community may not be known to all key informants. Careful purposive sampling is important in these circumstances.

A closely related problem is that of response bias. Not all persons identified as potential key informants will agree to be interviewed. Williams, Snider, and Ryan (Williams et al., 1994) encountered this difficulty in using key informants in support of community-oriented primary care

(COPC) at an inner-city health center. They were unable to interview any of the ministers suggested to them as key informants. Such a failure to interview a portion of the key informants carries the obvious danger of losing the unique perspectives and data from those informants. Furthermore, not all interviews are good interviews. The questions may not open pertinent areas for discussion; the informant may not be knowledgeable; the informant may not trust the researcher enough to reveal critical information; the researcher may not recognize the significance of information when given.

Although the researcher needs to be constantly aware of the limitations of sampling and questions, this should not diminish the value of the key informant method. Rather, it emphasizes the need for continuous efforts to validate or disprove the data being collected as described in the preceding section on corroborating/legitimating.

APPLICATIONS IN PRIMARY CARE

The key informant technique has a close kinship with clinical care. To quote Helman (1991), "every patient is an informant," and our access to the culture of a particular family is through our patient or "key informant." The interviewing and patient relationship skills so critical in primary care are a natural stepping stone into the use of key informants for any of several primary care or other clinical research purposes.

Indeed, many of the problems we confront professionally have been illuminated by such ethnographic studies as Bosk's (1979) study of mistakes, Smith and Kleinman's (1989) study of management of one's emotions in medical training, and Miller's (1992) elucidation of the taxonomy of office visits. Key informants may also inform study development, such as when informants pointed out the need to account for gender differences as a factor affecting participation in a cardiac rehabilitation program (Lieberman et al., 1998).

Another use of key informants is in the study of "critical incidents." In these examples, individual accounts of specific incidents provide a microcosm of other significant issues in the culture. Analysis of and reflection on the particular incident illuminate others. An example from primary care is a study of general practitioners' use of MRI. The requests for MRI highlighted the impact of personal, contextual, and biomedical variables on physicians' decision making and led to the development of locally informed consensus criteria (Robling et al., 1998).

Key informants can also be useful in research aimed at planning the delivery of primary care (Penayo, Jacobson, Caldera, & Burmann, 1988). Taken to the level of the primary care practice, key informant methods can provide information needed for answering pressing clinical and organizational questions (Gregor & Galazka, 1990; Williams et al., 1994). The method is readily adaptable to the practice setting and is particularly valuable in cross-cultural settings where key practice decision makers are not part of the community from which the patients come.

A variation on the standard key informant approach is the *"key informant network,"* also known as "key informant trees" and the "snowball" technique (Gregor & Galazka, 1990; Williams et al., 1994). After identifying an initial set of key informants, a network is built by asking these first key informants to suggest additional key informants for interview. The process is reiterated until either no new informants are suggested or the data becomes saturated (see Figure 4.2). A network approach is particularly useful in the practice setting because it facilitates the identification of key informants of whom the practice staff may be unaware.

Gregor and Galazka (1990) used key informant networks to understand the health care needs of the geriatric population living in the community served by their primary care teaching practice. Their initial key informant from a senior citizen housing complex suggested three other key informants, one of whom suggested two more key informants. Proceeding in this way, they built a network of 13 key informants. When it became apparent that this network was not adequately representative of the needs of the local African American senior citizens, a second network was built identifying key informants able to represent this segment of the community. Information from the two networks painted a composite picture of many needs (such as the need for increased mental health services, the inaccessibility of transportation, etc.) and resources in the geriatric community.

This use of key informant techniques in the practice of primary care may be an area of great potential. Costs cited in one study suggest it would be feasible to include it as a part of practice operations (Williams et al., 1994). Conducting the key informant network took approximately 6 hours of professional (physician or administrator) time and 8 hours of nonprofessional (clerical) time.

Another use of key informants in primary care is as part of community-oriented primary care (COPC). One of the goals of COPC is to use both qualitative and quantitative methods for understanding a community so as to provide the most appropriate primary care. As a component of this community assessment process, the data gathered from key informants is complementary to that gathered from other qualitative methods, such as focus groups. Key informants, as a sample, tend to differ from samples drawn for other qualitative methods, and the characteristics of their interview differ from the group dynamics of a focus group. Although major themes may be consistent across methods (and are validated by this consistency), nuances may vary. We have found key informants to be

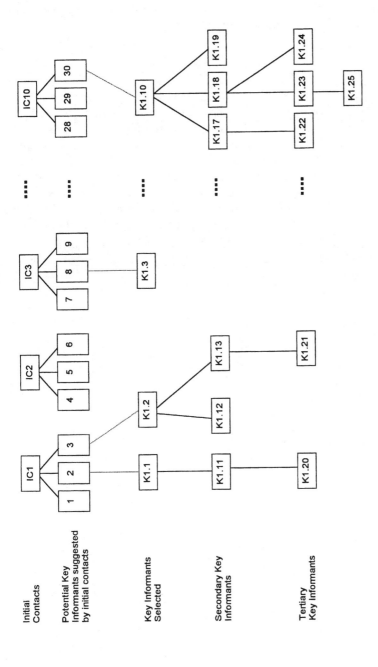

Figure 4.2. Schematic Diagram of a Key Informant Network

NOTE: Each key informant may or may not suggest further key informants, leading to the irregular structure of the network.

87

generally better informed about resources in a community than focus group members. Focus groups, on the other hand, may provide more emotional context to the topic of discussion than key informants.

SUMMARY

Key informant interviewing is an extremely valuable interpretive research tool for clinical investigators. It is an efficient way of obtaining information that is not readily accessible. All research is interpretive to some degree, but key informant interviewing involves the interpretive filters of the informant as well as that of the researcher and the interpretive process of translation. Thus, this method is most useful in conjunction with other methods, especially participant observation. Ultimately, the strongest understanding of any issue will arise from the multiple perspectives of many approaches. We urge the researcher to reject the tyranny of methodology and to use whatever method best answers the question at hand and to report honestly what is done.

5

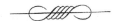

Depth Interviewing

William L. Miller
Benjamin F. Crabtree

Seeing, listening, and touching are primary sources of information about the world. The interview is a research-gathering approach that seeks to create a listening space where meaning is constructed through an interexchange/cocreation of verbal viewpoints in the interest of scientific knowing. Traditionally, research interviewing in primary care represented an attempt to "standardize" listening in an effort to mine the gold of information stored in the respondents. This narrow and limiting understanding is appropriate only within the paradigm of materialistic inquiry. Research speaking and listening occurs in various forms and includes listening as an unobtrusive outsider; actively participating in everyday conversation or therapeutic conversation (see Chapter 17); sharing and hearing within a study-specific, confidential, open-ended discourse; or confronting respondents with forced-choice questions. These latter two situations have been the most common ones used in primary care research. This chapter explores the interview as a partnership on a conversational research journey and details the depth interview as an example of one qualitative, semistructured (focused) interview approach to the gathering process in primary care research.

It's flu season; the waiting room is packed; staff are out sick; the doctor has a headache; the nursing home keeps calling to report more fevers. Into this maelstrom strides Carmelita. She is 39, a single mother of two, and has recently moved into the area. She is working two jobs, attending school, and has unrelenting hand, hip, and lower back pain not relieved by maximal dose nonsteroidals. She wants relief so she can remain in control of her life. Carmelita and the doctor meet. The doctor can't quickly identify a pathologic diagnosis and is worried about the possibility of addiction if she gives Carmelita narcotics, so she recommends a new nonsteroidal. The doctor also wants relief and to remain in control of her day. Carmelita is angry, leaves the office, and never returns. Both remain in distress and not in control. What is going on? Who are these people? What is important here? What meanings and practices occurred in this lived experience? Why did this occur as it did? What does pain mean to these two individuals?

How shall we seek answers to these questions? How do we investigate the relations of individuals and context? How do doctors and patients think about pain? Our present knowledge about pain informs us that seeing (observation, pain drawings) and touching (examination, experimental stimulation) are inadequate sources of data (Fields, 1987; Frank, Moll, & Hurt, 1982; Melzack, 1975). Pain is a physiosubjective experience. Understanding pain requires participating with and asking patients and physicians about their experiences of pain. Thus, how are we to listen? We can position ourselves within social situations where people are in pain and eavesdrop on the conversations that spontaneously arise, or we can casually enter into these same conversations. When pain is mentioned within the discourse, we can even interrupt and informally explore the topic further. These approaches are informative and work best within a participant observation/key informant interview framework (see Chapters 3 and 4). An alternative is to formally develop a common set of questions, lists, or ratings about pain and expose selected respondents to these same sets of stimuli (Melzack, 1975). This structured approach runs the high risks of phrasing the researcher's own concerns into the mouths of the respondents and never giving voice to the interviewee's own perceptions and meaning making about pain. It also ignores the role of the interviewer in this meaning-making process. Qualitative depth interviews are an option that accounts for these risks.

We used depth interviews to hear six family physicians and six paired patients from a small suburban community in north-central Connecticut. The goal was to identify and compare their understandings and experiences of pain. The depth interview is a powerful qualitative research tool when the focus of inquiry is narrow, the respondents represent a clearly defined and homogeneous bounded unit with an already known context, the respondents are familiar and comfortable with the interview as a means of communication, and the goal is to generate themes and narratives.

In the remainder of this chapter, we will demonstrate the "doing" of depth interviews, illustrating each step with the pain research outlined above. To provide a context for depth interviews, we will first give a brief overview of the interview as a partnership, as a communicative performance, and as a conversational research journey.

PARTNERSHIP, COMMUNICATIVE PERFORMANCE, AND CONVERSATIONAL JOURNEY

The traditional understanding of the interview in clinical research is that it is primarily a behavioral event consisting of controlled verbal informational exchange from a repository of personal knowledge to a skilled listener/recorder. The interviewer supplies a stimulus and the interviewee responds; each question and answer is independently meaningful and isolatable and can be coded and counted accordingly. It is becoming increasingly clear that all of these assumptions are false. In every interview, there are also nonverbal and emotional interchanges and a continuous exchange of multilayered messages being differentially perceived (Mishler, 1986). The questions/transmissions are complex, ambiguous, and jointly constructed from within the context of the discourse. Both the interviewer and the respondent have multiple social roles beyond their roles as interviewer and interviewee. These different roles influence the many different motivations each has for engaging in the interview. Some of these interactional goals include requests, performance/expression, politeness, persuasion, attention, exerting authority, therapy, ritual, evaluation, and/or reference to specific knowledge. The interviewer's goal may be a particular type of knowledge, but this goal may not be shared by the respondent.

The interview is better conceptualized as a special type of partnership and communicative performance or event. It is not political oratory, storytelling, rap, a lecture, a small group seminar, or a clinical encounter. Rather, it is a conversational research journey with its own rules of the road. Figure 5.1 depicts a simplified contextual understanding of the interview as a communicative performance (derived from Briggs, 1986; Gottlieb, 1986; Gumperz & Hymes, 1972). Interview discourse occurs within a specific social situation consisting of a physical place, actors, and activities. A second context for any communication event is the communication or discourse itself (the arrow in Figure 5.1). This includes the form of the message (verbal, gesture, facial expression, etc.), the actual message or sign, and the "something else" represented by the sign. This "something else" can refer either to some person, object, event, or process in the world (referentiality) or to some other index feature of the discourse itself, such as the meaning of "I" in a conversation (indexicality).

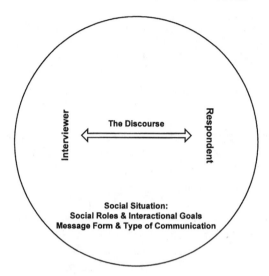

Figure 5.1. The Interview as a Communication Event
SOURCE: Briggs (1986), Gottlieb (1986), and Gumperz and Hymes (1972).

Sociolinguistic studies of the "conventional" interview reveal many cultural assumptions and expectations. Hierarchical interviewer-respondent role relations are presumed, and rules for introducing new topics, taking turns, and judging the relevance of statements are included. There are also expectations for etiquette, linguistic forms, and an understanding that the major purpose of the interaction is to provide referential information. When communicating in the interview or other interaction, the respondent talks the most, turn order is fixed, the length of exchange is specified, topics are fixed, and turn allocation and interview rapport are controlled by the interviewer (Sacks, Schegloff, & Jefferson, 1974; Werner & Schoepfle, 1987b). The research interview as partnership, communicative performance, and conversational journey recognizes this knowledge but expands on it and alters its meaning. Partnership reminds us that there are two active participants involved in "meaning-making work." Both are participants in an interpersonal drama with a plot that develops around the area of inquiry (Holstein & Gubrium, 1995). The journey does begin with a hierarchical relationship, as the interviewer initiates the process and sets the opening scene with a question. And the "rules of interviewing" noted above are initially in effect because they are usually shared cultural knowledge, due to the pervasive public presence of television "interview" role models such as Oprah Winfrey, Barbara Walters, and Ted Koppel. The metaphor of journey, however, also helps us open to change in the process as the two (or more) partners develop their relationship and construct meaning. The hierarchy may shift; rules may change; improvisation emerges.

DEPTH INTERVIEWS

A profound implication of understanding the interview as a communication event is the clarification of when and which interview to use as a data collection tool. The interview is appropriate only if interviewing is a known communication routine of the respondent and if it is a culturally appropriate communication form for the topic of interest (Briggs, 1986). The type of interview depends on the interviewer's and the respondent's preexisting shared level of knowledge and the culturally appropriate form of questioning related to the topic of interest (Werner & Schoepfle, 1987b). As Briggs (1986) notes, learning how to ask requires that we first identify the different ways in which people communicate and then decide on the appropriate research methods.

The depth interview is a particular field research data-gathering process designed to generate narratives that focus on fairly specific research questions. As such, it is not the "holistic" ethnographic approach most often used by anthropologists in which the details of all aspects of a *culture* or *subculture* are investigated. The depth interview concentrates on the figure at the expense of the ground—it focuses on facilitating a coconstruction of the interviewer's and an informant's experience and understanding of the topic of interest and not necessarily on the context of that understanding. The depth interview is personal and intimate, with an emphasis on "depth, detail, vividness, and nuance" (Rubin & Rubin, 1995, p. 76).

Depth interviews primarily use open, direct, verbal questions that elicit stories and case-oriented narratives. We chose this data collection tool in our pain study because (a) we know our potential respondents are familiar and comfortable with the interview as a communicative performance and event; (b) discourse about pain in the study community often takes the form of stories (by patients) and of cases (by physicians); (c) the discourse about pain between doctors and patients usually occurs within an interview format using direct, verbal questions; (d) our study is exploratory; and (e) our goal is to discover and cocreate individual perceptions and narrative understandings about pain.

The complete interview-to-transcription process involves a series of carefully designed steps. It starts with mapping the research topic landscape through a cultural, literature, and self-review. This is followed by a designing phase, which includes developing a sampling strategy; constructing an interview guide; and planning informed consent, confidentiality, and protection strategies. The next step consists of preparing for the interview.

**Designing: Selecting the Actors,
the Dramatic Outline, and Ethics**

Designing a depth interview study begins with developing a sampling strategy. Once the sampling frame is known and combined with the mapping information, it is then possible to create an interview guide. The final step in the designing phase is accounting for core ethical considerations, including informed consent and issues of confidentiality.

For depth interviews, respondents should be selected so as to maximize the richness of information obtained pertinent to the research question. As such, the *sampling* strategy should be purposeful and not random. Patton (1987) and Kuzel (see Chapter 2) discuss several types of purposeful sampling strategies, including extreme or deviant case, maximum variation, homogeneous, typical case, critical case, snowball or chain, criterion, confirmatory or disconfirming case, and sampling politically important cases. One or more of these can be used, depending on the particular research situation. Homogeneous sampling is particularly important in depth interviews because it is often important to account for cultural and contextual influences prior to the actual interview. Recall that depth interviews are usually not a good means for learning about cultural context; they focus on the relations of individuals to that context.

In our research on pain, we used a combination of homogeneous, criterion, and snowball sampling. We wanted folks from a homogeneous community with recent exposure to pain, and we wanted their family physicians. Therefore, we selected the first four family physicians from a small homogeneous community and asked them to provide the name of a patient over age 21 who had been discharged from the hospital within the previous 2 weeks. Two more pairs were identified later in the study to serve as disconfirming cases. When interpretation of those interviews revealed no new significant insights (data saturation), interviewing was stopped.

Depth interviews are organized around an *interview guide* consisting of some relatively closed identifying questions and a few (one to six) open-ended "grand tour" questions, with associated prompts/probes and follow-up questions. This guide outlines the dramatic format for the interview. The stage is set by rapport-building biographical questions, followed by the introduction of research themes through questions designed to elicit narratives detailing the informant's conception of the identified domains. Prompts and probes are used throughout to expand the rich context.

The first set of questions often consists of standard biographical ones that ask for short, structured, direct answers. These introductory questions serve the following seven functions: (a) establish interview style, (b) build rapport, (c) jog the respondents' memory, (d) build a bridge to intimacy, (e) "assign competence" to the interviewee (Holstein & Gubrium, 1995),

1. Would you take me through an experience that has influenced the way you deal with pain now?
2. From your experience, can you tell me about usual and typical kinds of pain?
3. Would you describe for me how you decide what to do when you have pain? (For patient interview: If a doctor has a patient with pain, would you describe for me how the doctor would decide what to do?)
4. From your experience, would you tell me about the usual or typical kinds of people with pain.

Figure 5.2. Grand Tour Questions From Interviews With Patients and Physicians in a Study of Pain

(f) provide context data for analysis, and (g) weave a discourse context for the topical research questions. These 10 to 20 minutes spent talking about birthplace, family, religion, and occupation create a climate of trust, communication, and self-disclosure. The interviewing couple is prepared for the grand tour. Because the introductory questions "condition the interview" (Holstein & Gubrium, 1995), there may be times when these identifying questions aren't asked until the end of the interview. This is especially true when you want the interviewee to take the lead in the interview.

Grand tour or main questions are open, easily understood, descriptive questions that seek to elicit understandings, feelings, key terms, and major features or attributes about people, acts, time, goals, expectations, motivations, and experiences (Spradley, 1979; Werner & Schoepfle, 1987b). They open a space for discovering what others (and yourself) think and feel about some aspect of the research topic (Rubin & Rubin, 1995). A good grand tour question engages the respondent in the topic of interest. To succeed, the question must be broad, use clearly defined terms, provide necessary time and space perspectives, supply needed facts, stimulate memory, avoid jargon and emotionally loaded words, be easily and clearly understandable, delimit the scope of the question, avoid suggesting an answer, and arouse the respondent's interest and motivation (Gordon, 1975). The grand tour questions are based on the categories discovered during the literature reviews and cultural category explorations. They are designed to provide answers that ultimately relate to the theoretical literature and yet are open to new meanings being made.

In our pain study, the four broad categories found in the literature review were consistent with those discovered in the search for cultural categories. Thus, four grand tour questions were developed for the interview guide based on these domains (see Figure 5.2). The final wording of each question followed lengthy group discussions. For example, the initial wording of question 3 was, "Would you explain your management approach to pain?" Group analysis revealed that this question presumes the respondent has already described the management and is now to explain why, when we really wanted a description about what they do. The word *management* represents confusing jargon from medical, political, and economic perspectives. The question is also not clear as to whose pain is to be managed and for whom the description is intended—the interviewer or some other audience. In response to these issues, the final question form is, "Would you describe for me how you decide what to do when you have pain?"

Once launched on the grand tour, the interviewer must be prepared to keep the story flowing and maintain narrative competence. This is accomplished through the use of "floating prompts." Seven such prompts include *silence,* or the permissive pause that gives control to the respondent, enhances spontaneity, and creates a thoughtful mood; *the attentive lean,* where the interviewer leans toward the respondent with an affirmative head nod; the *eyebrow flash; affirmative noise,* such as "uh-huh"; the *echo prompt,* or repeating the last word spoken by the respondent in an interrogative style; the *reflective summary,* where the interviewer summarizes the respondent's last statement; and *recapitulation* or re-presenting in summary form something mentioned earlier in the interview (Bernard, 1988; Gordon, 1975; Schatzman & Strauss, 1973).

A successful grand tour facilitated by strategically placed floating prompts elicits key terms and features, but not all of these terms are fully detailed. The details, depth, vividness, and nuances characteristic of depth interviews are obtained from minitour questions and probes. The most commonly used minitour questions are *category questions,* which simply seek elaboration and/or clarification of all the parts, settings, relationships, activities, and relative worth or value of the domain being discussed. These include the "what else," "where," "when," "how," "why," and "why important" questions. Another common type of minitour is the *contrast question,* which seeks to clarify the similarities and differences between two key terms or features: "What is the difference between ___ and ___?" (Fetterman, 1989; Spradley, 1979).

There are steering probes, depth probes, and housekeeping probes. *Steering probes* refer to gentle comments that keep the interview flowing into the mainstream. It is important to allow both partners in the conversation to explore upstream along many tributaries, some of which may initially seem like dead ends or unrelated. Steering probes that link the conversation back to the research question can help relate these sidelights to the main narrative; they become part of the meaning-making work of the interview. *Depth probes* facilitate expanding and deepening understanding of the coevolving narrative and can include the *hypothetical question, devil's advocate questions, special incident probes,* and *posing the ideal probes* (Bernard, 1988, 1994; Schatzman & Strauss, 1973). Finally, there are *housekeeping probes,* which enhance the details and nuances. These include *elaboration probes, clarification probes, continuation probes,* and *completion probes.* Figure 5.2 details the pain management grand tour question from our interview guide; however, the actual interview guide also includes associated probes that act as cues for the interviewer. Probes must be as carefully worded as the grand tour questions and must avoid "leading" the respondent. For example:

> **Interviewer:** Well, see if you can tell me. . . . Think of something that's. . . . And you can tell me as a story. I want you to start at the beginning and telling me like a tale, like, "I woke up in pain, etc.," or whatever the situation is.

> **Respondent:** Well, back then I'd be limited because there is nothing to tell there. I wake up and it's there. [story continues]

In this segment of the transcript, the interviewer is trying to get the respondent to recite a narrative about her experiences with pain; unfortunately, the respondent may have chosen this "wake up" story because the interviewer suggested it.

Once the initial sampling strategy is known and the first draft of the interview guide completed, one is ready to address three important *ethical considerations* in depth interviews. The first issue is informed consent, which is part of any institutional review board protocol. Depth interviews usually deal with personal, intimate material and stories. It is essential that potential interviewees clearly understand what type of relationship they are being asked to participate in and what the topics will be and how they can disengage from the relationship without risk. If tape recorders are being used, the respondent needs to be so informed and be able to turn them off if desired. It also means that the right to privacy, protection of identity, is assured and that all precautions are taken to protect the respondent from immediate or future harm.

Preparing: Staging the Scene

Once the dramatic outline is complete and the actors selected, final preparation for the interview begins. The dramaturgical metaphor is most applicable for this step because an interview is really a staged communication event; it is a purposefully situated process (Douglas, 1985). Each social situation or scene has its own culturally prescribed norms of nonverbal and verbal interaction that influence the interpretation of what is expressed

(Briggs, 1986). Thus the components of this step include setting the scene, learning the part, equipment checking, and practicing or doing pilot interviews. Preparing starts with *setting the scene*. This includes initial preinterview contact to set up the interview. This contact is usually by telephone. The goal of depth interviews involves maximizing narrative competence, so most such interviews should occur in a "grass hut" setting. "Grass hut" refers to the usual, everyday location where the research topic is discussed, as opposed to a "white room," or sterile context site (Werner & Schoepfle, 1987b). Good lighting (to facilitate observation of nonverbal communication), a minimum of external disturbance (sound or activity), privacy, a face-to-face encounter with a six- to eight-foot separation, and well-mannered informality are also helpful staging parameters (Douglas, 1985).

In the pain study, we elected to conduct the family physician interviews at the physicians' offices, where they routinely engage in interviews about pain with their patients. The patient interviews took place in the privacy of the patients' homes.

Once on the scene, the interviewer has six goals for the preinterview contact. It should (a) introduce the interviewer (i.e., identify role and give name), (b) identify sponsorship, (c) explain purpose, (d) explain selection of respondent, (e) assure anonymity, and (f) obtain informed consent. The interviewer may also wish to discuss note taking, recording, and the anticipated length of the interview (Gordon, 1975). It is usually better to have done all of this at least a day before the actual interview; this prevents any possible ego threat at the time of the interview. The preinterview contact also involves a negotiation type of discourse that is quite different from the interview discourse. In the pain study, this preinterview contact took place by telephone, usually a week before the interview.

There are three major aspects to *learning the part*. It is important to know as much about the interview partner and the local setting as possible. Who is the partner? What are the partner's patterns of identification (Levy & Hollan, 1998)? What are the local norms for presentation and speech? Spending time in the neighborhoods of your future interview partners and gaining linguistic competence is time very well spent. The depth interview is an "organized occasion" for constructing knowledge (Holstein & Gubrium, 1995), thus its success and quality are contingent on the nitty-gritty preparation work at learning the language of the partner. Idiomatic expressions and nuances of meaning that are not recognized or understood in the conversation become lost opportunities for sensemaking. For example, learning the metalanguage of doctors and nurses greatly facilitates depth interviews with them. The second and third aspects to learning the part are learning how to dress and learning how to define, present, and negotiate your role in the interview. These are especially important when interviewing across genders, across ethnic groups, or across social cleavages (Rubin & Rubin, 1995). Again, these issues are optimally addressed by doing some brief participant observation and key informant interviewing.

Always remember to do *equipment checking*. Before arriving for an interview, the interviewer must thoroughly check and clean all equipment, including changing the batteries in the tape recorder (don't assume AC will be available). Interviewers must have extra batteries, a supply of blank tapes, informed consent forms, and note taking materials. Nothing is more embarrassing, undermining of professional status, or disruptive of the interview journey than having equipment that doesn't function properly.

The final step in preparation is to conduct one or more *pilot interviews*, initially with friends and then with partners culturally like the actual people to be interviewed (Douglas, 1985). This process will help in finalizing the sequence and wording of the grand tour questions and will suggest additional minitour questions and probes. The pilot interviews also serve as a training tool for the interviewers. Finally, we recommend that the researchers themselves transcribe the pilot interviews. This process will help them appreciate the need for good recordings and will aid in deciding what style of transcription they want.

Interviewing: Let the Play Begin

As we have presented it, the depth interview is a constructed dialogue focused on a creative search for mutual personal understanding of a research topic. It is situated communication requiring sincerity, cooperative mutual disclosure, and warmth (Douglas, 1985). The discourse must be open; no two interviews are the same. Only the grand tour questions are "standardized," and even they may change from interview to interview. The goal is to seek deeper collective interpersonal understanding. The validity or quality of the interview craft is seriously jeopardized with further standardization (Kvale, 1996). Thus, the interviewer needs to love to engage the pain and uncertainty of self-discovery and human existence. The interviewer, not the research guide, is the research instrument. The interviewer's role is to assume a low profile but encouraging stance, to put the informant at ease, to acknowledge the value of the information and assign competence to the interviewee, to take on the role of the respondent (Holstein & Gubrium, 1995; Schatzman & Strauss, 1973), and to reinforce the continuance of the conversation—to facilitate improvisational story-telling.

In the actual interview, the attitudes expressed by the interviewer should reinforce the interviewer's role. The interviewer should display desired enthusiasm; be nonjudgmental; show interest in the information as it unfolds; be empathic; and avoid forgetting previous answers, condescension, and rigidity (Gordon, 1975). The organization of the interview guide is designed to assist in these efforts by beginning with biographical information that grounds the interviewer into a brief life history of the interview partner and places later conversation in a context.

The interview is as paradoxical a tool as the human existence it seeks to probe. Having just pleaded for the interviewer to engage his or her travel partner with warmth and intimacy, we now argue for the interviewer to manufacture and maintain distance within the interviewer-respondent relationship (McCracken, 1988). Phenomenologists refer to this distancing as "bracketing"—putting the self aside so a phenomenon can be experienced as it is (Denzin, 1989b). This process requires the self-understanding undertaken earlier when discovering cultural categories. The interview is a dance of intimacy and distancing that creates a dramatic space where the interview partners disclose their inner thoughts and feelings and the interviewer knowingly hears and facilitates the story and recognizes, repairs, and clarifies any apparent communication missteps. Humor, gentle surprise, and the use of metaphor (such as our dramaturgical one) are a few helpful techniques for manufacturing distance in an intimate and respectful way (McCracken, 1988). For example:

> **R:** I think losing a child must be, must be terrible, really terrible. I think a husband and wife always expect, some day you're going to lose each other. I would hope if I had to lose one of those four kids, I could handle that. They're nice kids, they really are. I sound like a mother! (laughs)

> **I:** (laughs) What are mothers for? Let's talk a little bit. . . . You were telling me about the pain if you lost a child or pain for a death. Could you tell me, from your experience, what the usual or typical kinds of pain are?

A good interview has a steady, slow, progressive flow and should maximize the facilitators and minimize the inhibitors of this flow. Gordon (1975) describes four inhibitors that limit the willingness or motivation of the interview partner to provide information: (a) competing demands for time, (b) ego threats (evasion, denial, minimization, confession, and depersonalization), (c) etiquette, and (d) recollection of a traumatic event. He also mentions four inhibitors that limit the ability of the partner to provide information: (a) forgetting, (b) chronological confusion, (c) inferential confusion, and (d) unconscious behavior. Note that all of these factors also pertain to the interviewer. Facilitators discussed by Gordon (1975) to maximize the interview flow include (a) fulfilling expectations, (b) recognition, (c) altruistic appeals, (d) sympathetic understanding, (e) new experience, (f) catharsis, (g) need for meaning, and (h) extrinsic rewards.

Judicious use of prompts and probes as the grand tour stories evolve is essential to maintaining the progressive flow of conversation. Two general rules of thumb are to (a) avoid dominance-submission or parent-child games (Douglas, 1985) and (b) use the least direct probe necessary. Begin with silence and slowly progress to self-disclosure. Paddling in the flow of interview discourse is much like paddling a canoe. In slow, smooth water, paddle harder with more directness; in choppy water, just use the paddle gently to maintain course (Whyte, 1984).

Not all interviews proceed smoothly. The interviewer should have several strategies for dealing with the different types of resistance that occasionally emerge. If a fearful respondent wants to know, "Why are you taking notes?" just tell them. For the commonly encountered, "I don't remember," a permissive pause often brings results. If the interview partner becomes tongue tied, use a reflective probe (immediate elaboration). Steering runaways back on course often necessitates a gentle change of topic (Schatzman & Strauss, 1973; Gordon, 1975). Gordon (1975) suggests that when a reluctant interviewee says, "I don't know anything," the interviewer can use retrospective elaboration and encouragement. In the following example, the respondent is having difficulty with a question eliciting information about what doctors should think about when dealing with pain (question 3b in Figure 5.2):

R: With a doctor relieving my pain?

I: Whatever occurs to you.

R: Um. Maybe I'm not getting the question right.

I: Could be. Let's start with. . . .

R: You mean if the doctor thought the patient might become addicted to a pain medicine, he might not give it to them? He'd have to know his patients pretty well. Still, I suppose he'd still have to give you something to relieve whatever you had. I don't know what to tell you on that one.

I: If you went to a doctor with pain, what would you hope that the doctor would do for you?

R: Well I would hope that if I went to him with pain, that he would give me something that would relieve it. And if it was something that was going to continue, that he'd tell me what he was going to do about it like an operation or something like that. I'd want it right away. I wouldn't want to stay on medication.

Here an encouraging reframe keeps the discourse flowing.

The alert interviewer also continuously evaluates the content of the ongoing conversation. The interviewer listens for key terms; watches for changes in the type of communication, such as switching from interview discourse to performative discourse; and listens for possible misunderstandings. It is also important to identify those times when the conversational partner is attempting to create an impression or self-presentational image. Similarly, it helps to recognize "positional shifts," such as when the interviewee shifts from speaking as a mother to speaking as an employee or as a daughter (Holstein & Gubrium, 1995). Every person has aspects of him- or herself that remain outside of self-awareness—what Douglas (1985) calls our personal "black holes." Sensitive interview partners will recognize the other's (and their own) black holes when they encounter persistent topic avoidance, exaggerated behavior/responses, or a culturally inappropriate lack of emotional display. These are signals to ease up and to go more slowly, to manufacture distance, and possibly to use self-disclosure, as in the following example:

> **R:** Well I think (laughs) you've brought back a few memories I'd forgotten I even had! The first time I ever had real pain was when I had the first baby. And Joseph was very. . . . He was the second one. Sue was a tough one. She was the last one. She couldn't make up her mind if she wanted to come out or not. (laughs) Like I say, I've never really thought of pain until this week when you called and asked me if I would talk to you and I thought, what can I tell her about pain? I don't even have headaches. So I guess there's a lot to be said about it.
>
> **I:** What's it like to think about it?
>
> **R:** I don't know because I never think about it.
>
> **I:** Now that you are thinking about it. (laughs)
>
> **R:** Yes, right. Um, I think even as much compassion as I have for Charlie, for all this length of time, I would even have a little more for him, because I know he doesn't have any pain with the ah, you know, the stoma and all that sort of thing. But I often think when I change it for him, if there's pain there he's not telling me about it. And once you've had cancer I suppose you always hope that there isn't a little bit floating around in there because you hear. . . . [story continues uninterrupted for several minutes]

Here the black hole of denial is gently and slowly entered with a touch of distancing humor.

During the interview, the interviewer is taking brief notes, referred to as "field jottings" by Bernard (1988) and Bogdewic (see Chapter 3). These notes include observations about the respondent (i.e., nervous or evasive), about the surroundings (i.e., temperature, noise, distractions), and about the interview itself (i.e., the number of interruptions, changes in type of communication). Notes to facilitate the remembering of key terms and names are also kept. As soon as possible after the interview, the interviewer expands on these jottings and dictates extensive methodologic, descriptive, and analytic observations for his or her field notebook.

When the official interview is over and the tape recorder is turned off, it is important to linger for 5 to 15 minutes of postinterview contact. This is the time for closing small talk that sets a tone of empowerment and good relations. This is also an opportunity to elicit your interview partner's impressions of the interview and to be alert for the unexpected moment when new information is revealed (Gordon, 1975; Werner & Schoepfle, 1987b). Say thank you!

There is no one way of doing depth interviews. It is a craft. The above discussion purposely avoided naming a series of steps, as that presumes more control and direction from the interviewer than we believe is appropriate in a quality depth interview. Both participants are active in the exciting and unpredictable world of collaborative storytelling. Thus we provided some helpful guides for the journey. Nonetheless, there is a common, implicit map to the depth interview process that can help you know where you are and where you may still need to go (Holstein & Gubrium, 1995; Rubin & Rubin, 1995). This path starts with *naturalizing,* creating a feeling of natural involvement for both participants, and often involves just chatting. The journey moves on to *assigning competence* and then to *activating narrative,* both of which are discussed above. Once the stories are flowing, you travel to *getting the details.* As comfort, trust, and intimacy increase, it becomes possible to ask the more difficult and sensitive questions; you have arrived at *getting deep.* Borrowing from the wisdom of the scuba diver, we recommend surfacing slowly from these depths. Thus the latter part of the interview process usually involves *toning down* the emotional level. The journey ends with *closing.* Just recognize that great adventures await those who journey afar and aren't afraid to leave the map. Have faith in your partner.

Transcribing: The Final Script

Before transcription, an interview needs to be evaluated for quality and then transcribed only if acceptable. This *evaluation process,* as discussed by Whyte (1984) and Werner and Schoepfle (1987b), is to ensure the quality of the tape, the overall quality of the interview, and the assessment of ulterior motives, possible distortions, and surprises. This screening prevents unnecessary transcription expense and is the first step in indexing the interview. Schatzman and Strauss (1973) also recommend noting the following for each interview: (a) length; (b) rate of speech; (c) number and length of silences; (d) length of preliminary and closing interchanges; (e) relative amounts of talking by each participant; (f) percentage of remarks couched as questions, and who asks; (g) who controls the interview and when; (h) who signals termination; and (i) tone of the conversation. Kvale (1996, p. 145) suggests six criteria for assessing the quality of an interview: (a) extent of spontaneous, rich answers; (b) longer responses than questions; (c) degree to which interviewer follows up and clarifies; (d) interpretation goes on throughout interview; (e) each partner attempts to verify his or her interpretations; and (f) interview is story in itself, is self-communicating.

Transcription involves the complicated process of translating from oral discourse to written language. The interview is an oral, visual, and kinesthetic dance between two living, active bodies with multiple levels of communication (see Figure 5.1). The transcription of this performance will never capture that reality. This must be remembered when using the transcriptions for analysis; they are frozen interpretive constructs. Thus, it is important to be clear about the *style* of transcription, about how the transcription is made (Kvale, 1996). There are several choices. Do I transcribe word by word, verbatim (see examples above)? Do I "clean it up" and formalize it? Do I include pauses, emotional expressions, intonations? How much detail? Do I summarize and condense? The answers are mostly dependent on the original research question and the evolving interpretations. Thus, transcription style can change during the course of the research; keep your original tapes until the research is finished. Actual transcription takes approximately 4 to 6 hours for every 1 hour of interview.

CONCLUSIONS

The creative depth interview is an entranceway to narrative understanding. It is a situated, encapsulated discourse balancing intimacy and distance, which opens the way to understanding how particular individuals arrive at the cognitions, emotions, and values that emerge from the conversational journey. It is an adventure in sense making. The purpose is to construct a metanarrative of the many stories heard from the many interview partners. This interpretive process is on-going and informs each subsequent interview. The artificial separation of gathering and interpreting present in this chapter is unfortunate. In actual field research, both of these processes occur in circular iterative fashion, as discussed in Chapter 7. Interviews are analyzed as they are collected, and modifications in the guide or changes in the sampling strategy are made before the next series of interviews. The understanding of "truth" emerges within the research process and not in a significance level at the end. Qualitative "truth" gives voice to the hidden, to the silent, to the noisy, to the unspoken obvious, to the hurt, to the joy. Good depth interview research preserves the multivocality and complexity of lived experience.

It's flu season; Carmelita and her family physician have met. Both were separated in distress and feeling out of control. Through depth interview research on pain, on their pain, we can connect with their distress, and the pain becomes ours. We risk being changed. Carmelita and her physician begin seeing ways of turning themselves around to each other again. We see ways of changing physician socialization and physician-patient communication (Miller, Yanoshik, et al., 1994). A new journey begins!

6

The Use of Focus Groups in Clinical Research

Judith Belle Brown

The qualitative method of focus groups has a more than 40-year-old history in the social science literature (Stewart & Shamdasani, 1990), most prominently in the arena of marketing research. In the last decade, focus groups have been successfully adapted to primary care research—pioneered and championed by David Morgan (Morgan, 1988, 1992a, 1992b, 1998a). After hearing Morgan present at the second Foundations in Primary Care Research Conference in February 1990, I was intrigued by this qualitative approach. Although a seasoned social work clinician, I was then a novice researcher in primary care—listening to Morgan helped bring the two worlds together for me.

Since that time, I have been involved in 10 studies that have used this technique as a means of data collection, either as the primary source of data collection or as a secondary source. Half of the studies have examined the patient's perspective on a number of topics ranging from the determinants of women's decision making in relation to initiating or remaining on hormone replacement therapy (Marmoreo, Brown, Batty, Cummings, & Powell, 1998) to the factors that contribute to patients' long-term attendance at a family practice teaching unit (Brown, Dickie, Brown, & Biehn, 1997). Other studies have explored the perspectives of health care professionals involved in primary care, most notably those of family physicians.

The topics covered in these focus group projects have included family physician identification and treatment of woman abuse (Brown, Sas, & Lent, 1993) and family physician care for patients with atrial fibrillation (Brown, Harris, & Sangster, 1997). Thus the topics have been broad and wide-ranging, with the intent of capturing the views and opinions of the participants in each area of inquiry. In many of these studies, focus groups have been the sole source of the data collection in examining a specific research question.

When the avenue of discovery has not yet been explored or well understood, focus groups have acted as a means of initial inquiry. In other instances, focus groups have served to supplement or enrich the study findings. Thus the use of focus groups can fulfill many needs in the research process.

This chapter examines the use of focus groups in primary care research, noting the various applications of this data collection technique in the advancement of primary care research. Throughout the chapter, I use two of my studies to illustrate how specific decisions are made in the use of the focus group technique, for example in the development of the research question, in sample selection, in recruitment, in the number of focus groups, and in the interpretive process.

In the first study, our intent was to explore the factors contributing to patients' long-term attendance at a family practice teaching unit, where they are constantly being seen by different residents rotating through the Center[1] (Brown, Dickie, et al., 1997). We conducted five focus groups, composed of patients who had been affiliated with one of the three practices at the Center for more than 15 years. In the second study, the objective was to identify barriers and facilitators to independence as perceived by seniors with chronic health problems and their informal and formal caregivers (Brown, McWilliam, & Mai, 1997). In particular, we sought insights into their experience with three aspects of care: medical, home-based, and public health services. We conducted seven focus groups, consisting of two groups of seniors, two informal caregiver groups, and three health care provider groups, representing each of the three primary care areas—medical, home-based, and public health.

Before embarking on a further description of the focus group method, I will briefly return to the history of focus groups in primary care. In preparing this chapter, and also to track the use of the focus group technique in primary care research from 1988 to 1998, I requested a literature search from the Canadian Library of Family Medicine of the College of Family Physicians of Canada. Because there is no medical subject heading (MeSH) term for focus groups, the search was conducted by identifying articles that contained the expression "focus group" or "focus groups" either in the title or the abstract. In addition, each article had to be relevant to primary care and/or family medicine.

The literature search identified 109 citations describing the use of focus groups in primary care research in the last decade. Space limits a report of all these publications, but it is noteworthy that the use of focus groups in primary care research spanned the globe. For example, there were studies from Africa (Barker & Rich, 1992), Australia (Temple-Smith, Hammond, Pyett, & Presswell, 1996), Canada (Brown, Dickie, et al., 1997; Brown, McWilliam, et al., 1997; Cave, Maharaj, Gibson, & Jackson, 1995; Cohen, Woodward, Ferrier, & Williams, 1995; Wood, 1993), Israel (Borkan, Reis, Hermoni, & Biderman, 1995; Monnickendam, Borkan, Matalon, & Zalewski, 1996), Scandinavia (Malterud, Baerheim, Hunskaar, & Meland, 1997), the United Kingdom (Roche, Guray, & Saunders, 1991) and the United States (Marchand & Morrow, 1994; O'Connor, Crabtree, & Yanoshik, 1997; Thom & Campbell, 1997).

The literature search also revealed diverse research topics, such as education—undergraduate (Burack et al., 1997; Frasier, Slatt, Kowlowitz, Kollisch, & Mintzer, 1997); postgraduate (Borkan, Miller, Neher, Cushman, & Crabtree, 1997; Butler, Seidl, Holloway, & Robertson, 1995) and faculty development (Baldwin, Levine, & McCormick, 1995); prevention (Cogswell & Eggert, 1993; Ornstein et al., 1994) and health promotion (Li, Williams, & Scammon, 1995); health care delivery (Brown, McWilliam, et al., 1997; Thornton, 1996); behavior change (Cave et al., 1995; Wood, 1993); guideline development (Fardy & Jeffs, 1994); and intervention strategies (Rodriguez, Quiroga, & Bauer, 1996). The studies explored both consumers' (Brown, Dickie, et al., 1997; Brown, McWilliam, et al., 1997; Liaw, Litt, & Radford, 1992; Mellor & Chambers, 1995) and practitioners' perspectives on primary care practice and health care delivery (Brown, Sas, et al., 1993; Cohen et al., 1995; Jackson & Yuan, 1997). This attests to the importance of focus groups in primary care research.

However, in reviewing these publications, and from my own experience and that of my colleagues, many questions arise: What are focus groups? When and why should you use focus groups? How do you conduct and analyze focus groups? This chapter will attempt to address these questions and guide the reader in the application of the focus group method in primary care research.

In our study on long-term attenders, four key themes were identified as the primary factors contributing to long-term attendance of patients at a family practice teaching unit: the relationship context, the team concept, professional responsibility and attitudes, and comprehensive and convenient care. How we crafted the research question, decided on the sample, conducted the focus groups, and organized the analysis of the data will be discussed later in this chapter. The findings of our seniors' independence study elucidated four main themes, characterizing the barriers and facilitators to seniors' independence: attitudes and attributes, service accessibility, communication and coordination, and continuity of care. How decisions were made in the design and implementation of this study will also serve to illustrate the application of the focus group technique.

Description of Focus Groups

Focus groups in clinical research generally consist of studies with four to 12 homogeneous or heterogeneous groups consisting of six to 12 participants. Focus groups are dynamic, spontaneous, synergistic, and fun. They are conducted by individuals who are most often trained moderators (i.e., familiar with groups process and group dynamics) and sometimes familiar with the topic of inquiry. Many studies use focus groups as the sole technique for gathering the data. Other researchers use focus groups as a means to generate information at the outset of the inquiry (Brown, Dickie, et al., 1997) or to complement or verify the results of a survey (Schattner, Shmerling, & Murphy, 1993). The latter use of focus groups can provide greater "depth" or richness to the results. Thus the use of focus groups is both flexible and diverse.

It is important to differentiate focus group research from other types of group interviews or activities. Focus groups are not designed to serve as a support group or psychotherapy session (Morgan, 1998a), although participation can often be therapeutic (Marmoreo et al., 1998) or educational (Brown, Sas, et al., 1993). Nor is it the goal of a focus group to promote consensus-building or decision making—by contrast, the intent is to gather information based on the participants' interactions (Morgan, 1998a).

The focus group technique also needs to be distinguished from other types of group interviewing, such as the nominal group technique, which brings together the ideas of individual participants; the Delphi technique, which relies on the collective opinion of an expert panel; and brainstorming sessions, which seek to generate new ideas and creative problem solving (Morgan, 1998a; Stewart & Shamdasani, 1990). Group interviews can also be a crucial component of participatory research, as described by Thesen and Kuzel in Chapter 15. In contrast to focus groups, this technique transpires in the naturalistic setting (Morgan, 1988), and the process is more observational than facilitative (Frasier et al., 1997).

Determining the difference between the focus group technique and other types of group interviews is essential to the research enterprise, as is the comparison with individual interviews. One primary difference is that the individual interview captures the sole story of one participant, in contrast to a focus group, which, via the dynamic and interactive exchange among the participants, produces multiple stories and diverse experiences. As Morgan (1998a) notes, the individual interview provides a detailed account of the person's unique and personal experience, whereas the focus group generates a discussion of similarities and differences among the participants. Also, in a focus group, contrary opinions can be explored and may generate new areas of inquiry (Schattner et al., 1993).

The use of individual interviews may be more appropriate when discussing sensitive issues or topics that require self-disclosure (Borkan, Miller, et al., 1997). Participants in a focus group may be reluctant to share issues of a deep and personal nature due to concerns of confidentiality and privacy (Frasier et al., 1997). Conversely, the synergy, spontaneity, and stimulation of the focus group process can facilitate both candor and emotionally provocative exchanges among the participants (Barbour, 1995; Stewart & Shamdasani, 1990).

The differences in the cost of conducting individual interviews versus focus groups and differences in the time required to collect the data using either technique has been debated (Morgan, 1988, 1998a). In my opinion, time and money should not be the criteria on which to base the decision to use the focus group technique versus individual interviews for data collection. Rather, the method of data collection needs to be responsive to the research question and reflect the most effective strategy for addressing the question. For example, in our study examining why family physicians practice palliative care, we used individual interviews because we were endeavoring to understand what personal and professional dimensions influenced their decision (Brown, Sangster, & Swift, 1998). The stories of personal loss and professional failures revealed during the interviews might have been "edited" in a focus group setting. Similarly, individual interviews were the data collection technique of choice in our exploration of the disempowering process of chronically ill older persons (McWilliam et al., 1997). Only a detailed account of the individual's personal experience could capture the process of disempowerment. In contrast, the choice of the focus group technique for the two studies described in this chapter was made on the basis that focus groups would generate rich and diverse views, opinions, and experiences from multiple participants.

With this overview in mind, let us examine the issues pertinent to focus groups, including the research question; sample selection; recruitment; conduct of focus groups (size, number, length); moderator role; interpretation of focus group texts; and reporting.

The Research Question

Studies that use focus groups begin with a clear and precise research question. The research question leads to design areas to explore such as,

Will the technique of focus groups answer the question? How will focus groups further the topic under exploration? What is the advantage of using focus groups versus another qualitative technique such as depth interviews or a quantitative approach such as a survey? Ultimately, the research question will direct the development of the interview guide to be used in the focus groups, as will be discussed later in this chapter.

For example, in our study of long-term attenders at a family practice teaching center, we were interested in understanding what factors influenced patients' decisions to remain patients at the Center for over 15 years despite the fact that the medical personnel—specifically, the medical residents—changed every 6 months. Because the research question reflected a new area of inquiry, the focus group method was viewed as an effective means to gather patients' reasons for continued attendance at a teaching center. The participants were being drawn from three different practices at the Center; therefore, mixing them in different focus groups provided an exchange of ideas and experiences about the Center. Individual interviews might have limited the participants' description to one specific practice. Thus the focus groups provided breadth to the discussion, and the group synergy expanded the participants' contributions.

It is important to note how our bias was embedded in the development of the research question. We assumed that the changing medical personnel would be a central issue. Thus, in creating the interview guide, conducting the focus groups, and interpreting the data, we had to exercise caution and prevent our bias from impeding the research process.

Several factors influenced the decision to use the focus group technique for exploration of the barriers and facilitators to seniors' independence. This study represented the initial springboard in a comprehensive research program on seniors' independence consisting of 14 studies being conducted in three sectors of the health care system (medical, home-based, and public health) involved in the care of seniors. Thus the study was viewed as an opportunity to establish a baseline perspective of the status of seniors' independence at the outset of the research program. Because we were charged with the goal of capturing the ideas and opinions of multiple stakeholders, including seniors and their informal and formal caregivers, the focus group method was a logical choice. In addition, we wanted to elicit as wide a range of barriers and facilitators to seniors' independence as possible. At this stage of inquiry, a survey could have limited the parameters of the research question and been contaminated by our own biases. It was essential that we first hear from the stakeholders themselves. Ultimately, the findings from the focus groups served as a template in the development of a prevalence study regarding the barriers and facilitators to seniors' independence that surveyed over 1,000 randomly selected seniors in the community.

In summary, the decision to use the method of focus groups as the means of data collection is determined by the research question. With that principle established, let us now examine the various steps required in conducting focus groups.

Sample Selection

In selecting participants for a focus group, several issues require consideration, including the type of individual being recruited; the nature of the group composition—homogeneous versus heterogeneous; the degree of familiarity among the participants—strangers versus friends, relatives, or colleagues; and the level of compatibility among the participants.

First, what constitutes a good focus group participant? In my experience, participants need to have some degree of personal or professional investment in the topic under examination—either as a consumer, provider, or policy maker. They also need to be articulate, have an opinion, and be at ease speaking in a group setting.

The choice of whether the focus group should be composed of homogeneous or heterogeneous participants has been debated (Barbour, 1995; Schattner et al., 1993; Tang, Davis, Sullivan, & Fisher, 1995). Again, the decision regarding group composition should be based on the research question. Homogeneous groups share a common background or experience (e.g., all members had been patients at the same family practice teaching center for over 15 years) that facilitates communication and an exchange of ideas and experiences. Similar contexts may also promote a sense of safety in expressing conflicts or concerns. However, there is also the danger of "groupthink."

In contrast, a heterogeneous group can bring together a more diverse set of participants, whose different experiences and viewpoints can stimulate and enrich the discussion. By introducing new ideas and potentially conflicting perspectives, speakers may inspire other group members to consider the topic under discussion in a different light. However, with diversity comes the risk of power imbalances and lack of respect for differing opinions. A highly opinionated and dominant participant can be destructive to the group process. Thus the decision to use a homogeneous versus heterogeneous group must take these issues into consideration.

Historically, it was considered best to have groups that were composed of those who were strangers to each other, to prevent preset assumptions, avoid editing or restricting discussion on emotional or highly charged topics, limit groupthink, and preserve confidentiality. Recently, Morgan (1998b) has noted that in certain situations it is not possible or feasible to generate a sample of strangers. The key point he raises is that the group dynamics change when the participants have a prior relationship, and this may necessitate higher moderator involvement to limit "side conversations" and assumptions about knowledge, experience, and opinions (Morgan, 1998b; Stewart & Shamdasani, 1990).

Finally, the issue of participant compatibility. In my experience, the issue of participant compatibility overrides the above and is based on Morgan's (1988) premise that "participants should really have something to say about the topic and they should feel comfortable saying it to each other" (p. 46). Furthermore, Stewart and Shamdasani (1990) emphasize that "compatibility does not necessarily imply homogeneity" (p. 43). Group compatibility may promote group cohesiveness, group satisfaction, and ultimately the group's effectiveness in discussing the topic under inquiry. The level of group compatibility will also influence the extent of the moderator's "control" over the group, as discussed later in this chapter.

If the views and opinions of one specific group are being explored, as in our long-term attenders study, then homogeneous groups are the most appropriate choice. In contrast, heterogeneous groups, reflecting a maximum variation sample with a potential range in age, gender, ethnicity, socioeconomic status, geographic location (urban versus rural), and/or disease category, effectively gather multiple perspectives on the topic under inquiry (Patton, 1990).

For example, in our seniors' independence study, the impressions and experiences of a variety of stakeholders were needed. To achieve this goal, we conducted seven focus groups. Two of the groups comprised seniors who ranged in age from 62 to 86 years; 80% had one or more chronic health problems. Because access to services for seniors was thought to be a potential barrier to independence, we made a deliberate effort to include seniors from both rural and urban communities. Informal caregivers composed two groups, and again, maximum variation sampling with regard to age, gender, location, and caregiving responsibilities was a major consideration in the selection of the participants for these focus groups to provide as wide a range as possible of experiences, ideas, and perspectives.

Each of the three groups of professional caregivers comprised health care providers from one of the three primary care components: public health, home-based care, and medical care. Each group was caring for a similar population—the frail elderly in the community—but their practice contexts and concomitant needs and experiences were different enough to warrant separate focus groups for each group of providers. Also, issues of group dynamics and levels of power and authority in the health care system supported the separation of the different professionals. In the public health group, the participants were, for the most part, public health nurses—however, they had a wide range of experience in caring for the elderly. The group of home-based professionals consisted of nurses, occupational therapists, physiotherapists, social workers, and homemakers, all with different responsibilities, roles, and levels of involvement in caring for seniors in the community. The diversity in this group provided various perspectives on the barriers and facilitators to seniors' independence. Medical providers, who comprised the final group, consisted of family practice nurses, family physicians, and geriatricians. Again, they reflected different levels of responsibility and expertise in the care of seniors.

In summary, one essential criteria is to include "information-rich" participants who have ideas, opinions, and feelings about the topic and are comfortable with voicing their views in a group setting. My two studies demonstrate how deciding to use homogeneous or heterogeneous groups is derived from the research question. Finally, participant compatibility promotes group interaction and cohesiveness.

Participant Recruitment

Participants may be recruited through a variety of methods, such as advertising through the local newspaper, contacting support groups or community groups, using established mailing lists of health care professionals, or purposefully selecting a group of individuals with a particular interest in the topic under discussion. During the recruitment phase, the researchers need to be mindful of the key issues presented in the section on sample selection described above. In addition, recruitment may take longer than anticipated and require the assistance of recognized leaders in the area of inquiry or community. Also, potential participants need sufficient time to rearrange their schedules or make necessary arrangements to attend the focus group.

For example, recruitment for the long-term attenders study was relatively simple, with names of potential participants being provided by the family practice nurses from each team at the teaching center. In the seniors' independence study, the recruitment process was more complex due to the number of stakeholder groups and the diversity needed within some of the groups. Consequently, a variety of recruitment strategies was used, such as accessing established mailing lists, contacting community agencies serving seniors, and advertising at senior centers.

In my experience, when recruiting certain populations, it is important to overrecruit. For example, health care professionals, especially physicians, are often detained or called away by emergencies. Also, with groups such as the frail elderly, illness or impairment may impede their participation on any given day. Therefore, to ensure eight participants at the focus group, I would recommend recruiting 12 to 15 individuals. Also, to ensure adequate numbers at the actual event, it is useful to contact participants by telephone the day before the focus group as a reminder of the time and place.

In summary, recruitment can occur from a variety of resources and can be conducted by the research team or recognized community leaders. Recruitment takes time and planning, with overrecruitment being necessary with certain populations.

Number of Groups

In my experience, if focus groups are the sole means of data collection, a minimum of 4 to 5 focus groups is required to reach saturation (also, see Chapter 2). As noted previously, a sole focus group can be used as a form of member checking or as a means to supplement the findings. There does not appear to be a consensus on the maximum number of focus groups that can constitute a study. The maximum number I have used is 12; however, Morgan (1992b), for example, has used up to 30 focus groups. In studies where I have used more than 5 groups, we were attempting to capture potential regional variations or to accommodate multiple stakeholders, as in the seniors' independence study. The central issue, in my opinion, is how many focus groups are required to reach saturation, and therefore the final decision on the number of groups is determined by this fundamental principle.

It is advisable to conduct a "pilot group" to determine the effectiveness of the interview guide in terms of both the content and process of the focus group. The pilot group is sometimes included in the data set, depending on the quality of the data.

Number of Participants

The debate continues about the number of focus groups conducted, but there is consensus regarding the number of participants required to compose a focus group. Six to eight participants represent the optimal number. If there are fewer than 5 participants, the interaction and dynamics of the group will be limited, and more than 10 participants will not allow enough "airtime" for all the participants to express their views. Again, this raises the issue of overrecruitment to ensure adequate numbers in each focus group.

Length of Focus Groups

Focus groups need to be 1 to 2 hours in duration. If a focus group is less than 1 hour, there is a risk of not fully exploring the topic under inquiry. However, if the focus group extends beyond 2 hours, fatigue or disinterest may set in for both participants and moderators (Tang et al., 1995). For example, during our focus groups with seniors, we were very cognizant of the time factor and the potential for fatigue. In addition, in the same study, we needed to be respectful of the time commitment being made by busy health care professionals and potentially overburdened caregivers.

The Role of the Moderator

The focus group moderator(s) play an essential role in the conduct of a successful focus group. Being a good moderator requires observational and facilitation skills. Engaging all the participants in the discussion, promoting a lively interchange, modulating conflict, and all the while following the interview guide is a demanding role for a focus group moderator. In all of my studies using the focus group method, I have employed two moderators. Often, one moderator has had specific skills and experience with the focus group process and the other moderator has expertise in the content area of the study. In the latter role, the moderator must be aware of his or her potential biases and not impose these on the group. The other caution for the "content expert" moderator is that participants may look to him or her for the "correct" answers or be reluctant to express their views for fear of being "wrong."

For example, in our study of seniors' independence, the moderators were health care professionals with recognized expertise in caring for seniors. Therefore, attention was given to our own potential biases and assumptions, as well as to promoting the exchange of experiences and expertise within all the focus groups. In truth, the real experts were the seniors themselves, who confronted the barriers and facilitators to living independently every day.

Another benefit of using two moderators is that one moderator can be observing the nonverbal communication taking place in the group. In addition, he or she can be making field notes during the group. Morgan (1988) has described how moderator involvement can vary in focus groups. In the long-term attenders study, the moderators' involvement was low, with their role being facilitation of the patients' stories and experiences of being a patient at the Center for more than 15 years.

In comparison, the moderators' involvement in the seniors' independence study was high, as they were searching for barriers and facilitators to seniors' independence from multiple stakeholders. All participants needed to be given an opportunity to express their views, but the moderators also had to explore whether or not the participants shared similar perceptions of the barriers and facilitators to seniors' independence, as the findings would have implications for implementing change at the individual level (i.e., altering attitudes like ageism) and the systems level (i.e., improving service accessibility for seniors).

Although it is preferable to have the same moderators conduct all the focus groups, this is not always possible, particularly if the focus groups are being held in various locations such as different cities or states. In this instance, training and standardization of the moderators is critical. Their role in the analysis is essential for promotion of the iterative process of the focus group technique.

In summary, as Krueger (1998) has noted, a focus group is only as good as its moderator(s).

Developing the Interview Guide

Essential to the focus group method is the careful development of a semistructured interview guide reflecting the research question. The interview guide should be reviewed for clarity and comprehensiveness by individuals familiar with the topic. For example, in our seniors' independence study, we had seniors and informal and formal caregivers comment on the proposed interview guide before proceeding with the focus groups.

It is important to begin with a broad, open-ended question. Again, an example from our seniors' independence study, where we began with the following question: "How does the health care system affect the independence of seniors with chronic health problems?" Often you need to begin with a question that defines the area under inquiry. Also, begin with low emotional intensity issues and then move to high emotional intensity issues. For example, the following question has higher emotional intensity, compared to the opening question described above, because it required the seniors to reflect on their own actions and personal responsibility: "What part do you play in maintaining your own independence, despite your health problems?" Finally, it is useful to have "probes" ready to prompt the focus group participants for further explanation or "depth" on the topic, such as "Can you explain in more detail?" or "Can you give us an example?"

In summary, the interview guide is just that—a guide, for the most part. Groups will generate substantial data, and the interview schedule provides the facilitators with a "map" to guide them through the process. Rigidly following an interview schedule may preempt the natural flow of the interaction among the participants. Instead, moderators should use the interview guide to help them "negotiate the terrain." Here Morgan (1998b) has the final say: More structured groups answer the researcher's questions; less structured groups help to reveal the perspectives of the group participants and may assist in the discovery of "new ideas and insights" (p. 47).

The Logistics of Conducting the Focus Group

There are several logistical issues requiring consideration when one conducts a focus group. Some of these are quite practical and basic, such as providing adequate parking, holding the group in a convenient location, collecting basic demographics, providing name tags, using a high-quality audio system for recording the focus group, and designating one moderator to record field notes regarding the tone and mood of the group as well as nonverbal behaviors. Documenting nonverbal communication is important, as it may serve as the only means to capture, for example, the head nodding of participants that signifies consensus on an issue.

Specific incentives may be used to encourage participation, such as providing child care, transportation, an honorarium, or light refreshments. For example, in accommodating the busy schedules of health care professionals, I have conducted the majority of the focus groups either early in the morning or at the dinner hour; thus providing a light meal was essential. Several authors (Morgan & Krueger, 1998; Stewart & Shamdasani, 1990) have provided comprehensive overviews of the logistics that need to be addressed in conducting focus groups.

In regard to the actual conduct of a focus group, I always begin with a preamble that includes welcoming the participants; outlining the purpose of the discussion; setting the parameters of the discussion (length, audiotaping, and transcribing); assuring confidentiality; and informing participants that there are no right or wrong answers—rather, their ideas, opinions, and experiences are important for us to hear. I then proceed with the semistructured interview guide. The key is not to be constricted by the interview guide but to allow it to serve as a means of organizing the data collection, which is the focus group discussion. As I near the conclusion of the focus group, I often ask if there are issues or concerns that require further discussion or have not yet been addressed. This acts as a form of member checking during the focus group.

Before embarking on the analysis, the following steps require completion. All the focus groups need to be transcribed verbatim. It is important to proofread the transcripts to check the transcriber's work, as he or she will miss words or names. If there are large sections missing in the transcript, or portions of the tape that were inaudible, the moderator may need to review the audiotape. Consequently, having two audio systems and detailed field notes is invaluable. Also ensure that the transcriber provides enough room in the right margin to make notes during the initial analysis.

In summary, addressing these logistical issues will facilitate the use of the focus group method.

Interpreting Focus Group Texts

The interpretation of focus group data is a rigorous process. I use the following central principles to direct the process. First, each focus group is the unit of analysis, not the individual participants. Second, team interpretation is imperative to ensure credibility and trustworthiness and to control researcher bias. Third, the interpretative process should occur along with the data collection. Qualitative research is an iterative process; thus the interview guide may be modified as the interpretation proceeds, with new questions or probes being added for exploration of concerns or issues that surfaced in prior groups. Fourth, the analysis should include both independent as well as team analysis.

Initially, each investigator independently reviews the transcript, searching for key words and phrases. I usually highlight pertinent sections, making notations in the right-hand column as themes emerge. Next, the research team assembles to discuss whether its members are hearing and experiencing the same thing. If not, they need to examine why this is not occurring, with the final goal being consensus. After the first focus group, it is important to ensure that the interview guide, as well as the research team's perceptions of the process, are "on track." At the outset of the analysis, it is important to clarify that the research question is being adequately addressed by the focus group process.

In the initial organizing phase of the analysis, there will be numerous categories or ideas that surface. As the analysis cycle proceeds, these will begin to cluster under major themes until there are no more themes emerging—hence, saturation has been attained. Throughout the analysis process, it is important to look for within-group and across-group differences and similarities. For example, in the seniors' independence study, the multiple stakeholders and three areas of primary care under examination made this a challenging but essential step in the analysis. It became evident that although the seniors viewed transportation and inclement weather as serious barriers to independence, the informal and formal caregivers did not raise these issues to the same extent.

In the long-term attenders study, we assumed at the outset of the project that access to comprehensive and convenient care would be the major factor influencing the patients' decision to remain at the medical center for more than 15 years. However, what emerged in the interpretive process, across all the focus groups, was the powerful impact of the patients' relationships with the medical team and how this influenced their decision-making process.

The research team session can be a face-to-face meeting with all the investigators or a meeting via a teleconference call. The latter is a bit more cumbersome but still effective, and it is essential if you have investigators located in various geographic locations. For the final analysis cycle and report preparation, I have found it to be important to have a face-to-face meeting.

Three additional points about interpreting focus group texts: In recent years, a number of computer software programs have become available to assist in qualitative analysis. These programs are particularly useful in organizing the data if you have a large number of focus groups such as eight or more. The key point is that computer programs can help organize the data, but they cannot think for you. Second, and to reiterate, the focus group discussion is the data. If the analysis gets sidetracked or you begin to doubt or question the trustworthiness of the themes, return to the raw data and listen carefully to the participants' stories. The final point is, when do you reject the data from a focus group to maintain quality control over the data? This is a difficult issue and requires attention to potential research bias. What is relevant to the participants may not be relevant to the research team, and vice versa. What needs to be determined during the team analysis is when certain data are serving as extraneous "noise" or opening up a new vista of inquiry. Only then can a decision be made as to whether to include or delete the data from the interpretive process.

At the conclusion of the process, the central themes reflecting the focus group discussions will have emerged. These should be illustrated by relevant quotes. This often represents a challenge, as there will be many rich and thoughtful comments, but space and readability of the final report restrict the number of quotes that can be included. This leads me to the final section of this chapter—reporting the findings.

Reporting the Focus Group Findings

As qualitative research (and, in this case, the focus groups technique) has entered the mainstream of clinical care research, more journals are welcoming qualitative manuscripts for publication. Some journal editors have developed guidelines for qualitative submissions, assisting both researchers and reviewers. However, others have not—leaving the responsibility for maintaining scientific rigor to the investigators. All the steps required for successful implementation of the focus group method, as outlined in this chapter, need to be addressed in the manuscript: everything from the statement of the research question or study purpose to the final interpretation of the key themes.

In reporting the two studies that I have used as illustrations throughout this chapter, I had two key goals. The first goal was to tell the participants' stories—allowing their "voices" to be heard. The second goal was to help their stories make a difference, whether that was removing barriers to seniors' independence or promoting relationships between patients and their primary care providers.

CONCLUSION

Focus groups are a valuable and effective qualitative technique in primary care research. They are interesting, dynamic, and often yield unanticipated findings. To avoid abusing this important research method, follow the suggestions provided in this chapter and those of other authors (Morgan & Krueger, 1998), and always be guided by your research questions.

NOTE

1. Because of the need for this organization to remain anonymous, it will be referred to here only as "the Center."

PART III

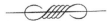

Interpretation

Strategies of Analysis

7

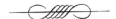

The Dance of Interpretation

William L. Miller
Benjamin F. Crabtree

W elcome to the big dance! Move your body, feel the music, hear the sounds, see the excitement, smell the aromas. Embrace your partner, the texts you've collected, and start the interpretive dance toward "sensemaking" (Weick, 1993). This chapter will provide an overview of how a team of qualitative researchers (or a single investigator) approaches and makes sense of all the data it is gathering and accumulating.

WHERE ARE WE?

In earlier publications (Miller & Crabtree 1994a, 1994b), we describe the use of four analysis styles—quasi-statistical, template, editing, and immersion/ crystallization. This simplified typology was useful as a way of introducing qualitative analysis to primary care research initiates who had neither the time nor background to wade through the waters of complex, historically based qualitative methods and their jargon. The typology enabled beginning clinician researchers to start doing qualitative studies and to apply them to their experientially based questions. This was especially true for primary care medical researchers, who understand their discipline as more empirical and craft based than theoretical. The approach was successful (see the introduction to this book for more detailed explanation); however,

127

it is now time to advance to the next level of our apprenticeship in the craft of qualitative analysis. This chapter presents a next step in our development.

This revised approach features six enhancements. Most significantly, the dynamic and iterative qualities of the whole research design, including analysis, are more fully highlighted. In harmony with a more expansive perspective, we now speak of the larger interpretive process of which analysis is a part. This interpretive process encompasses the intimately related operations of analysis and of presenting the results and connects the analysis process with data collection. "Analysis styles" are redefined as organizing styles within a larger analysis process, and their iterative and changing aspects are highlighted. The quasi-statistical style is not discussed because it is rarely, if ever, used by qualitative researchers. The relationship of numbers to qualitative research is better discussed in the context of multimethod strategies (Miller & Crabtree, 1994a; Stange, Miller, et al., 1994). A fifth enhancement is the conspicuous recognition of the important role of paradigms and theory in qualitative research in general and the interpretive process in particular. Finally, the contributions of multiple disciplines and qualitative research traditions are acknowledged.

This chapter begins with a brief overview, depicting the interpretive process as a "big dance." This is followed by a closer examination of the texts engaged in interpretation and some of the implications of this engagement. The third section is the largest and describes how to dance, including discussions of five phases of the interpretive process and the three organizing styles. A brief exploration of some of the decision-making issues in analysis and a diagrammatic tool for describing the organizing aspects of analysis follow. The roles of theory, disciplines, traditions, and the experience of clinical reality in the interpretive process are then discussed. The chapter concludes with a summary of some of the common principles, pitfalls, and pearls of interpretation. Let the dancing begin!

INTERPRETATION AS DANCE

Interpretation is a complex and dynamic craft, with as much creative artistry as technical exactitude, and it requires an abundance of patient plodding, fortitude, and discipline. There are many changing rhythms; multiple steps; moments of jubilation, revelation, and exasperation; and, always, like high school prom night, the process is a sweaty, physical, experienced one. Interpretation is like a night at the big dance. The dance begins with an invitation to attend. These invitations state the intent, establish the context, determine the guests, suggest what to bring and wear, and propose boundaries for what to expect. It's a senior high school prom, or it's a community contra dance. This is the initial descriptive phase of interpretation. It's depth interview data about physicians' pain experiences, or it's field notes about being on call as an intern. Once at the dance and with the fun under way, however, the dance often changes. New partners appear, the music shifts, the unexpected happens, you and some of your closest friends change, and new relationships form. You must keep redescribing and adjusting, gathering new information; this is the iteration between data collection and interpretation. There is an opening dance that sets the tone for the evening, much as the initial organizing style frames the interpretive possibilities. The big dance event ends with a closing dance that, one hopes, resolves the evening's tensions. Many qualitative analyses will end with a code-book style exploration for disconfirming evidence or alternative explanations. In between, over the course of the evening, is a series of small dances, some slow, some fast, some intimate, some distant, some frenetic, some tightly stepped, which mark many of the moods and stories being lived. Similarly, the interpretive process will experience many iterations and shifts and will often necessitate changing organizing styles and analytic approach.

The health care practitioner is also a craftsperson and artist, and the clinical process is also like a dance. How a clinician makes sense of a patient's story parallels how qualitative researchers make sense of their data. Both have to dance with their partners, whether the partners be texts or patients and their families. Both have to be iterative and responsive. In other words, dancers, doctors, nurses, and qualitative research interpreters all have to decide how to relate to each partner, how and what to observe and what to pay attention to, and how to interpret what is said and done to complete a good dance, working diagnosis, assessment, or account. All three dances begin with knowing who are the dancers.

Who Are the Dancers?

The dance of interpretation is a dance for two, but those two are often multiple and frequently changing, and there is always an audience, even if it is not always visible. The two dancers are the interpreters and the texts. The simple definition of a text is that something which is the basis for analytic work. "That something" could be typed transcripts from key informants, focus groups, audiotaped clinical encounters, or depth interviews. It could be health care records, minutes from hospital meetings, or photographs of a neighborhood. It could also be field notes from observations or life space drawings or genograms resulting from interviews or videotapes. Whatever physical things the researcher uses as interpretive materials are texts.

What is important to notice is that *all* texts are derivative. Just as all dance partners come to the dance from somewhere else, so also do all analytic texts. The texts derive from some field experience. This experience may or may not have involved some member(s) of the interpreting research team. Thus, all texts are already representations/interpretations of some source experience (see Chapters 3 through 6 for more details on the gathering processes that produce some of these texts). The researcher/ interpreter also comes to the dance from the world of his or her life experience and cultural milieu and from some relationship with the field experience that is the source of the analytic texts. As a result, the self can be partially understood as text. It is the analysis of self as text that is partly meant by reflexivity. This is one reason why we believe that working with a team is so important to good qualitative research. Team members can be very helpful with each other's self-analysis. In addition, it is common in clinical research for some of the team members to be the primary field workers and for others to be more involved in the interpretive process. The field workers then become "living texts" for the other team members (for example, see Chapter 16, where a field worker is hired to spend extensive time in family practices to collect data).

In the dance of the interpretive process, there are many audiences. Each research team member has the audience of each other and of participants in the field. They also have a larger audience of academic peers, family, funding sources, and any intended audiences for the final account. The field experiences behind the analytic texts also have their own respective audiences. The interpretive dance is a very large one, indeed, to which many are invited.

HOW TO DANCE

The qualitative research interpretive process is a creative, artistic craft situated within a diverse knowledge-defining community. Anticipating going to the big dance can be both frightening and exhilarating, and it can seem daunting. Do I have the right clothes? Will I choose the right partners? Do I know enough dances? Will I recognize the music? Can I really attend the big dance? Do I know how? This section will help you to be ready to waltz and twist and tap your way through the fun and discovery of the interpretive process. Start the music.

The interpretive process consists of five phases through which one iteratively spirals and shifts throughout the process (see Figure 1.4, p. 16). These five phases are (a) describing, (b) organizing, (c) connecting, (d) corroborating/legitimating, and (e) representing the account. Organizing, connecting, and corroborating/legitimating are the actual analysis part of the larger interpretive process. The describing phase serves as a link to the data collection process. Redescribing after each round of analysis serves as an interlude or pause between dances to reflect and plan the next iterative steps for both new data collection and new analysis. How is the night going? Similarly, the representing the account phase stays linked to the analysis.

We hope that it is now apparent that qualitative interpretation usually consists of many iterative cycles. There are four different types of iterations that occur. The first is the iteration between data collection and data analysis, which is facilitated by the describing phase. Then there is within-analysis iteration, in which organizing, connecting, and corroborating/legitimating iterate as a spiral, possibly several times, before reconnecting with describing and the collection/analysis iteration. Third, representing the account and analysis iterate to varying degrees—some research teams begin developing the account or story along with the analysis, connecting them almost like a double helix. Others periodically intersperse writing the account up between cycles of analysis. What is not recommended is waiting to share the research results, to tell the story, until after the analysis is done. Finally, there is the self-reflection loop, the iterative cycle of reflexivity. The research team and each member of the team are also learning about themselves as they are learning about the research topic. This loop connects with all parts of the field research process. The interpretive process is constituted by these four iterative loops, which periodically feed back to each other.

The relationships of the members of the investigative team to the data and its sources can be characterized by the tightness of the coupling among these four iterative cycles. Multiple variations are possible. Some team members may be closely coupled to the collection/analysis iteration but much less so to the representing the account/analysis iteration or the within-analysis iteration. For example, in Chapter 16, the field workers work very closely with the analysis team, making it possible to feed back to the collection process but much less so to telling the story. These variations are types of *primary analysis* as long as the questions and interpretation derive from the originating data and there is some coupling. *Secondary analysis* occurs when original data is revisited and there is no coupling of the three iterations. An important methodological issue for future research is to better understand the implications of the various loose and tight couplings between different team members and the four different iterative cycles. We are now ready to begin stepping through the five phases of the interpretive process, beginning with that part of the qualitative research process we have named describing.

Describing

The interpretive process, just like the larger research design process, starts with the researchers and describing. Describing is a reflective phase in which the research team steps back from the field and analysis and reviews what is happening, how what has gone on has influenced the interpretation (reflexivity), and what should happen next. Describing begins with revisiting reflexivity and the paradigm question. Who are we? How have we been changed and influenced by the collection process? How have our earlier assumptions and fantasies been challenged? How is our language and culture influencing, shaping, and limiting our imaginations? What are the strengths and weaknesses of our group process? Investigators working alone should ask, What methods am I using to challenge my thinking? These are some of the critically important reflexivity questions that need to be explicitly answered by the research team when the interpretive process is initiated and whenever describing is revisited in the iterative cycles.

The paradigm question is equally important. What is the operating paradigm? Are the collection methods and the proposed analytic approach consistent with it? A common error in clinical qualitative research is switching from a critical or constructivist paradigm back to a materialistic, positivist paradigm part of the way through the research process, most often at the interpretive moment. The cultural forces pushing and pulling toward universal, reliable, and valid "truths" with generalizable, predictable, and controllable outcomes is subtle, persistent, and powerful. For example, you are moderating focus groups with the intent of better understanding parents' lived experience of caring for a child with severe asthma. You are operating within Shiva's circle of constructivist inquiry. While reading the transcripts, you hear two very different experiences. Sharing this interpretation with some peers, you are challenged to give more "objective" evidence of your sensemaking. You think about counting some key words associated with the two styles of experience or even counting the number of individuals with each style in all the focus groups and correlating the experience style with asthma outcomes. Beware! You are slipping into the trap. Stay within the constructivist paradigm and build your case there (see Chapter 1). The gathering and interpretive processes are too closely linked to be able to shift paradigms when moving from one to the other. If you must, design a different study using materialistic inquiry to answer these new questions. The holy, materialistic, research trinity of reliability, validity, and generalizability is tough to overcome. Only by paying attention and re-asking the paradigm question frequently can this temptation be successfully resisted.

There are a host of other, more mundane, but important questions in the describing phase. Most of these act as reminders of what needs to be considered in doing analysis and interpretation and as helps in decision making. What is the question and/or focus? What are the boundaries of the question domain? Where is the field from which the texts derive? What kinds of texts do we have? What intentions motivated their production? Do they represent processes, context, behavior, and/or perceptions? What is the quality of the texts? What are their limitations? Is the analysis primarily driven by clinical experience and considerations or by theoretical or tradition-based concerns? Another set of questions relates to future data collection. These questions focus on asking what additional data need to be obtained to enhance emerging understandings, test alternative ones, or explore newly revealed possibilities. All of these questions and others that may arise need to be reviewed not only at the start of interpretation but periodically, after one or more passes through the analytic cycle.

Organizing

The actual analysis begins with selecting appropriate *organizing styles,* some scheme for approaching and relating to the analytic texts. We have identified three idealized organizing styles for qualitative analysis—template, editing, and immersion/crystallization (see Figure 1.5, p. 22). These styles are similar to idealized dance forms such as ballet, tap dance, and free-form dancing. They are forms or styles that guide but that also serve as bases for creating, innovating, and bringing alive. We have named these styles *organizing* because they give structure to the analytic process: They help sift, prioritize, and form the interdependent texts and investigators into a whole. We considered using the word *classifying,* which means organizing by classes or categories, but found this to be too limiting. Immersion/crystallization, for example, may move from text to interpretive statement without ever developing explicit descriptive categories; nevertheless, there is organizing occurring within the investigator through the prolonged immersed engagement within the field of research.

The organizing process has been described by many others. Some examples of their schemes will help clarify our concept of organizing styles. Miles and Huberman (1994), who make extensive use of explicitly structured data matrices and formats, present an interactive model consisting of data reduction, data display, and conclusion verification. Dey (1993), who explicitly links his analysis scheme to the use of the computer, presents the task of organization as four steps: creating categories, assigning categories, splitting and splicing, and linking data. A different approach is taken by Mason (1996), who views the organizing phase as a more closely interwoven process of sorting, organizing, and indexing. She describes three different approaches to this process. The first is "categorical or cross-sectional indexing," in which an indexing (or coding) scheme is applied to the texts as a whole. Another is "non cross-sectional indexing," in which different schemes are used for different parts of the data. She also describes the use of diagrams and charts as aids in organizing the data. Ely,

Anzul, Friedman, Garner, and Steinmetz (1991) present three components of the organizing process: applying thinking units (originally defined by Lofland & Lofland in 1984) such as meanings, roles, groups, and so on; establishing categories; and creating organizing systems.

Our own approach to the organizing phase of analysis is to conceptualize a continuum of three different idealized organizing styles, with permeable, fluid boundaries capable of changing over the course of any given study. These styles incorporate all the aspects of organizing mentioned by the authors above. One advantage of distinguishing three different styles is the ability to recognize how each limits, alters, and disrupts the natural stream and structure of the text. This recognition reinforces the suggestion to use multiple organizing styles over time. More important, we hope the three styles, and our description of their use over time, help display and promote the dynamic, creative, iterative, yet disciplined craft of qualitative interpretation.

Template, editing, and immersion/crystallization each characterize a particular manner and stance for acting and for entering the texts and getting to the phase of connecting. They are idealized metaphors of how qualitative analysts reduce, highlight, arrange, and rearrange the data so that connections are made and new sense is created at any particular time in the overall interpretive process. They provide formalized ways for thinking about how to identify the meaningful units and developing analyzable categories for later connecting and corroborating/legitimating and, finally, for representing an account. These three organizing styles are not comprehensive analysis schemes; they are no more or less than different ways of organizing the texts. The analysis and interpretive processes involve much more than this activity. It is important to remember that they are also idealized. Any particular study may move from one style to another, mix styles, and alter styles to fit particular needs and opportunities. Chapters 8 through 10 provide several illustrations of the dynamic and complex use of these styles. The three organizing styles are distinguished by the timing of classification and by the process of organizing. The template style refers to entering the text with a classification scheme, whereas the editing style refers to entering the text and only later developing a classification or coding scheme. A specific classification scheme either will never be defined or will be defined only at the end when using an immersion/crystallization style. The process of organizing when using the template style involves using initial codes or categories to interact with the text; additional categories can emerge or old ones changed based on that interaction. Using the editing style, the analyst identifies new categories through direct interaction with and sifting and sorting of the text. The immersion/crystallization process moves directly from entering the text to making connections, without development of explicit categories or codes.

The *template* organizing style uses a template or code manual as the organizing system for entering the text and identifying units of interest for further analysis and interpretation. The specific template used can range from very broad categories, such as the "thinking units" of Lofland and Lofland (1984), to very detailed code manuals (Willms, Best, et al., 1990). The organizing scheme is generally derived prior to entering the text and can come from multiple sources. These include the literature, self-analysis, research team discussions, prior research, or the results of earlier analyses in the present study using other organizing styles (see Chapter 9). Connecting and making interpretations is performed on already explicitly sorted information. The code manual or indexing system should stay open to constant revision throughout the analytic process.

The *editing* organizing style enters the text in a different way. It is the interpreter, acting as an editor, who is the initial organizing system. The interpreter enters the text and begins to segment the data by identifying the information most pertinent to the research question and then categorizing, cutting, pasting, splitting and splicing (see Dey, 1993), much as an editor does. The code book, or organizing scheme, is thus created after entering the text and results from the ongoing interaction with the text and the organizing process. Ethnography, grounded theory, and hermeneutics often incorporate this style into their interpretive processes. What distinguishes their use of this style is what constitutes a meaningful unit. Traditional ethnographers focus on cultural descriptive units such as kinship or material goods; grounded theorists generally search for theoretical units such as social process; hermeneuticists often seek experiential and/or metaphorical units.

The *immersion/crystallization* organizing style is significantly different from the other two. In this style, the interpreter, as an intuitive participant, serves as the organizing system. The analysts' intuitions and team reflexivity work as they are engaged with the data are the primary source of interpretation. The phases of organizing, connecting, and corroborating/ legitimating are collapsed into an extended period of immersion in the texts, out of which interpretations are crystallized. Reflexivity is especially critical when using this organizing style.

Connecting

Analysis involves the ongoing iterative spiral of organizing, connecting, and corroborating/legitimating. Once an organizing approach for entering the text is determined, sensemaking continues at a new level, and the connecting phase is soon entered. Sometimes the connections come as spring blossoms of inspiration. More often, they result from critical and patient reflection and persistent engagement with the text, one's analytic memos, sorted segments of text, team discussions, and disciplined organizing.

Connecting is that phase that specifically refers to the discovery of themes and patterns, to making linkages between categories, to developing models, and even to generating new theory. There are many techniques for facilitating this process, and some of them are described in the next four chapters. Particularly helpful ones are briefly mentioned here. Creating maps and diagrams can help display information and suggest new connections and patterns. Visualization of concepts and categories is a powerful and creative tool (for example, see the use of practice genograms in Chapter 16). Similarly, the use of data matrices, as described by Miles and Huberman (1994), can also be helpful in making connections. Writing short stories or developing vignettes from your data can help new connecting metaphors and relationships emerge.

Corroborating/Legitimating

The third phase of the tightly linked analysis process is corroborating/legitimating. This phase has also been referred to as "uncovering" (Heidegger, 1927/1962; Packer & Addison, 1989) and also as *verifying* or as *determining validity*. We have concerns with these latter two phrases because of their close association with materialist inquiry and their deep connotations of universal truth within the clinical research traditions. Corroborating means to make more certain and to confirm. These meanings are less rigid and more consistent with the intent of qualitative research. The corroborating/legitimating phase consists of re-viewing the texts after initial or later analysis, seeking to corroborate the multiple "truths" or perspectives voiced in the texts and by the analysts to confirm internal consistency of interpretation and to explore the relationship of the interpretations to the empirical world as experienced by all the research participants. This re-viewing is consistent with the concept of *uncovering*. Uncovering refers to the interpretive act of evaluating an account, examining whether it answers or provides a solution for the anomaly or confusion that motivated our inquiry (Packer & Addison, 1989). Many strategies for doing this have been devised. Several are discussed in each of the other chapters, and most are summarized in Chapter 18. For this particular phase, these strategies include searching for alternative explanations, disconfirming evidence, negative cases, and member checking. A template organizing style can often be helpful here, especially toward the end of the interpretive process. A code book based on the emergent understanding is applied to the original text or to newly derived texts with the intent of searching for confirming or disconfirming evidence.

This phase is also referred to as *legitimating* because that term signifies several other important aspects of this phase of the analysis process. The interpretations will ideally be viewed by multiple audiences, each of whom has different expectations and criteria for believability and utility. The research team needs to be aware of these legitimating criteria and explicitly address those that it can. The four most obvious audiences with whom legitimacy needs to be negotiated include the research team itself, the audience of other researchers, clinicians, and the people and "worlds" who were in the lens of the researchers. This is often very difficult and sometimes impossible. This crisis of legitimacy is seen by Denzin and Lincoln (1994) as one of the two defining crises in qualitative research at this time. The second defining crisis is that of representation, part of the last phase of the interpretive process.

Representing the Account

The final phase of the interpretive process consists in sharing the new understandings and interpretations, finding some way to represent an account of what has been learned in the researching. What form the account takes will depend on the audience, your skills, and the nature of the findings. It could take the form of a traditional research report for some trade journal or a more extensive monograph or even a book. Sometimes, however, creating a performance, writing a story or poem, or presenting at town meetings can be more appropriate accountings. In each case, the challenge is to find a way to honestly represent the process, the participants, and the many interpretations generated yet also recognize the political realities and the limitations in understanding. This is another place to remember your operating paradigm. If it is not materialistic inquiry, and most qualitative research isn't, then beware of slipping back into the positivist tar pit; that is not where you wanted to be. Both constructivist and critical/ecological inquiry insist on iteration and honor the multiple voices in the texts. At the same time, however, two of the important audiences for primary care researchers are clinicians and biomedical researchers, both of whom often define science only in terms of materialistic inquiry. Clinically rich descriptions with clearly articulated clinical relevance will usually hold the attention of clinicians. Our own response to the biomedical research community is to emphasize the different standards of quality and to apply them explicitly and rigorously.

This phase completes the interpretive process and needs to be part of the other four phases. In some cases, the representation is developed as the analysis unfolds. This is illustrated by Richard Addison in Chapter 8. In other cases, the story isn't put together until much later in the interpretive process. It is, generally, not a good practice to wait until the very end to begin preparing an account, as this limits one's ability to obtain feedback along the way. Part of representing the account is describing the process of analysis and the analysis decisions made along the way. The next section discusses these decisions and presents a tool for visualizing part of the process.

TOOLS FOR THE DANCE

Returning to the big dance metaphor can help us imagine the many decisions and changes that occur throughout the interpretive process. The question then becomes, "How do I map the big dance?" One approach is to see the dance as a "set," with a repertoire of many songs and their different associated dances that are cocreated by the dancers and the musicians over the course of a night. This score of music and choreography could then be mapped or diagrammed, providing one image of the big dance. The dance of interpretation between any two partners, a particular text and its interpreter, can be mapped on an analysis grid in a similar manner. Creating this analysis grid for each text helps outline the decision making and illustrates the organizing flow of the analysis (see Figure 7.1). The horizontal axis refers to time and the vertical axis refers to the three organizing styles. This creates an analysis space within which one can map key steps in the analysis part of the interpretive dance (see Willems & Rausch, 1969, for concept of analysis space).

The organizing styles point toward how one enters the text and organizes the search for meaning; they describe what type of dance is being performed. But who leads the dancing as text and interpreter move across the space? Jennifer Mason translates this question into knowing how one wishes to read the text (1996). She suggests three options. The text can be read literally, interpretively, or reflexively. "If you are reading your data *literally*, you will be interested in their literal form, content, structure, style, layout, and so on" (p. 109). In other words, the text leads in the dance. A *reflexive* reading locates the interpreter within the text and explores his or her role in the process of data generation and interpretation. The interpreter leads in the reflexive dance. The text and researcher dance in partnership with many "natural" lead changes when reading the text *interpretively*. In this case, an interpreter reads the data to construct what he or she thinks the text means, what it is trying to say, what he or she can infer. The use of "sensitizing concepts" can be helpful when reading the text in this manner (Blumer, 1954; van den Hoonaard, 1996). The actual marks or nodes on the analysis grid denote whether the text is read literally (L), interpretively (I), and/or reflexively (R).

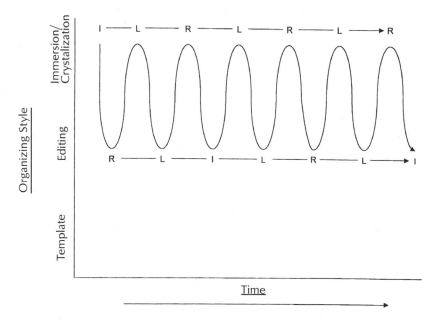

Figure 7.1. Analysis Grid for Richard Addison's Study (Chapter 8)

Figure 7.1 depicts the choreography of Ritch Addison's study, described in detail in Chapter 8. He begins using an immersion/crystallization (I/C) organizing style in partnership with the text and field. He continues using I/C throughout the study but alternates between reading his text literally and reading it reflexively. Shortly after starting, he also begins using an editing organizing style that he continues to use throughout the study. With this style, too, he alternates between literal and reflexive readings, with an occasional interpretive reading. The analysis grid illustrates this fluid, dynamic, and iterative flow of analysis.

Figure 7.1 also demonstrates how the organizing styles often change over time, how the way the text is read changes over time, and how the whole interpretive process is repetitively iterative. The process is energetic and vital, its many twists and turns based on changing data, changing self-analysis, and changing interpretation.

At least four ways of categorizing the use of organizing styles over time can be identified. A *single style* can be used for the whole study. The depth interview study of pain experiences described in Chapter 5 and in Miller, Yanoshik, et al. (1994) is an example in which only an editing organizing style is used; however, all three ways of reading the text are done over time.

Phased styles is illustrated by the three studies described in Chapter 9, where a template organizing style is used with other styles, but they are sequenced over time. Figure 7.1 specifically visualizes *fluid styles,* where two or more organizing styles weave back and forth in dynamic interplay and are often being used simultaneously. *Layered styles,* a fourth category of organizing style use, pertains most commonly to case study designs (see example 1 in Chapter 9 and see Chapter 16). In this situation, there can be styles for particular types of texts, such as one style for field notes and another for interview transcripts. There can be styles for organizing the case as a whole, styles for comparing cases, and styles for comparing types of text across cases. This pattern of organizing style use is much harder to illustrate on the analysis grid, but it is possible if you use different types of lines for the trajectory of a particular text and different colors for particular cases.

Selecting the Tools

The analysis grid depicts decisions already made. For all of us either planning a new study or stuck in the middle of a data pile, the challenge is how to choose an appropriate organizing style and way of reading the text. Each of the next three chapters discusses the decision-making processes for the particular studies being described. Several common factors and questions to consider are highlighted here.

Several of the questions asked during the describing phase of interpretation are noteworthy (see pp. 131-133). Reflexivity and *self-analysis* are a good starting point. There are multiple ways of knowing, and we each have preferential styles and aesthetic styles. Some of us work best with structure and deductive logic; a template and/or formal editing organizing style fits well here. Others prefer intuitive approaches, which fit immersion/crystallization. The researcher must also examine the *question and aims* of the study. If the goal is exploration, discovery, or understanding the lived experience of others, a more open approach such as editing or I/C is helpful. If the goal is theory testing, however, a template organizing style, with the theory shaping the template, may be a viable option early in the interpretive process.

Another important consideration in analysis decision making is the amount of *prior knowledge* already in hand about the question or domain of interest. If there is much existing literature, especially good qualitative literature; knowledge from prior research; and/or much existing theory, then using an a priori code book based on this literature and/or theory as an initial organizing style may be of much assistance. Who the possible *audiences* are is another factor. Using a more explicit structure, such as a template, somewhere in the interpretive process may be helpful for legitimating your study with a clinical audience. On the other hand, allowing the research participants' voices, what Mishler (1986) calls the "voice of the lifeworld," to be more active in the interpretation may also be an important consideration if they are a significant audience or if one is using a participatory approach. Thus it can be helpful to include an editing or I/C organizing style in the process. The advantage of using several styles in the course of a study should now be clearer.

A final consideration addresses one's *relationship to the text*. This refers to the three ways of reading the text discussed earlier—literally, interpretively, and reflexively. We believe all three are valuable at different times in the analysis. A literal reading is helpful near the beginning and again near the end, where you want the text, the data, to lead. Interpretive readings provide much of the core interpretations, and reflexive readings help clarify the reader's role in the emerging interpretations. Any one of the three organizing styles can be read in these three ways.

RESTORING THE ANCESTORS

In the past, we often downplayed the importance of the many disciplines and traditions from which qualitative research approaches derive and in which they are used. A primary reason for that omission was the fear that our research peers in clinical medicine would be unwilling and, often, unable to struggle through the jargon jungle of that literature. As a result, little qualitative research was being done; therefore, we simplified the language. Now the situation is different. Much qualitative research is taking place in all the clinical disciplines. A common problem we are finding, however, is that the interpretations in a significant portion of the research suffer from premature closure and remain too superficial. They are stuck in description and in need of theory. The time has come to restore the critical importance of our ancestors and to expand our community to include all the other qualitative researchers struggling with similar questions and methods from multiple other perspectives and theoretical persuasions (see the appendix at the end of Chapter 1).

The process of interpretation nearly always implies a theory. The medical world often forgets its theoretical and cultural moorings and assumes it speaks only of facts. The result is that participant observation is sometimes used without regard to "culture," which is central to the integrity of the method. It is critical to preserve the richness of the qualitative disciplines and traditions. Sometimes the research may be primarily data driven. When clinical relevance is the primary goal, one option is to interpret back to the clinical situation and limit the results or final interpretation to its clinical significance and not to its theoretical or scientific significance (Thorne, 1997).

In this edition, we have included many examples of clinical research that make extensive use of theory and traditions. Malterud (Chapter 17) has her research interests triggered by a personal clinical anomaly. "What is going on with the many women I see who have medically unexplained symptoms?" She finds helpful theory from the tradition of linguistics, which helps guide and powerfully inform her research. Addison (Chapter 8), on the other hand, initiates his research already steeped in the traditions of hermeneutics and grounded theory. These overtly shape his research design and interpretation. Early on in the iterative interpretive process, he recognizes the need to use socialization theory from the disciplines of psychology and sociology, which influence and provide context for his later interpretations.

Willms (described in Chapter 9) enters the research process explicitly using his background in the tradition of ethnography and the discipline of anthropology. Toward the end of his research, he discovers how his emerging interpretations connect with existing theory about the patient-centered clinical method (Willms, Allan, et al., 1991). Finally, Miller, Crabtree, McDaniel, and Stange (described in Chapter 9) begin their research with little explicit theory; however, when the data defy interpretation beyond mere description, the "discovery" of complexity theory is an "ah ha" experience and the interpretive process is accelerated forward (Miller, Crabtree, et al., 1998). Complexity and systems theory go on to explicitly shape and inform the follow-up comparative case study discussed in Chapter 16. The ancestors are restored. We all need to be at the dance.

PRINCIPLES, PITFALLS, AND PEARLS

Before closing, we want to share some principles, pitfalls, and pearls from our own and others' (many key informants') past experience. They serve as guideposts for the interpretive process just described. Think of these as rules for the dance. The following are eight principles for the interpretive process:

- Know yourself, your biases and preconceptions.
- Know your question.
- Seek creative abundance. Consult others and keep looking for alternative interpretations.
- Be flexible.
- Exhaust the data. Try to account for all the data in the texts, then publicly acknowledge the unexplained and remember the next principle.
- Celebrate anomalies. They are the windows to insight.
- Get critical feedback. The solo analyst is a great danger to self and others.

- Be explicit. Share the details with yourself, your team members, and your audiences.

The following are 13 pitfalls and pearls to help improve your dance of interpretation, with the first six coming from Silverman (1993):

- "Don't mistake a critique for a reasoned alternative." (p. 197)
- "Avoid treating the actor's point of view as an explanation." (p. 199)
- "Recognize that the phenomenon always escapes." (p. 201)
- "Avoid choosing between all polar oppositions." (p. 203)
- "Never appeal to a single element as an explanation." (p. 205)
- "Understand the cultural forms through which 'truths' are accomplished." (p. 208)
- Do not go native. Be wary of overidentifying with research participants.
- Watch for elite bias. Recognize that you prefer some people more than others and compensate.
- Do not stereotype.
- Avoid the holistic fallacy. Not everything makes sense.
- Beware of premature closure. Keep searching.
- Avoid overly delayed closure. Good enough is good enough, never perfect.
- Avoid overdoing data shuffling. If stuck, stop fiddling and go collect more data or go dancing.

Welcome to the big dance of interpretation!

8

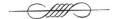

A Grounded Hermeneutic
Editing Approach

Richard B. Addison

Good qualitative analysis is not easy. Later in this volume (see Frankel, Chapter 18), you'll read about standards or criteria for evaluating qualitative research (Packer & Addison, 1989). The focus of this chapter is analysis: specifically, one of Crabtree and Miller's four organizing styles of analysis of qualitative research—what they call "editing." To illustrate this style, I will use an example from one of my own qualitative studies on the socialization of family physicians.

In its more mundane form, the word *editing* conjures up images of a balding man with visor, cigar, and pencil marking up a text, working late into the night, surrounded by blue billowing clouds of smoke, trying to meet a deadline for next morning's edition. Of course, all card-carrying qualitative analysts know that even though the cigar and visor are required accouterments for carrying out qualitative analysis, these days a computer may be substituted for the pencil (see Meadows & Dodendorf, Chapter 11, for more on software recommendations for systematic editing analysis).

AUTHOR'S NOTE: This chapter is a revision of my chapter in the first edition of this book. The title and some of the content have been changed.

On a more scholarly note, the word *edit* is derived from the Latin *editus*, from the verb *edere*, meaning to give forth. It is also related to the Latin verb *educo*, to lead forth, or to educate. So in its higher form, editing can be thought of as an organizing style of analysis that helps to bring forth greater understanding of or meaning from text or data.

The fundamental task of any analysis is to make sense out of or bring some comprehensible and illuminating order to the complex set of human practices and interrelationships that are usually the object of inquiry of qualitative research. The world is an incredibly complex place. Good analysis is rigorous, complex, and challenging work. Good analysis can also be a creative, intense, and satisfying endeavor.

In an attempt to simplify qualitative analysis and make it accessible to interested researchers, the editors have differentiated four organizing styles of analysis. However, as they pointed out in the preceding chapter, very few studies limit themselves to using only one organizing style. For example, although I rely heavily on an editing style in the research study described in this chapter, I also employed aspects of an immersion/crystallization style (see Borkan, Chapter 10) at various points in my analysis. If editing is the bread-and-butter style of qualitative analysis, immersion/crystallization is the creative, generative, synthesizing style of analysis that suggests that bread and butter might taste very good together. To limit oneself to one style of analysis is a mistake of oversimplification for any qualitative researcher.

**Examples of the Editing
Organizing Style of Analysis**

Many studies in health care have relied on the editing organizing style for analysis of their data. For example, Bob Dozor and I used a very similar approach to the one I describe later in this chapter of how family physicians coped with dying patients and their families (Dozor & Addison, 1992). Also, Susman, Crabtree, and Essink (1995) carried out a study on how rural family physicians reacted to depressed patients. An evaluation of a standardized preventive program for family physicians also used a comprehensive editing analysis schema (McVea et al., 1996; also see Chapter 9). O'Connor, Crabtree, and Yanoshik (1997) used a similar editing style of organizing their analysis to look at different responses of diabetic patients to treatment interventions.

For the purpose of this chapter, I will discuss a specific case study. The approach to analysis used in the study, what I call a grounded hermeneutic approach, is a rigorous, comprehensive, and illuminating approach that incorporates the editing organizing style for a major part of the analysis.

The Circular Character of Good Analysis:
Describing the Background Context

I want to emphasize that analysis is not just one step in a linear progression that comes soon after data collection and sometime before writing up the results. Good qualitative research is always more of a circular process than a linear one. Analysis does not fall outside this circular or spiral form. Analysis is part of a larger interpretive process. For instance, interpretation begins in the formulation of the problem and the method of investigation. In circular fashion, I return to refine my analytic procedures as I begin to collect data. My developing analysis helps direct my further data collection. The circle of interpretation continues to spiral.

Analysis is also circular in regard to assumptions and biases. First, I get as clear as possible about my assumptions about physician socialization before I begin my investigation. Then as my research proceeds, I learn more about my assumptions. This process of reflexivity is circular in that what I "discover" is colored by my initial conscious, acknowledged, or foreground assumptions, and as I learn more about physician socialization, I find out more about my unconscious, unacknowledged, or background assumptions. So in effect, my assumptions become clearer or more fleshed out as the circular movement spirals on. I address the specific way this occurs later in the chapter.

Similarly, my background in hermeneutic philosophy and my training as a clinical psychologist and a grounded theory researcher colors the way I look at the data I'm analyzing (as well as the way I initially conceptualize the problem to be investigated). Therefore it is important for me to be as clear as possible with myself and my readers about my background way of looking at and carrying out my analysis. In a circular or spiral fashion, as my way of analyzing and thinking about my data changes, I begin to adjust my way of carrying out my research.

Hermeneutic analysis is a necessarily circular procedure. Even now, as I attempt to describe this process by writing words, sentences, and paragraphs that follow one another in linear fashion, I am aware of the difficulty of communicating the circular feel of my research procedure. While I was still immersed in observing resident practices, taking notes, and recording interviews, I began analyzing the notes and interviews. I moved back and forth between collecting, reflecting, analyzing, reflecting, and writing in a way that cannot be laid out or predicted in advance. At the same time, all of the collecting, coding, and analyzing follows from the practical research problem: the problematic aspects of becoming a family physician. I will show in more detail how the circular character of the research is exemplified in the actual analysis later in the chapter.

This circular or spiraling form of interpretation is one of the central features of a hermeneutic approach. The discussion that follows will allow the reader to gain a good feel for the editing style of analysis within a hermeneutic framework. Attempting to clarify the background understandings and assumptions that the researcher holds is an essential part of any good qualitative analysis, so I will begin by addressing the assumptions and practices of the hermeneutic tradition of research.[1]

Hermeneutics

Hermeneutics is an awkward word with a long tradition. It simply stands for the business of interpretation. The word is thought to derive from Hermes, the Greek messenger god and trickster, who carried messages from the gods to the people. His role was to interpret these messages from the gods and to make them understandable to humans.

The central task of hermeneutic analysis is "the process of bringing a thing or situation from unintelligibility to understanding" (Palmer, 1969). Trying to understand, take meaning from, or make intelligible that which is not yet understood is not only the central task of hermeneutics, it is an essential aspect of our being in the world (Gadamer, 1976; Heidegger, 1927/1962). As an approach to understanding written texts, hermeneutics has long been applied to fields as diverse as biblical exegesis, legal interpretation, and linguistic and literary analysis. It was not until the end of the 19th century that a hermeneutic approach for studying the human sciences began to gain prominence (Bleicher, 1980; Palmer, 1969). In hermeneutic research, there is no absolute standpoint from which the researcher can determine the truth value of a theory or account. Hermeneutics talks about the "coconstitution" of foreground and background, parts and whole, interpreter and interpreted, researcher and research participants, data and theory in a circular or spiral form, what Gadamer calls the "fusion of horizons" (Ashworth, 1997b; Bernstein, 1983; Bleicher, 1982; Caputo, 1987; Dreyfus, 1986, 1991; Habermas, 1968, 1977; Koch, 1995; Lather, 1986; McCarthy, 1978; Packer & Addison, 1989; Rabinow & Sullivan, 1979; Ricoeur, 1981).

Grounded Theory

For my qualitative investigations, I rely heavily on the methodology of grounded theory. The readers of this chapter are probably far more familiar with grounded theory and the constant comparative method of analysis, popularized by Glaser and Strauss (Glaser, 1978, 1992; Glaser & Strauss, 1967; Strauss, 1987; Strauss & Corbin, 1990) than with hermeneutics. Grounded theory is a methodology used widely in sociology, in nursing, and now in other health care research. It entails a rigorous method of editing analysis that I will illustrate later in my case study on physician socialization. For the reader interested in more theoretical discussions of the methodology of grounded theory, see Annells (1997a, 1997b) and Ashworth (1997a). Although grounded theory now does a bit better job of theoretically acknowledging the prejudiced stance and practices of the researcher, it is still often employed in a too technical and nonhermeneutic fashion, without regard to the researchers' assumptions and practices to adequately incorporate reflexivity. Ashworth (1997a) states,

> Because of its relative clarity, grounded theory, whereby the discovery of a "theory" governing some social phenomenon is made inductively on the basis of the painstaking analysis of data, is coming to be a favorite form of qualitative research. . . . However, there is a very real danger that grounded theory can be taken as a technology for doing qualitative analyses. Non-positivistic qualitative research cannot be, and ought not attempt to become, a mechanical process akin to experimentation. (p. 218)

This is a danger that many grounded theory researchers do not consider in their research practice.

An Approach to Research

I do not think of a grounded hermeneutic approach as a method in the sense of a prescribed set of techniques that can be applied to a research project. A grounded hermeneutic approach cuts below specific methods or techniques. For the research described in this chapter, I chose a grounded theory method, specifically the constant comparative analytic method of grounded theory, on a more comprehensive hermeneutic framework. I call the hermeneutic approach described in this chapter "grounded" for several reasons: first, it seeks to illuminate social, cultural, historical, economic, linguistic, and other background aspects that frame and make comprehensible human practices and events; second, it is grounded in the everyday practices of individuals in ongoing human affairs (Kuzel, 1986); and third, it employs the constant comparative method of analysis as well as other aspects of grounded theory.

Assumptions of a
Grounded Hermeneutic Approach

A grounded hermeneutic approach embodies certain assumptions or understandings about the world, the people in it, research activity, and the relationships among these. Briefly, these assumptions and their implications for qualitative analysis are as follows:

- Understanding begins in misunderstanding. When something is missing, wrong, absent, or doesn't make sense, analysis must address the misunderstanding or not-yet understanding. This is the beginning of hermeneutic inquiry.

- The behaviors of research participants have meaning. Good qualitative analysis aims at understanding these possible meanings or helping the research participants understand the meaning of their behavior.

- Meaning is not only that which is verbalized; meaning is expressed in action and practices. To understand human behavior, it is important to look at everyday practices, not just beliefs about those practices. Therefore, interview studies, focus groups, and self-report surveys should ideally include an observational component to ascertain whether people do what they think or say they do.

- Meaning gains greater focus when background conditions such as immediate context, social structures, personal histories, language, shared practices, and economic conditions are illuminated. Data must always be analyzed with these background conditions in mind.

- The meaning and significance of human action is rarely fixed, clear, and unambiguous. Meanings are not limited to preestablished categories. Meaning is being negotiated constantly in ongoing interactions. Meaning changes over time, in different contexts and for different individuals. Therefore, the categories of analysis cannot be rigidly fixed in advance of analysis and data collection.

- Interpretation is necessary to understand human action. Truth is not best determined by how closely beliefs or actions correspond to some fixed reality. It is never possible to achieve an objective, value-free position from which to evaluate "the truth of the matter." Facts are always value laden, and researchers have values that are reflected in their research projects. Any interpretation must attend to how researchers' biases color the framing of the problem, the data selected, and the analytic decisions made.

- Research can accelerate change. Researchers must be conscious of the way their research practices affect the research participants and the research situation. Follow-up is often indicated.

These assumptions will be illustrated in the case study.

Central Practices Of
Grounded Hermeneutic Research

Even though a grounded hermeneutic approach is not a method in the sense of a set of techniques, it is possible to list the following seven practices that are central to grounded hermeneutic researchers:

1. immersing oneself in the participants' world to understand and interpret the participants' everyday practices;
2. looking beyond individual actions, events, and behaviors to a larger background context and its relationship to the individual events;
3. entering into an active dialogue with the research participants, research colleagues, research critics, the account itself, and the researcher's own values, assumptions, interpretations, and understandings;
4. maintaining a constantly questioning attitude in looking for misunderstandings, incomplete understandings, deeper understandings, alternative explanations, and changes with time and context;
5. analyzing in a circular fashion the progression between parts and whole, foreground and background, understanding and interpretation, and researcher and narrative account;
6. offering a narrative account of the participants' everyday practices that opens up new possibilities for self-reflection and changed practices; and
7. addressing the practical concerns of the researcher and the research participants against a larger social, cultural, historical, political, and economic background.

Accordingly, grounded hermeneutic researchers approach a particular problem from a concerned, involved standpoint; immerse themselves in the participants' world; analyze human actions as situated within a cultural and historical context; offer a narrative account of how a problem developed and is maintained; and offer directions for positive change. These practices will also be illustrated in the following step-by-step discussion of my research practices.

Framing the Substantive Problem

For many years I had been interested in the long and arduous education and training involved in becoming a physician. I saw this intense, stressful process as a problem for the trainees, their families, and their patients. I wanted to better understand what becoming a physician was like for the individuals involved, how the practices of resident physicians became problematic, and whether positive alternatives were possible.

Choosing an Approach to the Problem

The method of inquiry and interpretation must fit the problem and goals of the research question. To address the questions detailed previously, I knew that questionnaires or self-report surveys would be inadequate for capturing the complexity and richness of the everyday practices of individuals as they became physicians. I wanted to understand what they actually did as they began their residency, not just what they thought they were doing, believed they were doing, intended to do, or said they did. I knew I needed to have a strong observational component to the research.

Clarifying Initial Understandings: Describing Reflective Reflexivity

Because I was working alone, I narrowed my focus to one university-affiliated family practice residency program in a semiurban county setting. Again, good analysis begins before data is collected. Therefore, before beginning my observations and data collection, I tried to clarify my initial understandings about the problematic aspects of family medicine and residency training. These understandings centered around two issues. First, increasing technological expertise was demanded of physicians who had chosen family medicine; this would create a contradiction for them in their training if they envisioned themselves as healers rather than technicians. Second, stress and impairment in physicians, as evidenced by poor patient care, burnout, dropout, marital problems, substance abuse, depression, and suicide, seemed to be far more problematic than ever before.

I decided to focus most of my efforts on the first year of residency, long recognized as most stressful in terms of its encompassing demands and most significant in terms of inculcating attitudes, beliefs, values, and practices (Bloom, 1963; Mumford, 1970). Habits and patterns of behaving and interacting that are forged at this time often extend beyond internship and residency into personal and professional lives. I narrowed my focus to gain as thick and comprehensive an understanding of their everyday existence as possible.

I presented myself simply and straightforwardly as a psychologist and researcher who was studying how individuals become physicians. I followed nine first-year residents solidly for a year and intermittently for the next two, observing them in almost every aspect of their lives. I followed some more closely than others, as I found some residents more welcoming of my presence, some more verbal, and some more critically reflective. I openly recorded observations about what I saw, what I felt, how I was doing research, what I understood and did not understand, and what I thought was important. I interviewed the residents, their spouses, and others associated with their education and training, asking questions about what I observed. I read the enormous volume of memos, schedules, and documentation that was churned out by the hospital, the residency, and the residents themselves. (For a more detailed description of participant-observation research, see Bogdewic, Chapter 3; for a more detailed description of key informant interviewing, see Gilchrist and Williams, Chapter 4).

Immersing myself in the everyday activities and practices of the residents was important for me to develop an understanding of what these activities meant to them. Analysis occurs while observations are being made and data are being collected. For example, when I accompanied them to their first surgery conference, the surgery coordinator made them stand up and recite differential diagnoses. He called on one of the first-year residents who was very uncomfortable talking in front of groups. She sounded unsure of herself, hesitated, and the coordinator quickly moved on to someone else. I sensed her embarrassment; it reminded me of how my seventh-grade teacher ridiculed me in front of the class because I spoke my answer too softly. When I later interviewed the resident, I told her that I imagined how she must have felt at the moment. She went on to talk about a wealth of similar experiences in medical training when she had felt embarrassed, chagrined, abused, and demeaned. Attuned to her feelings, I noticed that she sometimes did not attend conferences taught by certain physicians. My own experience helped me to understand her reaction to being *pimped* by the attending physician and her resulting avoidance of his teaching. I saw these dynamics repeated with other residents and their attending physicians. Out of this, I came to an interpretation about the importance of such interactions in constituting residents' practices, such as *isolating*.

This type of analysis is essentially and necessarily a hermeneutically circular process: I immersed myself in the residents' everyday existence, wherein I developed an experiential understanding of their practices. I then made this understanding explicit in the form of an interpretation of the meaning of their practices. These fuller interpretations helped me decide where to concentrate my further observations and immersion to understand more or different aspects of their existence.

Concurrently Collecting, Fixing, and Analyzing: Editing as an Organizing Style

Again, the collecting, coding, and analyzing were carried out with an eye to the practical research problem of becoming a family physician. My selection of data to gather and analyze was determined by this focus.

I had my notes and interviews transcribed onto only the left half of the page, saving the right half for text analysis. I treated the social action I observed as a type of text (Ricoeur, 1979). Even though social action is fluid, dynamic, and ongoing, I "fixed" events, behaviors, interactions, dialogues, and practices in the form of a text so that I could interpret and analyze them. Although texts are usually thought of as written material, audiotaped and videotaped material also have been used as texts, usually along with a transcript of the tapes. Thus, the typed transcripts of my audiotaped interviews, my handwritten notes, and my reflections on both of these became the text for what Miller and Crabtree (Chapter 7) call an editing organizing style.

I used two different ways of analyzing the transcripts for developing my account. The first type, often referred to as "in vivo" coding (Strauss, 1987), consisted of selecting from transcripts residents' words or phrases that stood out to me as potentially significant for understanding how the residents were becoming family physicians. For example, I coded such words and phrases as *learning the ropes, punting, pimping, dumping,* and *surviving.* These were terms residents used that later became categories in the developed account. I used as much in vivo coding as possible.

I also used a second and more global type of analysis. This type of analysis was like the reflective process notes I take after seeing psychotherapy clients. In this latter type, I recorded comments and notes on what the residents' words or practices reminded me of, on what I felt to be significant, on what I thought their practices meant and were connected to, on what I did not understand, on how I thought my presence influenced their practices, and on the implications of their practices for their professional socialization. For example, one of my reflective process notes read:

> I went up to see [a 21-year old patient who was dying]: the guilt of not spending enough time with him, and the discrepancy I noticed between the people around him who know he's going to die, and his not talking about death, or not having anyone to talk to about dying. . . . I feel guilty at not spending enough time with him, and I'm sure the residents do too.

This note developed into an analysis of residents' difficulties in dealing with dying patients, and it was the impetus for a later study on death and dying (Dozor & Addison, 1992).

Again, collecting, coding, and analyzing data occurred concurrently. Interpretation and analysis began as soon as I started observing residents and collecting data. For example, one of my early notes read: "I sit at the nurses' station . . . trying to hide out and write my notes. I am feeling absolutely overwhelmed with the amount of input." Another note read: "I feel tired, not at my best, even though I got five hours sleep, considered a good night on call (white cloud). The residents must get used to this." Again in circular fashion, my reactions helped me understand their existence: how "totalizing" their lives as residents were.

I started to put all of these codes and notes on index cards. I cut up relevant sections of my transcribed notes and interviews that were too long to fit on index cards. I began to sort the hundreds of cards and longer selections into piles that seemed to have a common thread. I looked for patterns and relationships between cards and piles of cards. I looked for themes that organized piles of cards. Every horizontal surface above floor level was filled with cards and cut-up transcripts. I began to see progressions and flows. I started making lists of groups of practices, people, reactions, and events and connecting these lists on big sheets of white paper. No horizontal surfaces were left, so I removed pictures and prints and tacked these lists and categories onto walls.

A Thunderbolt: The Beginning of Connecting

Suddenly, 3 or 4 months after beginning, out of this wealth of seeming chaos, I had a flash of clarity: The central organizing theme for the residents as they began the residency was *surviving*. It seemed to both describe and unify their practices in a way that made sense. On finding such a unifying theme, I set out to learn how they survived and how they did *not* survive that first year of residency. Thus a detailed, line-by-line editing analysis was complemented, focused, and directed in future analysis by the thunderbolt. Another way of interpreting my research endeavor was that immersing myself in the residents' existence allowed the emergence and crystallization of the central unifying theme of my analysis. In this way, my immersion and systematic editing laid the groundwork for the subsequent crystallization of a central theme. A strong case can be made for analysis that combines editing and immersion/crystallization (see Borkan, Chapter 10, for more on the immersion/crystallization style).

Diagramming

I then began to reanalyze my transcripts, interviews, notes, and index cards with reference to surviving. I began seeing a different, more cohesive organization, which seemed to incorporate previously scattered experiences and practices. I constructed a diagram that encompassed most of the lists and categories from my wall charts. This beginning diagram, or attempted pictorial whole, of what happened to these individuals as they began their residency, looked something like a child's drawing of an extraterrestrial's digestive system. It was the first of many such attempts to make diagrammatic sense out of their existence.

Understanding and Interpretation

The progression just described again illustrates the circular or spiral movement of hermeneutic research from understanding to interpretation to deeper understanding to more comprehensive interpretation. After immersing myself in the residents' lives (the felt experience of lived understanding), I began to analyze my notes and interviews (conscious, cognitive, intentional interpretation) to make sense out of them. My flash of (deeper understanding of) how *surviving* played such a central role for the residents led me to reanalyze my transcripts, diagrams, and models in light of the centrality of *surviving* (more comprehensive interpretation). Following this, I returned to observe and interview the residents (aiming for greater understanding and even further development of the interpretive account). Thus, as I spiraled around the hermeneutic circle, my understanding continued to deepen, and my account became more coherent, cohesive, and comprehensive.

Questioning the Account: Corroborating/Legitimating

A very important phase in any analysis is that of invited reflection and criticism. When working with a team of researchers, this is easily initiated in team meetings. When working alone, as I did in this study, I tried always to keep my critical voice active, questioning my notes, looking for contradictions, inconsistencies, gaps, omissions, and ambiguities in the developing account. For example, I knew that two strategies the residents employed for surviving, *helping* and *isolating,* were only part of a larger story. It was not until I questioned the conditions under which residents *survived* by *isolating* themselves and the conditions under which they *survived* by *helping* that I was able to push the account further.

This is only one example of how questioning an account serves as a key element of hermeneutic analysis. It is essential for developing and refining any account of human practices.

Entering Into a Critical Dialogue With Other Researchers

Because I worked alone and was not part of a research team, I joined a weekly analytic seminar of other health care student researchers led by a sociologist and health care researcher (Strauss, 1987). I presented my research to the seminar for questions and criticism. At various stages, I also presented the developing account to other colleagues and teachers. One mentor (an educational sociologist) cautioned me about identifying too strongly with the residents' plight and encouraged me to expand my interpretations. Bonding or identifying too closely with the research participants is a frequent occurrence in participant-observation research. Although my bonding with the residents helped me understand their everyday practices, I also needed to stand back, reflect on, and question my understandings. Another mentor (a psychologist and behavioral scientist) filled in valuable pieces of local history. Another primary care physician and researcher pointed out logical inconsistencies in my account. In this way, I created my own research team to help me critique my developing account.

Showing the Account to Research Participants

When I felt ready, I tried to explain the working diagram to the residents. I received many helpful comments and questions about various aspects of the diagram. I was also greatly surprised at the initial reaction I received: No first-year resident could sit through my brief presentation of the account without either crying or becoming extremely anxious. One spoke of his reaction upon hearing the account:

> I had an incredible amount of anger about everything that was on that sheet. I mean, everything that was bothering me was on there in some way . . . and all the arrows went exactly the way the arrows in my brain were going . . . but I was unaware of a lot of them at the time. . . . And I looked at them all and . . . within fifteen seconds my eyes were just welling up with tears. . . . It just made me feel so uncomfortable. (Addison, 1989b, p. 49)

I took this reaction to the diagram as a sign that the account was a powerful one; it had some significance for the residents. I also interpreted this type of reaction to mean that they had no broader understanding of what was happening to them as they carried out their everyday tasks and responsibilities. This understanding of their limited range of reflective vision became a central element of the developed account. Additionally, their reaction told me that I needed to be sensitive and careful about those to whom I presented the account, when I presented it, and how I presented it. I needed to think through the implications of showing the account to individuals already experiencing enormous stress.

Reflexivity: Reflecting on Initial Understandings

One of the essential elements of hermeneutic research is the inclusion of the researcher in the hermeneutic circle. As no privileged position exists from which to observe human behavior, researchers' beginning understandings inevitably influence how researchers carry out their observations, what questions get asked, what data get selected, how data get interpreted, and what findings get reported.

An example of how these early, sometimes taken-for-granted understandings can affect the course of inquiry (and how understandings can change during the course of inquiry) involved the residents' choice of specialty. As noted previously, when I began my study, I was very interested in the split between why I thought individuals chose family medicine (because they wanted to be healers) and what they would be doing as they learned family medicine (learning the technology of medicine). I thought this split would be the central contradiction in their everyday existence. Through the research, I came to understand that although this contradiction was important to the residents, it was not nearly as central as I thought. I learned that individuals chose family medicine for a variety of reasons: because they thought it would be challenging, because they would meet interesting people, because they thought it would allow them to perform a great variety of procedures and give them a vast breadth of knowledge, because they thought they would not be accepted in other specialties, and because they saw themselves as altruistic healers. I only came to this fuller interpretation after I reflected on *my* professional choices: I became a psychologist instead of a family physician and a psychotherapist who eschews technical or cookbook approaches to psychotherapy. This was biasing my perception of the residents' choice of family medicine. Once I saw how my professional choices affected my developing understanding of the residents, I began to see some of the other reasons why the residents had chosen family medicine. At the same time, the split I had identified as central (technician-healer) became far less central. By moving in a circular fashion between reflecting on my evolving account and my developing understandings, these reflexive understandings changed as my interpretation of the residents' everyday practices evolved.

Continued Observations

At the same time, I continued observing and interviewing to flesh out underdeveloped portions of the account and to correct aspects that were not yet coherent or cohesive. For example, the residents were troubled by their outpatient clinics, the kind of setting in which they would be spending most of their time after residency. One of their complaints about their clinics was that they had too many patients to see; they always felt rushed and harried. When I questioned the faculty as to the rationale for the number of patients residents were required to see, they replied that residents needed to learn how to see patients quickly and efficiently now for them to earn a decent living after residency. After continued questioning of other medical educators, I identified another and perhaps more important reason for the number of patients in the residents' clinics: The outpatient facility needed the income from these visits.

In addition to showing the value of continued questioning, the example just given illustrates how it is impossible to interpret sufficiently the significance of a singular event without reference to the larger context within or on which the event took place. I moved back and forth between foreground (the residents' dissatisfaction) and background (the economics of the clinic and hospital). Again, this circular, back-and-forth movement is central to a hermeneutic approach to analyzing research data.

Revisiting the Problem

From my thorough immersion and analysis, I constantly returned to the problem at hand: how individuals became family physicians. I wanted to make sure the account addressed this question directly and did not wander off on interesting and important points that were not quite relevant to my specific question.

Refining and Representing the Account

As I began to fill in the gaps, inconsistencies, and mistaken under-standings of the developing account, my diagrams changed, looking less indigestive and otherworldly, more digested and cohesive. I grew more confident of the account and began to write it up as a narrative whole. Even at this stage, I saw aspects of the account that did not quite hang together. I had to go back and reinterview and reobserve to fill in missing connections or sections that were unworkable. Knowing what was missing would probably not have been possible without careful, rigorous, reflective analysis of what fit and made sense as well as what did not fit nor make sense. Interpretation continued well beyond the coding and cutting and pasting phase.

The Account Itself: Surviving the Residency

The focus of this chapter is the process of interpretation using an editing style, so I will provide only a brief summary of the account. A more detailed narrative can be found elsewhere (Addison, 1984; Addison, 1989b).

In studying how individuals became family physicians, I found "*surviving*" to be the unifying theme of their everyday practices. As they began the residency, they were confronted by certain immediate issues (work and information overload, time pressures, sleep deprivation, inexperience, responsibility, control, and dying patients). They encountered different groups of people (other residents, nurses, receptionists, faculty, attending physicians, and significant others) whom the residents sometimes found helpful and sometimes found to be sources of abuse. In response, residents adopted certain strategies for dealing with these stressful issues and inter-actions. Strategies ranged on a continuum from *helping* to *isolating* and included *learning the ropes, forming teams, covering, punting, dumping,* and *pimping*. These encounters took place against a background of conflicts and contradictions in the fabric of the residency.

These contradictions occurred in two arenas. I called the first arena *spheres of existence*. It consisted of three spheres: *work, education,* and *life outside of residency*. As residency progressed, the purpose and balance of the spheres changed radically. Work became all-encompassing, education became defined as doing procedures, and life outside became negligible.

I labeled the other arena of conflict and contradiction *models of medicine*. Although residents entered the residency hoping to learn family medicine, they soon found themselves torn among the medicine practiced and taught by specialists and subspecialists in the life-and-death atmosphere of the hospital, the medicine practiced and taught by general practitioners in the harried atmosphere of the clinic, and the medicine taught by behavioral scientists at irregular intervals. They found no family medicine role models, especially in the hospital where they spent most of their time. Their ideals and their everyday practices were in conflict.

At times they found themselves *Covering-Over* these conflicts and contradictions; at times they found themselves *Over-Reflecting*. When they became buried in the covering over mode, they barreled through their work, forgot their ideals, and lost sight of their own place in the process of becoming a family physician. When they became paralyzed in the overreflecting mode, they became overwhelmed, had difficulty becoming involved in learning family medicine, and thought of quitting. Residents bounced back and forth between these two extremes in a jarring fashion without seeing what was happening to them. They defined the whole of their existence by the mode they found themselves in. What was missing was the opportunity to perceive the larger picture of this movement, to reflect on the disparity and contradiction between their ideals and their everyday practices, to learn to move more flexibly between covering over and over-reflecting, and eventually to begin to integrate these two disparate modes into one workable mode of being a family physician (Addison, 1989a).

The Hermeneutic and
Narrative Character of the Account

The product of my analysis is a comprehensive hermeneutic and narrative account grounded in the everyday practices of the residents. I do not believe that the account corresponds with, represents, or reconstructs "reality." Rather, I generated an interpretive account that looks at a crucial period in the process of becoming a physician; provides an interpretation of how distress developed and was maintained; describes the conditions, context, and problematic atmosphere of the process; discusses the costs and significance of the process for residents, their families, and health care; and suggests directions for improving physician training. The account can and should be modified as time, social conditions, and individuals change.

CONCLUSION

Grounded hermeneutic research that includes a thorough and rigorous editing style for organizing data is an extremely well-developed and powerful approach to meaningful, difficult, and complex human research questions. It addresses practical concerns of the researcher and research participants. It aims to describe and uncover significant background conditions, understandings, and practices that contribute to the problem at hand. It takes into account the values, attitudes, beliefs, and practices of the researcher. It can produce a cohesive, interpretive account of research participants' everyday practices. Such an account can open up new possibilities of self-reflection and action for the participants. It is my hope that this chapter will encourage researchers to recognize its value for addressing primary care research questions.

NOTE

1. Readers who are familiar with this tradition should feel free to skip to the step-by-step description of the research itself.

9

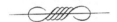

Using Codes and Code Manuals

A Template Organizing Style of Interpretation

Benjamin F. Crabtree
William L. Miller

Qualitative research often results in large volumes of textual material that must be analyzed and interpreted using one or more organizing styles, as discussed in the overview in Chapter 7. Text data may include field notes from participant observation (Chapter 3) and key informant interviews (Chapter 4), transcripts from depth interviews (Chapter 5) and focus group interviews (Chapter 6), and stories and narratives (Chapter 12). Often the researcher is confronted with combinations of these types of data, particularly in case study research, as in Chapters 14 and 16, and in ethnography. In this chapter, the process of using a template in the form of *codes* from a *code manual* is described as a means of organizing text as part of the larger interpretive process. This style is illustrated by contrasting three research investigations of primary care preventive services delivery that used participant observation field notes and/or interview transcripts (Crabtree, Miller, et al., 1998; McVea et al., 1996; Willms, Best, et al., 1990).

The chapter begins with some considerations for selecting an organizing style or combination of organizing styles when constructing an interpretive design. This section emphasizes a comparison of the template organizing style and the editing organizing style discussed in Chapter 8. The chapter then moves into an overview of some of the important mechanics of constructing codes and code manuals and approaches for coding, sorting, and connecting segments of text. With some of these important features highlighted, the chapter then presents three published studies, each of which uses a template organizing style in different ways in the overall interpretive process.

THE USE OF CODES IN TEMPLATE
AND EDITING STYLES

Just as the researcher must construct an overall research design, it is also necessary to develop an analytic strategy within the interpretive process. The analysis process remains fluid in the same way that sampling/collecting evolves so that multiple organizing styles may be used in the overall analysis. Constructing a particular analytic process depends on a number of factors, ranging from the goals of the analysis and the stage of the research to the background and comfort of the researcher with a particular style. For example, researchers wishing to confirm an already well-defined hypothesis, test a theory, or explore a limited facet of the data may construct an analysis process that begins with more structure, such as that provided by a template organizing style that uses code manuals. This might later be followed by an immersion/crystallization of retrieved coded segments. On the other hand, if the researcher is faced with an initial exploratory task, he or she may elect to begin with an immersion/crystallization organizing style. Some researchers may be more familiar with or comfortable with a particular tradition, for example grounded theory, and may elect to use editing as the primary organizing style in their analytic design.

The use of a template or code manual may be more focused and time efficient than the other organizing styles. In all three organizing styles, it is necessary to read all the text; however, with the template organizing style, the interpreter is able to focus on particular aspects of the text and, generally, does not delve into the tedious effort of intense line-by-line scrutiny called for in the editing style or into the time-consuming prolonged immersion necessary for immersion/crystallization (I/C) until after coded segments have been identified and sorted. Admittedly, this can make it more difficult to discover new, unanticipated insights. The template process reduces the amount of data being considered at any one time and brings together related pieces of text earlier in the process, which can facilitate making connections.

The template organizing style described in this chapter differs from an editing style (Chapter 8) primarily in the explicit use of "codes" as the starting point of the process. When using a template, the researcher defines a template or codes and applies these to the data before proceeding to the connecting and corroborating/legitimating phases of the analysis process. The template or codes can be constructed a priori, based on prior research or theoretical perspectives or created on preliminary scanning of the text (Miles & Huberman, 1994). Researchers using an editing style, on the other hand, generally begin more directly with the text, make observations during a systematic reading of the text, and then organize these observations into categories, or *codes,* which are then re-read for further interpretation, as illustrated by Addison in Chapter 8 (also see Glaser & Strauss, 1967; McCracken, 1988; Strauss & Corbin, 1990). For comparison, the editing and template styles are schematically presented in Figure 1.5 of Chapter 1. Note that, in the editing style, the researcher makes interpretations (observations) of segments of text, and these interpretations are then used to make further abstractions; the researcher using a template style identifies segments of original text that are sorted and used to make further abstractions (note where the recursive arrows occur in each).

EXAMPLES OF TEMPLATE
ORGANIZING STYLE

Perhaps the most widely used template has been the *Outline of Cultural Materials* (Murdock et al., 1950), which guided the work of anthropologists for many years. This categorization scheme guided ethnographers into minute details of cultures being studied, including details of postmarriage residence patterns, inheritance, birthing practices, healing techniques, and food-gathering strategies. The codes from the *Outline of Cultural Materials* are readily apparent in many ethnographic accounts and facilitated the collection of apparently comparative data. Contemporary ethnographers have raised serious concerns about this "reductionistic" approach and view use of this outline as "ethnography in a form disembodied from that of lived social world in which actors still exist" (Vidich & Lyman, 1994).

A less apparent template is the sociolinguistic approach described by Spradley (1979) in *The Ethnographic Interview,* in which the analyst applies semantic criteria to interviews in the search for domains and relationships. The goal of the analysis is to create taxonomies of cultural themes and domains such as drinking at a street corner or seeing a patient. The researcher looks at the text (field notes or interview transcripts) for key terms and, using a funnel approach, slowly narrows it down as close as possible to what the "natives" actually mean and intend (Cicourel, 1964).

Other major proponents of a template organizing style have come from educational research, particularly in the work of Miles and Huberman (1984, 1994). Much of the focus is on reducing the data through a coding process so that they can be displayed in an explicit form for interpretation. Miles and Huberman (1994) are very clear about their belief "that social phenomena exist not only in the mind but also in the objective world—and that some lawful and reasonably stable relationships are to be found among them" (p. 4). They are concerned about transcending the historical, social, and meaning-making processes that lie at the center of knowledge and phenomenological experience. Their aim is to construct (with care) explanations that can account for the processes in plausible ways (Huberman & Miles, 1998). Therefore, they emphasize explanatory structure and careful, deliberate, and explicit description.

THE MECHANICS OF A
TEMPLATE ORGANIZING STYLE

The template organizing style involves coding a large volume of text so that segments about an identified topic (the codes) can be assembled in one place to complete the interpretive process. Once similar segments are assembled, there are several strategies for making further interpretation and ultimately representing the account. The template organizing style, as part of the larger interpretive process, consists of a series of steps that begin once the field notes, transcribed interviews, or other form of qualitative data become available, often in the form of text in a text analysis software program or in a word processor printout (refer to Chapters 3 through 6). The template organizing style immerses the researcher in the often massive and confusing jungle of text, with the set purpose of identifying "chunks" of text so as to facilitate future data retrieval and analysis. The complete analysis process of organizing, connecting, and corroborating/legitimizing involves (a) creating a code manual or coding scheme, (b) hand or computer coding the text, (c) sorting segments to get all similar text in one place, and (d) reading the segments and making the connections that are subsequently corroborated and legitimized. The interpretive process is then completed with telling the story or representing the account.

There are a number of descriptions of the process of developing and applying codes and code manuals to text data. Tesch (1990) provides some guidance in constructing codes and overviews several software options that, unfortunately, have now become largely outdated. The workbook originating from educational research published by Miles and Huberman

(1984, 1994) is probably the most complete description. The workbook is somewhat limited for health care researchers because the examples come from an educational context that does not readily transfer to health care settings, and the workbook does not effectively integrate the template organizing style with other styles. Dey (1993) provides several chapters on creating and applying categories and on connecting processes that are quite helpful. Other sources include the manual for THE ETHNOGRAPH® software program (Seidel, Kjolseth, & Seymour, 1988), which provides a useful description from the anthropology and sociology traditions; a chapter by Bee and Crabtree (1992), who describe an application of coding with THE ETHNOGRAPH; and a brief summary by Altheide (1987) of an approach he refers to as "ethnographic content analysis."

Approaches for Developing a Code Manual

There are several approaches one can use to create a code manual or coding scheme to serve as a template for organizing the data. On one hand, the researcher or research team can rely on predefined or a priori codes, generally based on understandings from prior research or theoretical considerations. On the other hand, the researchers can develop codes only after some initial exploration of the data has taken place, using an immersion/crystallization or editing organizing style. A common, intermediate approach is when some initial codes are refined and modified during the analysis process. The approach often reveals the paradigmatic assumptions of the researcher, with those feeling more positivist pressures being more comfortable using a structured approach, and constructivists and critical ecologists leaning toward cocreated codes.

The code manual is a data management tool; it is used to organize segments of similar or related text for ease in interpretation and to search for confirming/disconfirming evidence of these interpretations. Before beginning, the researcher must decide on the level of detail to be coded, the decision generally related to the type of data (e.g., field notes versus interviews), the goal of the research (e.g., exploration versus description), and the level of previous understanding. How detailed the code manual becomes is often a function of where the researcher is in the research process. For example, preliminary studies may require a much broader net to catch alternate explanations than a study designed to enlighten several specific hypotheses emerging from earlier research. It is important to note that in constructing a code manual, the researcher is always walking a fine line between premature closure and creating codes so encompassing that every line of text requires coding. The advantage of using broad categories is that large amounts of text can be rapidly coded and that coded segments are longer, with broader context preserved, allowing the researchers to access more text for interpretation with a given search. The disadvantages are almost the same. There are many coded segments of peripheral use that would not have been captured with more specific codes. Some coded segments are very long, making reading tedious, and a given segment may contain multiple ideas, which makes later sorting more difficult.

A preliminary code manual is often based on an initial conceptual model and/or a literature review. Sometimes it is not necessary to make significant changes to this initial a priori code manual, as in the first example used later in this chapter (McVea et al., 1996), which was only slightly expanded based on initial readings of the text. Miles and Huberman (1984, 1994) offer some useful suggestions for the development of a code manual, including having individual members of the research team independently coding a number of pages of text to test for both intercoder reliability and the utility and appropriateness of the codes. The code manual can then be modified to correct for deficiencies. This is the approach that is used in the second example in this chapter (Willms, Allan, et al., 1991). Miles and Huberman (1984, 1994) have suggested test coding a number of pages of text and modifying the code manual accordingly, making it possible for many codes to originate from interpretive observations.

Coding Text

Once a code manual has been prepared, there are different approaches for using it. Before the advent of computers and text analysis software programs, text was hand coded, cut from the original, and then often pasted onto 3" × 5" index cards. This is the approach used by Addison in Chapter 8 as part of the editing organizing style. It is important to keep in mind that the codes can and usually should be flexible and open. There are times when the analyst will want to split codes and further refine them, and there will be other times when the investigative team will want to splice certain codes together. Dey (1993) describes a process of "splitting" and "splicing" the text in categories in which the investigator looks for subcategories in similar sorted segments. This is similar to the hierarchical approaches used by Richards and others who use the computer software NUD*IST® (see Chapter 11). This and other computer software programs now make the sorting, cutting, and pasting operations more efficient, although it is still necessary to "mouse code."

Computer coding of text entails telling the software program where each segment begins and ends. This is generally "mouse work" and can be done directly on the screen; however, many will find long hours looking at a computer screen to be very tedious and more likely to cause eye strain and/or headaches. Thus many researchers advise initial hand coding of a hard copy (printed version) with a pencil or highlighter (Bee & Crabtree,

1992; Miles & Huberman, 1984, 1994; Seidel, Kjolseth, & Seymour, 1988; Tesch, 1990). Code manual in hand, segments are then marked in the margins or highlighted with markers. Further details on the use of computers for coding, sorting, and retrieving text can be found in Chapter 11.

Another simple, but elegant, approach is to use different color highlighter pens on printed text. This works particularly well when there are relatively few codes in the code manual. This was used in a study of case managers conducted by Wetle and colleagues (Clemens, Wetle, Feltes, Crabtree, & Dubitzky, 1994; Feltes, Clemens, Wetle, & Crabtree, 1994). In this analysis of depth interviews of case managers, the researchers developed a simple code manual from the text in which pink indicated ethical concerns, green meant a client type, orange represented a communication among providers issue, and blue marked a case manager management strategy. After marking the printed version of the transcript, the investigators used multiple copies of the computer text and deleted everything except the text for a particular highlighter color. Thus, for each transcript there were four files, each with only those segments pertaining to a particular code.

Sorting Segments

With the template organizing style, sorting segments is a relatively simple process of having the computer software search for and print selected coded segments. It should be noted that there will be some variation in what text is retrieved depending on the software program (see Weitzman & Miles, 1995; also Chapter 11). The first two examples in this chapter both use computers to sort and print segments. When using an editing organizing style, on the other hand, the process is more like a pile sort of cards in which the stacks of cards themselves become the codes (see Chapter 8).

Another approach performed by some researchers uses counts of codes as a sorting approach that is very similar to quantitative or basic content analysis (Morgan, 1993). The researcher codes the text and then counts the frequency of different code occurrences as a means of identifying key areas that form the basis of the analysis. Codes with a larger number of segments become the focus of the analysis and are used to make connections. Examples of this approach to sorting segments in the health care literature are seen in the focus group work of David Morgan (Morgan, 1993).

Connecting and Corroborating/Legitimating

After each phase of organizing or reorganizing the data, the task switches to connecting and corroborating/legitimating. Having the data categorized into empirically based and meaningful segments through the use of templates can greatly facilitate both of these analysis phases. Two approaches to connecting are commonly used: *chunking* and *displaying*. *Chunking* refers to examining chunks of related texts together. Chunks are segments of text that are several paragraphs or pages in length. Initial or later use of a template will sometimes identify large chunks of similarly coded text. An immersion/crystallization organizing style can then be used to identify themes within those text chunks or even to develop vignettes or chunk summaries. These can then be used to search for further connections, patterns, and other associations. As part of a research team, several members can analyze the same chunks and their summaries or findings, then compare and contrast them in a group meeting. This process can help prevent both over- and underinterpretation and should be reported in the final account, noting any interrater reliability and/or whether there was a consensus process.

Displaying data is another powerful means for discovering connections. Maps and matrices are the basic tools of this approach. Both maps or diagrams and matrices facilitate seeing different coded segments of text next to each other. Miles and Huberman (1994) present, in great and helpful detail, a cornucopia of possible *matrices* that can be created from textual data based on sorted codes. Tesch (1990) refers to this type of connecting as "recontextualization." The matrix displays can be ordered or arranged by cases and/or by categories such as time, social roles, or concepts. Examples of concepts include attitudes about health prevention or barriers to providing immunizations. Matrices can also be based on relationships between categories, thus providing an easy way to explore possible links and/or associations between code-sorted segments of data. Examples of such links include x explains y, x is part of y, x shares part of y, x supports y, x frustrates y, and so on (Spradley, 1979). Another helpful connecting strategy is to create a context chart, which is a hybrid of mapping and matrices. All the components and known relationships between them for any given context, such as an office waiting room, are listed and/or drawn. This enables the researcher to see what is missing or what other connections may exist or have been overlooked.

Maps are another basic tool for displaying template sorted text (Dey, 1993; Mason, 1996). Different shapes can represent different categories, with the size of the shapes indicating frequency of presence in the text or scope. Lines with arrows can point in the direction of a relationship between categories, with the thickness of the line showing the strength of the relationship and the length of the line indicating the intimacy or distance of the relationship. A plus or minus sign above or below the line can refer to the value of the relationship. Space on the map can represent time. Some computer software programs, such as NUD*IST (Chapter 11), are now able to greatly facilitate this type of mapping once the text is coded. There is still value, however, in hands-on scissors, note card, and tape techniques of mapping. Addison (Chapter 8) created a wall-size display of his emerging interpretation using such methods.

The template organizing style also aids the corroborating/legitimating phase of analysis. *Fabricating evidence* is a surprisingly common problem in the process of interpretation (Dey, 1993). The issue is not so much intentional creation of false data as the unintentional, usually unconscious "seeing" of data that we expect to be there, even though it's not. The use of a research team certainly helps keep everyone honest. But also helpful is keeping a clear and evident trail of analysis and interpretation, an audit trail that can be reviewed by an outside auditor and by the team itself as a means of internal replication. Use of templates greatly facilitates this process. *Discounting evidence* is another source of error. One means of overcoming this is to intentionally analyze the gaps, the uncoded text, for exceptions or possible new interpretations. *Misinterpreting evidence* is a third source of error, which is partly reduced through member checking: having the research participants review the interpretations. This process is often easier if the participants can see the way coded segments were connected. They may sometimes reveal different ways through the maze of possible connections.

TEMPLATE ORGANIZING
STYLE IN ACTION

To illustrate the use of the template organizing style, we look at three studies that took different approaches to integrating the template organizing style into the interpretive process. The "Put Prevention Into Practice" evaluation study published by McVea and colleagues (1996) at the University of Nebraska began organizing observational field notes with an a priori set of codes that had emerged from the literature and from other research being conducted by the research team. At the same time, depth interview transcripts were analyzed with an editing organizing style. An immersion/crystallization organizing style was subsequently used to further organize the emerging categories and to make connections. In contrast, the study by Willms and colleagues (Willms, Best, et al., 1990; Willms, Allan, et al., 1991) from McMaster University began with an immersion/crystallization organizing style that was used to identify codes, which were then used to code the text. In a third study, Crabtree, Miller, and colleagues (1998) used an immersion/crystallization organizing style as the primary style in the analytic process and only developed the coding as a corroborating step to confirm or disconfirm the connections discovered in the initial analysis.

The "Put Prevention Into Practice" (PPIP) Evaluation Study

In 1993, the American Academy of Family Physicians (AAFP) took the responsibility for marketing and distributing a new and innovative office system designed to increase the delivery of preventive services among their membership. It was hoped that this system, the "Put Prevention Into Practice" (PPIP) program, would substantially change practice patterns. Researchers from the University of Nebraska Medical Center contracted with the AAFP to evaluate the effectiveness of the materials in "real world practices." The long-term goal of the study was to understand how office organizations change so that new innovations are more effectively introduced to family practices. This research goal asks for description, meaning, and an answer to the generic questions, "Who are these people and what are they doing?"

To address the research goal, a comparative case study design was used to discover the extent to which the new office system was adopted by family physicians and why the adoption did or did not take place. The study used a combination of participant observation, depth interviews, and chart audits collected at eight purposefully selected community-based family physician practices that had purchased the materials. A second-year medical student spent several days at each practice actively participating in the activities of the office by following the physicians during patient encounters and informally talking with staff. Observation field notes were dictated each evening by the field worker and later transcribed. An audiotaped individual depth interview was conducted with the practicing physician who purchased the PPIP materials, and this was also transcribed. Charts of a sample of patients from each practice were abstracted to determine levels of preventive service delivery, with the data entered for statistical analysis into SPSS.

The interpretive process involved the simultaneous analysis of each of the three types of data—field notes, interviews, and chart abstractions—followed by a final analytic process to connect the preliminary themes from the initial analysis. Three teams with overlapping membership were initially charged with separate analytic processes.

The team working with the observational field notes was given the task of looking for aspects of the office operations, level of office organization, existing office systems, relationships among practice participants, and use of PPIP materials. Each member was given a particular area to code, and a highlighter was set up in Folio Views® for coding each (see Chapter 11 for description of Folio Views). For example, all text about office operations, such as approaches for charting, patient scheduling, and other office systems related to preventive services delivery, was coded blue. Similarly, text about the use of PPIP was coded in lavender. This included text about barriers to PPIP, opportunities for PPIP, the physician's role in PPIP, and the staff's role in PPIP. Once the text had been coded, Folio Views was used to search for and print each of the segments. For example, a segment of text about office operations included the following:

> Jane is working on the phones today. She has a stack of charts in front of her and several loose sheets of paper. She starts to sort through the papers. She appears to be prioritizing the sheets of paper. She picks up the phone and calls the first person. She is telling this mother that she will consult with the doctor and get back with her about the treatment. She continues to call the people on the list. (Original field notes)

There are many such segments in each of the broad codes. Once printed, the coded segments or chunks went through another analytic process using an immersion/crystallization organizing style. Segments were read thoroughly and discussed in detail until the group was able to "crystallize" key concepts or themes from the field notes from each practice. This is an example of using chunking as a means of connecting. Key concepts included such things as "the practice places its emphasis on acute care visits, and prevention is only addressed during scheduled health maintenance visits," or "this practice has developed its own systems and that PPIP does not offer any advantages to its existing systems."

The team working with the depth interviews followed an editing organizing style much like that presented by Addison in Chapter 8. This organizing style was deemed desirable because it allowed an open exploration of the perceptions of the physicians who purchased the PPIP materials. Individual team members read each transcript, highlighted text they felt was relevant, and made interpretive notations or observations in the margins. The team members then discussed each interview in detail to identify salient themes. Themes identified for individual physicians in this analysis cycle included "the physician defines prevention in terms of screening tests and does not see his role as a prevention counselor" and "the physician wants to learn and knows he needs help, but doesn't know how to change."

The team working with the chart audit data had a relatively easy analytic process that consisted primarily of providing summary statistics of preventive services for each practice. This included "hit rates" for screening tests (cholesterol and women eligible for mammograms), immunization (tetanus), and counseling (smoking cessation). These were put in tabular form for each practice and provided to the larger research team for consideration in the next iteration of the analysis.

Once the three initial analyses were completed, the research team initiated a second stage with an immersion/crystallization organizing style guiding the analysis process. The investigators had access to the organizing categories from the initial analysis cycle described above, as well as the full range of primary data. In a series of group meetings, the research team systematically considered all the data and identified several overall themes that were presented by McVea et al. (1996). A key finding was the discovery of the role that organization and disorganization play in a practice's ability to initiate change. This interpretive process also identified the concept of the "bee in the bonnet" that has become a prominent feature of subsequent work (Crabtree, Miller, et al., 1998; Miller et al., 1998).

Patients' Perspectives of a Physician-Delivered Smoking Cessation Intervention

Smoking cessation efforts by family physicians received a major boost in the late 1980s with the development of nicotine replacement in gum form. Nevertheless, it was not clear which ingredients of an effective clinical prevention program were most effective and how patients perceived these interventions. Dennis Willms and his colleagues at McMaster University were offered the opportunity to conduct an ethnographic research project as a side study to a large clinical trial called the Family Practice Smoking Cessation Project (Wilson et al., 1988) to investigate specific features of a smoking cessation intervention that were effective from a patient's perspective. The primary data were a series of interviews with individual participants in the clinical trial and field notes recorded by the interviewer immediately after the interview. Two interviews were scheduled to occur before the participant's quit date and then once a week for the 4 weeks after the quit date. Follow-up interviews were scheduled monthly for the following 6 months, with a final interview after 1 year.

The interpretive process for the whole project included four stages; that is, the data were subjected to four different analysis cycles (Willms, Allan, et al., 1991; Willms, Best, et al., 1990; Willms & Stebbins, 1991). The first stage was the iterative process, which occurred as the data were collected and the interviewer had a chance to reflect between interviews. This immersion/ crystallization process was used primarily to ensure completeness of the data. Once the data were completed, three separate analysis processes were used to subject the data to different interpretive perspectives.

One of the analysis cycles used a template organizing style to understand issues and themes that seem to apply to a patient's experience with smoking cessation. Using a group process and an initial immersion/crystallization of the data, the research team constructed a list of themes, issues, and actions that were felt to be relevant to both the smoking experience and the cessation process (Willms, Best, et al., 1990). The researchers designed their own computerized software program, called Ethnographic Theme Search (this was long before existing excellent programs were available), and coded the entire data set with blinded coders. The code manual was very complex and included more than 100 separate codes (see Willms, Best, et al., 1990, for the complete code manual and details of the analysis process). In one analysis, the investigators focused on all the segments retrieved that pertained to the participant's perception of the doctor (Willms, Allan, et al., 1991). Further analysis of these coded segments, using an immersion/crystallization style, suggested that the most significant component of the physicians' intervention was the kind of support given. It was noted that although patients expect a certain amount of biomedicine, successful interventions needed a personalistic component to be successful.

Further interpretation of these data were performed with an immersion/crystallization organizing style in which case studies or life histories of individual participants were constructed and interpreted (Willms & Stebbins, 1991). The objective of this analysis was to understand the social and cultural context of the individual, including the uniqueness of the individual's experience and the authenticity of his or her story. By reviewing the case histories of participants, while still reflecting on the original data, the investigators discovered that the decision to quit smoking was predicated on more than the single issue of whether or not to smoke. Smoking was part of a particular way of living, and giving up smoking symbolized a new stage of life. The author discusses the implication of this symbolic use of cigarettes on smoking cessation efforts.

The Direct Observation of Primary Care (DOPC) Study

The Direct Observation of Primary Care (DOPC) study was designed as a large descriptive study of the patient care process of family physicians, with a particular focus on preventive service delivery. Much of the data collection centered around obtaining detailed quantitative data about the clinical encounters using the Davis Observation Code (DOC) (Callahan & Bertakis, 1991) and structured patient questionnaires. Research nurses spent a total of 4 days with each physician observing patient encounters and conducting chart audits. As part of this larger descriptive study, the research nurses were asked to dictate their subjective impressions of the physician and the office at the end of each day. These data were initially very impressionistic and focused on describing the practice in terms of key features such as location, office relationships, physical layout, prevention activity/materials, physician characteristics, and how the practice worked.

In the study design, these data were primarily intended to serve as a context for the more comprehensive quantitative data, but after an initial immersion/crystallization of preliminary field notes, the research nurses were trained to record more detailed and systematic observations. Over the course of 2 years, the research nurses spent 4 days of observation with each of 135 family physicians in 84 practices in northeast Ohio. Stange, Zyzanski, Jaen, et al. (1998) provide an overview of the methods for the complete study.

Once the dictated field notes were transcribed, they were imported into Folo Views for further analysis. The 4 days of contact time with each physician provided brief descriptive "snapshots" of physicians and their practices at different points in time that eventually totaled more than 1,000 pages of text. The analysis was initially done using an immersion/crystallization organizing style in which one member of the research team completed an independent analysis of the data. After reading all the data and identifying important categories, written case summaries were constructed on a purposeful sample of 18 practices selected to maximize variation in terms of practice size (solo versus group), physician gender, and practice location. All three members of the interpretation team then independently reviewed the case summaries and developed preliminary interpretations, which included important features, processes, and relationships in the practices. These were then used to construct a code manual for subsequent analysis using a template organizing style to cross check against the original data. The researchers used a purposeful sample of original field notes from the remaining practices for coding in a process designed to search for disconfirming evidence and to refine the interpretations.

This interpretive process led to two publications in a special issue of the *Journal of Family Practice*. Crabtree, Miller, et al. (1998) found that primary care practice is much more complex than research and transformation efforts generally acknowledge. The data suggest that efforts to alter practice behavior need to account for a diverse set of factors, including cognitive and behavioral components of physician philosophy and style; technical aspects of how individual physicians integrate clinical models of care and supplementary tools into patient care; and features of the practice organization such as office efficiency, clarity of staff roles, communication patterns among physicians and/or staff, and approaches to using office protocols. Miller, Crabtree, et al. (1998) expanded on this by seeing that primary care practices are best understood as complex adaptive systems and that the particular shape of each practice is determined by attractors, which can include income goals, practice vision, "bee in the bonnet" for particular aspects of practice, and patient/community expectations. This model suggests new strategies for promoting change at both the practice and practitioner level.

DISCUSSION

The template organizing style has several advantages that make it an attractive approach in the interpretive process. Making the code manual and coding the text is relatively quick, reproducible, and easy to grasp for those skeptical of qualitative research. On the down side, when used alone, there is a potential for missing information, especially if the code manual is produced in a completely a priori manner. The interpreter also runs the danger of not looking beyond the codes. These concerns can be overcome by using multiple organizing styles in different cycles through the iterative processes of analysis and interpretation.

The interpretation of a mountain of information-rich, purposefully sampled, qualitative texts can easily appear insurmountable and quixotic, especially to researchers proficient in quantitative methods. This is reason enough to pause and briefly tremble. However, the template organizing style described in this chapter is one specific way for quantitatively trained primary care researchers to take the first step into qualitative analysis.

10

Immersion/Crystallization

Jeffrey Borkan

Once a great master sat on a hill and listened to the birds
and the wind singing around her. She drank in her
surroundings, immersed herself in the setting, took careful
notes, and after a time, insights began to crystallize out as
dew drops, brilliant and translucent. With her new wisdom,
she returned to her village and spoke great wisdom.

So now you have the data—what do you do with it? This chapter
examines an organizing style within the qualitative interpretive process
that has the potential to be widely applicable, emotionally and intellectually
stimulating, and highly productive. Immersion/crystallization (I/C) consists
of cycles whereby the analyst immerses him- or herself into and experiences

AUTHOR'S NOTE: I would like to acknowledge the incisive contribution to this endeavor
made by my scholarly informants, all veteran qualitative researchers, who were able to
articulate the secrets of their craft: Professor Anne E. Becker, Department of Psychiatry and
Department of Social Medicine, Harvard Medical School; Professor Benjamin Crabtree,
Department of Family Medicine, University of Nebraska Medical Center, Omaha; Professor
Arthur Kleinman, Chairman, Department of Social Medicine, Harvard Medical School;
Professor Howard Stein, Department of Family and Preventive Medicine, University of
Oklahoma Health Sciences Center, Oklahoma City and Enid; Professor Carol L. McWilliam,
Centre for Studies in Family Medicine, University of Western Ontario, London, Ontario,
Canada; Professor William L. Miller, Vice-Chair and Program Director, Department of Family
Medicine, Lehigh Valley Hospital, Allentown, Pennsylvania; Professor Norma Ware, Department
of Social Medicine, Harvard Medical School.

the text, emerging after concerned reflection with intuitive crystallizations, until reportable interpretations are reached (Miller & Crabtree, 1992, 1994a, 1994b). Although the term was initially coined by Miller and Crabtree (1992) as one of the four idealized analytic styles, it is solidly in the mainstream of qualitative research and is congruent with multiple other analytical techniques—those with names such as *heuristic* (Moustakas, 1990), *hermeneutic* (Addison, 1992; Bleicher, 1980), *phenomenologic,* and those without proper titles. Similar methods may be found throughout the humanistic and social sciences, from communication to education and evaluation. Much of anthropological writing is based on this type of analysis; however, the masters of this discipline rarely detail the intricacies of their methodology. Rather, it is left in the realm of the unspoken, the secrets of the craft.

This chapter attempts to elucidate the topic and make it accessible to researchers from a range of disciplines. After reading this material, the investigator should be able to differentiate it from the other organizing styles (editing and template) and be able to consider using it in his or her own research endeavors. For a further discussion comparing styles, refer back to Chapter 7.

When I was considering how to frame this subject, the difficulty of describing the I/C process became apparent. Immersion/crystallization cannot be reduced to a cookbook formula. Its successful execution may be more akin to artistic expression. Just as making a painting is more than applying brush to canvas, I/C is a process that cannot be easily explicated. To assist with this task, I enlisted several veteran "masters of the art" to share the secrets of their I/C or I/C-like analytic skills. These key informants included Anne E. Becker, Benjamin Crabtree, Arthur Kleinman, Carol McWilliam, William Miller, Howard Stein, and Norma Ware (see acknowledgments). Throughout this chapter, I draw frequently from the informal interviews I had with them.

Where does I/C fit into the qualitative research cycle? Like other organizing styles, it provides a means to move from the research question, the generated text and/or field experience, and the raw field data to the interpretations reported in the write-up. However, I/C, unlike other more formally schematic methods such as the template style or perhaps some computer-assisted management strategies, is more intuitive, more engaged, more fluid during all research stages, from conceptualization to data collection to write-up. This method also uses more of the researcher, often requiring cognitive and emotional engagement of the self to get beyond the obvious interpretations to hear, see, and feel the data. This conceptualization is consistent with the definition of data analysis as linked subprocesses of data reduction, display, conclusion drawing, and verification that "occur *before* data collection, *during* study design and planning; *during* data collection as interim and early analyses are carried out; and *after* data collection as final products are approached and completed" (Huberman & Miles, 1994, p. 429, italics in original).

The Requirements

What is needed to undertake immersion/crystallization? The critical tool is not the fastest computer or the newest qualitative research software; rather, it is the *self*, particularly an openness to *uncertainty, reflection,* and *experience.* The Greek philosopher-scientist Archimedes may have been the first and ultimate adherent to this technique. While taking a bath, he was suddenly struck by the concept of buoyancy. More recently, in a personal communication, Will Miller noted: "Essentially the analysis is to immerse yourself in the data. . . . If you are analyzing an interview text, become alive through the text." Howard Stein (1994) mirrors a similar attitude when he encourages researchers to use the self in creative and constructive ways to progress beyond obvious messages and interpretations. This may require processing one's own emotional responses, using one's being as both recorder and filter:

The way I interpret Slovak American steelworkers' life or Oklahoma wheat farming family life is that I look at myself as I look at them—not through some kind of "anthroscope." I let them enter into my imagination. I don't remove myself, I engage myself. We [the researchers] do record raw data, we filter and record through our selves. . . . The only way to understand a person is with your whole self.

The other requisites are fairly straightforward:

- *Data:* well-recorded data from interviews, focus groups, participant observation, texts, or other sources (including existing documents) is required. The format for this information may be written, audiotaped, or videotaped. Arthur Kleinman admonishes the researcher to remember that "Primary knowledge is not just interviews, it is also the researcher's inter-subjective experience with the field from having conceptualized the study and collected the data." I/C most intimately combines your field notes *and* your experience.
- *Personality type congruent with the demands of the method:* This includes an ability to be contemplative, a sense of rigor, and a facility to "listen deeply" (Stein, 1994) to individuals, organizations, and to the data itself.
- *Time and patience:* The insights may not be able to be forced; rather, one must often wait for them to arise. I/C may require some significant time input, either in blocks or longitudinally.
- *Reflexivity:* This is the ability to reflect back on one's role and involvement and how it influences the data and the process of analysis.

- *Process-orientation:* Attention must be paid to each step along the path and to the overall design of the analysis, but getting there is half the fun!
- A *mentor and/or some experience:* This type of analysis may be daunting to the novice, so guides and prior knowledge of the route may be reassuring.

The Nature of the Process

On a conceptual level, what is immersion/crystallization? Although one may view it simply as an organizing style involving repeated delving into and experiencing of the data, leading to the emergence of insights and interpretations, many who experience I/C discover it to be a contemplative and artistic process. It may enlist both right- and left-brain processes, processing information that is both block and sequential over time. Stein referred to the technique using musical metaphors, a process that involves "not just knowing the notes."

[It is] the same way as with music—I hear the music play me and I convey this to the orchestra. There are people with stick technique who come off dead—others do it and you can hardly tell what they do—it's more than having a precise beat.

Ben Crabtree sees I/C as an awareness of patterns and connections:

We do it in every study, it's the real brainwork. Even if we use a fairly structured codebook, we still have to think about the segments of coded text. It's about finding patterns.

Some spiritual and philosophical components may also be present. As Stein describes:

It becomes almost a religious experience. All understanding is revelation . . . there is an opening of yourself to hearing. . . . The process is more important than the way station—the journey is the destination.

THE CORE PROCESS

In describing the core process of immersion/crystallization, one must answer two fundamental questions:

- What are the content and constituent elements?
- When does it begin?

Although best considered an immutable "whole," the nature of the process can be divided into several parts, with multiple points of entry and exit. Relying heavily on prior work by Moustakas (1990), Miller and Crabtree (1992, 1994a), Huberman and Miles (1994), and personal experience, I have outlined the elements as follows. Please note that the process is much more iterative or recursive than linear, more like a multileveled roller-coaster than a staircase.

- Initial engagement with the topic/reflexivity
- Describing
- Crystallization during data collection
- Immersion and illumination of emergent insights from collected data and texts
- Explication and creative synthesis
- Corroboration/legitimation and consideration of alternative interpretations
- Representing the account/reporting

Initial Engagement With the Topic/Reflexivity

Classically, we often think of data analysis starting *after* material has been collected. However, for some, the process starts at the very beginning of the iterative research cycle, *before* the first data have been gathered. When each of us approaches a problem or topic for research, we often begin with various biases and hunches as to what the investigation will yield. As we begin to develop a theme or issue into a researchable question, we draw on our past experience, our reading of the literature (both specific and general), and our past research. This often prolonged process is accompanied by multiple starts and stops, free-floating ideas and advice—both from within ourselves and from friends, family, and colleagues. For example, in a study on low back pain (LBP), the personal, family, and professional biases and experience of the investigators became the backdrop for the investigation (Borkan, Reis, et al., 1995). The research group wanted to study a common medical problem from a patient-centered perspective. After considering several ideas, we chose LBP. The impetus for this decision arose largely out of the frustration of the family physicians in the group with the inadequacy of treatments for this ailment. In addition, one of the researchers had become convinced of the unpredictable nature of LBP after watching his father get off the operating table just minutes before a planned orthopedic surgery, cured forever from his "intractable" LBP.

Moustakas (1990) uses the term *initial engagement* (p. 27) to describe a process of self-dialogue and discovery of an intense and passionate concern that calls out to and engages the researcher: "During the initial engagement the investigator reaches inward for tacit awareness and knowledge, permits intuition to run freely, and elucidates the context from which the question takes form and significance" (p. 27). Rather than relegate such material to the dark recesses of the mind, these bits can be garnered, developed, and duly recorded for later use. The recording of a priori biases has the special advantage of allowing us to consider the influence of our own background on the final results and interpretations. I personally open a file at the beginning of every research project where such insights can be stored for later reflection.

Crystallization During Data Collection

Insights may also crystallize *while* the first data are being collected, assisting with the identification of early patterns. As Norma Ware mentioned, "Some things emerge from the interview process—as you go along and talk to someone, something strikes you, an insight, an epiphany, an *Ah Ha*—the realization." Carol McWilliam has developed a method to encourage and harness the insights that arise during this stage of the research:

> I guess it begins the minute I ask a question and they start answering, I am trying to analyze what are the basic concepts, thoughts, key points that are coming out. I go after whatever really stands out for me—whatever appears to be important. I try to probe more in-depth right then at that time, I immerse myself a bit further.
>
> At the end of the interview it is my practice to try to summarize what I understood from what they [the interviewees] said. . . . I present what stands out, what are the real key points and then get their reaction . . . it is part of the analysis process.
>
> Then I go away and listen to the tape and read my notes and see if that jogs more key messages or thoughts and if it does, I write it down then and there—I try to do this as soon as possible after the interview—the same day. For participant observation—I might even sneak away to write.
>
> Then I go to bed and sleep on it—sometimes I wake up with an idea and jot it down. . . .
>
> Then I go on and do more data collection, put my previous thoughts on the back burner. When I talk to or listen to other people, I try to do it with an open mind. . . . If [previous ideas] come up, then I confirm or disconfirm any parallels.
>
> I go through the same process after every interview—by then I will have a batch of interviews or field notes from participant-observation and I look at the notes as I go along for any links.

A technique for recording such interview insights that has worked for me involves dividing notepaper by thirds, leaving two thirds for the interviewee's or group's words and one third for insights that arise during the data collection process. Meadows and Dodendorf describe this same process using computer software in Chapter 11. In addition, at the end of every interview or focus group, all those present from the research team discuss the new material, both summarizing its content and reflecting on any interpretations (also see Chapter 5). These are used immediately to help focus and improve data collection. Such discussions can be tape-recorded for later transcription, to be reflected on later in the research process. A similar technique can also be done during participant observation (see Chapter 3) or even while conducting quantitative research.

Unlike in experimental designs, changes in observational or interview protocols during a field study are likely to reflect a better understanding of the subject and the setting, thus heightening internal validity (Huberman & Miles, 1994). For example, during recently conducted fieldwork at a family practice residency, I continually updated the focus group moderator's guide and interview topics after reviewing the data collected on previous days. These early "in process" analyses of the material allowed me both to sharpen my focus during subsequent interviews and to recheck the validity of insights with informants.

Immersion and Illumination of Emergent Insights From Collected Data and Texts

Most who do I/C begin by reviewing the data they have *already* collected. Whether or not you use the interviewing phase as an opportunity for early I/C, the critical phase of I/C involves the systematic review of accumulated data, texts, and preliminary analysis notes. This is the stage when the researcher or team commits substantial concentrated time and focused mental energy to reading, rereading, and immersing themselves into the data. Anne Becker describes this need for time:

> I get very immersed in the data and won't do it unless I have several days. The immersion is necessary to get into the mind set and get comfortable with the language—to get into the language and the cadence.

Moustakas (1990) breaks down this stage into two separate processes of *immersion* and *illumination,* whereby insights occur "naturally when the researcher is open and receptive to tacit knowledge and intuition." Once you are ready, you are admonished to live the topic or question in all waking, sleeping, and even dream states. Preparing oneself for this stage by providing the right setting, freedom from outside interference, and an effective method for recording the outcomes may be essential to the process.

Horizontal Versus
Vertical Passes of the Data

When faced with the task of analyzing the mounds of qualitative data researchers are apt to collect, two strategies may be chosen: reviewing all the material from multiple horizontal "passes" or analyzing one section vertically from start to finish and only then moving on to the next. Will Miller describes his procedure for reading notes or transcripts from beginning to end in repeated horizontal passes. In his techniques, the investigator does serial readings of the whole body of text, searching for different types of evidence or perspectives on each pass.

The *first* time I just read [the data] without any preconceptions, I just read it and look at key *themes, emotions,* and *surprises.* "What is it about?" "Who is speaking?" and "What are they trying to say?" "What pops up, what is the overall story?". . . I reflect back on moments where I was surprised, said "Oh Wow." I note the big picture . . . the big themes . . . and where did I notice emotions in myself.

In *second readings,* I specifically read for those themes [I noticed in the first pass], the evidence that supports those themes, that is against those themes, and those places where I was surprised. I am looking to better understand what is going on there during this in-depth reading. I will go back . . . to see what surprised me, what might it be that elicited that emotion—part of the reflexivity to identify what it is in me that triggers what is going on in me that is triggered by the text.

In the *third readings,* I will go back again to see if there is anything else important that I missed—something that didn't refer to themes or surprises that are in the text.

In the *fourth reading,* I force myself to come up with one, two or three alternative understandings. . . . Fourth readings force me to take on other personas—would I have a different perspective if I were another person.

Fifth readings: If I come up with discrepancies [during the fourth readings], are there ways to link them together?

The technique of vertical passes concentrates on one portion of the data or one data type (in instances where there are multiple data sources or collection techniques) with prolonged review and analysis before moving on. Such a technique may be particularly useful when evaluating data produced through different collection techniques, when the enormity of the amassed materials precludes reviewing the total data set at one time, or when using a computer program to sort and print similar text. In addition, vertical review may be efficacious when conducted during data collection. Insights gathered during this stage may be fed back into the data

TABLE 10.1 How to Get Unstuck If the Insights Aren't Coming

Distancing from the material
Altered states of consciousness
 • Meditation
 • Psychoanalytic hovering
 • Sleeping/dreaming
 • Relaxation
Group analysis
Giving the material to others to review
Gathering insights from informants
External stimuli
 • Go to a lecture
 • Go to the literature

collection process, sharpening the focus of the whole research endeavor, as described earlier.

When Do The Insights Arrive?
And How to Get Unstuck if They Are Not Arriving

The process of I/C may appear rather mystical at first—you make the proper preparations, immerse yourself in the data, and wait around for the "wisdom" to crystallize. However, how do you ensure that the insights just keep pouring in and that the process does not become a fruitless and frustrating exercise, a "Waiting for Godot" who never arrives?

In talking to informants, and in personal experience, I find that insights come at various times. This may include while sitting at a desk concentrating on the topic, while taking a break, while engaging in entertainment, while going to a lecture, or even during sleep. The key is being open to them and chronicling appropriately. As Norma Ware mentioned, "It might hit me while running or driving home from the interview—I will try to record them [as soon as possible] even on the Dictaphone while driving."

My informants often noted that although it is possible to set the stage for insights to crystallize, the results cannot be coerced. As McWilliam notes, "It does not come to me by forcing it—if I force it I don't get much more." Moustakas (1990) gives the examples of remembering where a misplaced house key is or recalling a forgotten name—although they evade the seeker who is totally preoccupied with finding them, as soon as his or her consciousness is absorbed in something else, the key is found and the memory reappears.

As with finding the lost key or forgotten name, there are multiple techniques and tricks for enhancing the success of the process (see Table 10.1).

Distancing

Distancing yourself from the material, retreating from intense concentration on the question may be one of the most effective techniques for augmenting I/C. Anne Becker chooses to wait to analyze her data:

> The kind of data analysis I do is more intuitive—pattern recognition and taking a step back and letting it process—I like to sit on data. . . . I like to collect it myself, transcribe it and read through it in a week or a month, I like to let it filter, percolate.

Whether called distancing, percolation, or incubation, this stage involves a process of retreating from intense concentration on the question. During this process, you cease involvement with the topic, the collected texts, the people or places associated with the investigation. Nonetheless, this is not a period of dormancy. Rather,

> The period of incubation allows the inner workings of the tacit dimension and intuition to continue to clarify and extend understanding on levels outside immediate awareness . . . [achieving a] receptive state of mind without conscious striving or concentration. (Moustakas, 1990, p. 29)

A seed has been planted and undergoes silent care and nourishment, producing "a creative awareness of some dimension of a phenomenon or a creative integration of its parts or qualities" (Moustakas, 1990, p. 29).

Distancing yourself from the research may be particularly helpful when you are stuck. On one particular study, I found it difficult to assemble the big picture; I was continually being distracted by particular thorny issues that had great emotional weight, both for me and for the rest of the research team. Only after putting down the material and stepping back for many months was I able to gain a perspective that allowed me to see the forest, despite the trees. The long lists of individual categories, exclusions, and exceptions fused into a synthetic understanding that had eluded me previously and allowed the successful analysis of the material (Borkan, Miller, et al., 1997).

Altered States of Consciousness

As mentioned above, intense concentration and prolonged analysis do not always yield the desired results in I/C. Approaches that involve mental states other than directed consciousness may be more helpful. For example, McWilliam advises that "Meditation is one way to help it along—put yourself at peace—get rid of the pressure to achieve an outcome." Stein notes that "It is not simply that I sit down and inspect the [data] sets and look for this or that. It is very psychoanalytic in spirit—like hovering attention or free floating attention." Similarly, Becker describes a process of attentive inattentiveness: "I sit at my computer and listen to tapes and do something else at the same time—I don't want to rush it."

Dream states and other altered states of consciousness may also be harnessed by the enterprising and experimental investigator. McWilliam describes:

> I may get panicky because I am not getting the big picture sometimes. I am an outcome driven person—which I say only blocks my mind. I put [the analysis] on the back burner and some more will come to me, either in the middle of the night after 2-3 hours of deep sleep or in the morning.

Finally, although I am not advocating the use of drugs or alcohol during I/C, one research team with which I have worked for 10 years nearly always opens sessions with a good meal and a vintage bottle of wine. (Be sure to have a "designated note-taker," however, so insights are not forgotten before the night is over.)

Getting a Group Together or Giving the Material to Others to Review

Gathering a group of colleagues together for an interactive analysis session may be one of the best methods for moving I/C forward. Similarly, textual material may be shown to others for their review and insight. The coinvestigators need not be experts either in the field of study or in qualitative methods. Significant others, children, parents, students, and friends may provide unexpected insights, drawn from their own differing life experience, that may provide new inroads and perspectives. Although some researchers always work alone, many agree that richer insights and more varied alternative hypotheses are achieved with groups. I always have a few outside judges read over a sample of transcripts to suggest categories, interpretations, or hypotheses that may have been missed. Other qualitative researchers have been know to show videotapes, audiotapes, or texts to colleagues and students (with or without prior explanation or direction)—nearly always with impressive results.

Gather Insights From Informants

Sometimes, insights that elude researchers are apparent to the informants. As McWilliam admitted in regard to the analysis of a project on breast cancer, "[the interviewees] integrated the process more than we did! . . . A lot of the fine tuning of the impressions came from the participants." The informants, whether they have suffered from a particular illness, worked in a specific business, or raised their children in a certain town, have often had time to process their experience and gather extensive information and insights. For example, not infrequently, the parents of children with unusual illnesses come to know more about the disease and its physical, social, and familial ramifications than those who provide their medical care. Insights from informants can be gathered during initial interviews, even bouncing initial interpretations off them, as described earlier. I often try to present my findings back to informants before publication. At these sessions, I make sure to allow time for informants to give their opinions, reactions, and clarifications. These are duly recorded and incorporated into the final report or manuscript.

External Stimuli

Researchers are frequently influenced by what they see and hear during the course of their investigations. Each of us has had a "spark" set off by something heard or read. Such stimuli can be harnessed systematically by recording insights that occur while hearing a lecture or reading the literature. Kleinman, an adherent of the use of theory during analyses, believes that one can augment one's analyses by going both to the literature in the direct area of investigation and by going further afield to the broader literature of the sciences, the humanities, and the arts.

VARIATIONS OF I/C

The insights that come during the I/C process do not appear *de novo* without any basis or bias. Rather, they form on a prefixed matrix, which assists their crystallization and gives it a certain underlying structure. The two dominant methods for doing this are working from the foundation of *theory* or from the content of one's *data.*

Content-Driven I/C

In this type of I/C, the researcher attempts to let his or her data stand alone, without a "filter" based on other investigations or theoretical structures. Some will even avoid reading the literature, so as not to be influenced by the findings. Although there is some artificiality to this approach, as no investigator can be truly independent of his or her scientific tradition, the "baggage" of such traditions can at least be partially minimized.

Theory-Driven I/C

The approach that amasses the insights on the bedrock of theory starts from the explicit assumption that the research and the researcher are not an unformed and uninfluenced tabula rasa. Some say that an approach that claims to be "purely empirical" is both uniformed and naive, because this would require a separation of the research and researcher from the society and schools of thought in which they are posited.

Kleinman, an adherent of the theory-driven approach, believes that "What is most exciting is to be rich empirically and rich theoretically and to bring the two together. . . . The only way this gets done is to stay theoretical." He believes in the triangulation of several sources, including the data, literature in the field, the broader literature, and insights from members of one's research group.

Becker describes a slightly different use of theory during the analytic cycle. In her method, there are repeated cycles wherein the researcher "goes to theory, looks at the data, goes to theory."

Some caveats should be mentioned, however. As Huberman and Miles (1994) have noted, there is a "darker side" of theory that allows the same data to be interpreted in vastly different ways, owing largely to the investigator's allegiance to a preexisting body of thought. Wolcott (1995) reiterates the threat of the "darker arts" in field work and analysis that may stem from *superficiality, obviousness* (of either methods or results), *self-serving* conclusions (that serve best those who conduct the research), *lack of independence, deception,* and *betrayal* (of those we have studied).

Gender Differences

Much has been made of the different "ways of knowing" between men and women. In a process so cognitively based as I/C, the influence of gender is likely to be felt. Depending on the goals of the study, this may be another argument for including a mixed-gender team approach in the analytical process.

PITFALLS

Premature or Delayed Closure

As in any analytic method that uses a great deal of interpretation, there are risks of either prematurely drawing conclusions or, conversely, being unable to reach closure, frozen in indecision as to what the data mean. The first pitfall can inadvertently occur with great ease, as you can begin analysis even during the period of research conceptualization. Stein relates how he was once challenged by a young family medicine resident about his insights and conclusions regarding their lives. After further thought and analysis, he realized that the young physician had been right; he had prematurely drawn conclusions without either considering all his data or reflecting back his findings onto his informants. Such pitfalls can be avoided by taking a fresh look at the whole data set, involving others in the analysis, and bouncing conclusions off of those studied.

Inability to reach closure, on the other hand, may be overcome by setting deadlines for interpretations, letting the material incubate more fully, or, as with premature closure, involving others. The key, however, as in writing an article or painting a picture, is knowing when enough is enough. Here experience and a mentor may be extremely helpful.

Inexperience

For truly effective I/C-type analyses, experience is required—either personal or that of a mentor. As McWilliam describes it, "[Immersion/ crystallization] happens with experience. The first couple of times I did it, I was panic struck that I would not achieve an interpretation. . . . I have had masters' students in tears because they couldn't do it."

Issues of Corroboration/Legitimation
and Consideration of Alternative Interpretations

As described, the process of I/C may be long and laborious. How can you be sure that what you accomplish with I/C is actually meaningful? What gives your version any special legitimacy or value? How are your results any more well grounded, sound, or insightful than those of any passive bystander, journalist, or folklorist? Validity is often the Achilles' heel of qualitative research. As Moustakas (1990) writes:

> The question of validity is one of meaning: Does the ultimate depiction of the experience derived from one's own rigorous, exhaustive self-searching and from the explications of others present comprehensively, vividly, and accurately the meanings and essences of the experience? This judgment is made by the primary researcher, who is the only person in the investigation who has undergone the heuristic inquiry from the beginning formulation of the question through phases of incubation, illumination, explication, and creative synthesis not only with himself or herself, but with each and every co-researcher.

The issue of validity in qualitative research is a thorny one, particularly because much of the argument has either been formulated or expropriated by positivism and quantitative science. Positivism, the philosophical, methodological, and theoretical perspective that has justified the use of quantitative methods in both the social and natural sciences, has opted for the perspective that "validity," the accuracy and truthfulness of the findings, can be based on notions of "reliability" (repeatable, generalizable), or the stability of methods and findings (Altheide & Johnson, 1994).

Qualitative analytical methods rarely have the luxury of deductive universal categories, numerical proofs, or statistical generalizability. The fact that qualitative research is conducted by human beings tied to particular contexts has raised the specter that such work is, by nature,

> not only "nonobjective" but partisan, partial, incomplete, and inextricably bound to the contexts and rationales of the researcher, contexts he or she may represent (albeit unknowingly) and the rhetorical genres through which the flawed ethnographic reports are manifested and held forth. (Altheide & Johnson, 1994, p. 487).

In this light, qualitative researchers have had to take different tacks in attempting to make assertions of validity. Efforts have been multiple, but some of those that make the most sense in terms of I/C include the following:

- Reflexivity
- Depth of description
- Accuracy
- Rigor
- Intellectual honesty
- Searching for alternate hypotheses and interpretations

Analyses based on incomplete or inaccurate data are bound to fail in their task of providing valid information. Qualitative research reports are basically grounded in descriptions that are provided either by informants and/or the investigators themselves. The *depth of description* is critical both in avoiding superficiality and in ensuring that the issues, concepts, and contextual realities have been suitably explored. *Accuracy* is a primary responsibility of the investigator. The importance of accuracy is underscored by Hammersley (1992): "An account is valid or true if it represents accurately those features of the phenomena that it is intended to describe, explain or theorize" (p. 69).

Validity in qualitative research is also inexorably tied to notions of *rigor* and *intellectual honesty*. The reader must be certain that the investigator has been tireless in recording, examining, and interpreting the data and in searching for alternative hypotheses. All of this must be done with the utmost integrity, straightforwardness, and adherence to accepted norms of research.

Searching for alternative hypotheses implies that the investigator leaves open the possibility of other interpretations of the data. In regard to this, Stein suggests:

> I am wary of my own understandings, lest I see only what I want to see, or to see only as far as my favorite theory allows. I still allow the possibility that there is meaning in addition to what we initially generate. Under-standing is like marination; it is rarely instant. . . . We must be able to tolerate our own anxiety, to understand it, in order to let the data speak.

Kleinman warns us to be aware when "information presses up against the categories and won't shoehorn in." In such cases, we must be aware that other interpretations may effectively summarize or synthesize the data.

Reflexivity refers to the technique by which researchers turn the focus back on themselves to evaluate their influence on the findings and inter-pretations. Miller stresses the critical nature of this exercise:

> There is great importance to reflexivity. As much as possible, you must know yourself and your place in the data. You must be aware of the influences of you being part of the data and whatever comes out the result of this interaction [between you and the data].

Overall, immersion/crystallization should be well within the reach of any researcher willing to invest the time and energy, providing endless challenge and reward. Equipped with a clear mind, adequate resources, and prior awareness of both the analytic style and possible pitfalls, you are certain to succeed.

Final Plea: *Listen to your inner voice, experiment, experience!*

11

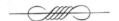

Data Management
and Interpretation
Using Computers to Assist

Lynn M. Meadows
Diane M. Dodendorf

INTRODUCING COMPUTERS
TO QUALITATIVE RESEARCH

Qualitative data interpretation is a rewarding and challenging undertaking. Regardless of the organizing style adopted or the derivative texts that are the subject of the research team's interests, interpretation, even with computer assistance, is a personal experience. There is still resistance among some qualitative researchers to using computers as a tool in analysis and interpretation, stemming from a fear that the process will be become too far removed from the researcher as expert or that the analysis will resemble a point-and-click quantitative analysis that yields results but no meaning. It is more likely, however, that the iterative process of analysis and interpretation, when aided by a computer program, will draw the analysts into the data with such appeal that enforcing or acknowledging closure becomes the most difficult task of the project.

Tesch (1989) noted 10 years ago that using a computer to facilitate analysis can save time, reduce drudgery, "make procedures more systematic and explicit, insure completeness and refinement, and permit flexibility and revision in analysis procedures" (Miles & Huberman, 1994, p. 44). Qualitative analysis software is a fast-moving field that has received increasing attention since Tesch's observation. In recent years, the field of qualitative research has moved from add-on discussions of qualitative methods and methodologies to texts, special journal issues, and regular articles on qualitative analysis and interpretation. These publications have helped move qualitative researchers away from colored pens and pencils, highlighters, and massive amounts of photocopying to a computer-assisted environment. Software programs that facilitate computer-assisted analysis allow the research team to go beyond sorting cards, multiple photocopies, and file drawers stuffed with derivative texts to small amounts of space on a hard drive or numerous zip diskettes. Initially, programs that were used in analysis drew features from word processing—the ability to "count" the number of occurrences of a word in the text or to search for a certain term. Programs are now increasingly sophisticated, with their components either adapted for qualitative analysis or specifically developed to aid in that process.

Excellent and thorough reviews of the many qualitative analysis software programs that exist are available elsewhere (Miles & Huberman, 1994; Weitzman & Miles, 1995). In a review of 22 software programs that existed in 1994, Miles and Huberman identified three types of programs that can be used for qualitative analysis but were not developed for that purpose and three others that are qualitative analysis specific. They note that word processors, word retrievers, and text-base managers can perform basic useful functions in the process of data analysis. Other programs, such as code and retrieve programs, theory builders, and conceptual network builders have been developed specifically by qualitative researchers or by those with whom they work and are intended to be used in that context.

Data management is a necessary and integral part of doing a qualitative research project. Data management has been defined in terms of "The operations needed for a systematic, coherent process of data collection, storage, and retrieval" (Huberman & Miles, 1994, p. 428). Good data management facilitates interpretation just as good orchestration facilitates good dance music. Systems of data management are resources that assist researchers in their task of data interpretation, no matter their actual approach (Bassett, Cox, & Rauch, 1995). Therefore, computer-assisted data analysis implies and should include the ability of a program to organize the derivative texts with which the research team are working so that the analyses can proceed with relative ease and the ability to document that process.

In this chapter, we will briefly illustrate how various features vary across the program types and mention how they might be useful for different interpretive approaches using different organizing styles. These include the template organizing style, editing style, and immersion and crystallization style (refer to Chapter 7). The chapter then concludes with a more in-depth look at NUD∗IST 4.0® and Folio Views® and concluding comments. Folio Views is particularly helpful with complex data management; NUD∗IST allows the researcher to proceed all the way to theory generation if desired.

Types of Software Programs

Word processing programs are primarily used for the production and retrieval of text. As such, they are useful for transcribing interviews, field notes, writing notes about the research under way, and generally creating text. These programs, available on both PC and MAC platforms, can be useful in identifying key words, in searching for strings of text, and generally in working at a find-and-count level of analysis. Currently, Microsoft Word® and WordPerfect® are two of the most common programs. Word retrievers are generally used to find instances of words, phrases, and combinations of them. Examples of those programs include Metamorph®, Sonar Professional®, and WordCruncher®. It is possible to do content analysis with some of these programs through generating lists of words and phrases in the context in which they occur. Again, these are fairly basic functions and not specifically intended for qualitative analysis.

Text-base managers can perform basic useful functions in the process of data analysis. They are used to organize text for better retrieval of information from internally or externally stored text. Folio Views, ask-Sam®, MAX® and ZyINDEX® are examples of text-base managers. These programs organize text into "records" consisting of specific cases of data and "fields" that organize information that is numerical or text from each case. These programs can search and retrieve memos made about the data, coding in the data, and words or phrases that are sought.

Researchers who have worked extensively with qualitative data have been instrumental in the process of improvement through discussion and development of computer programs more specifically designed to handle and help organize derived text in many forms (for example, Fielding & Lee, 1991; Richards & Richards, 1994a, 1994b). *Code-and-retrieve programs* assist in coding chunks of data and grouping them. Among those programs are HyperQual®, NUD∗IST, QUALPRO® and the Ethnograph®. One useful feature of these programs is the function that allows coded data to be displayed as the coded groupings or a combination thereof. *Theory builders* move beyond code-and-retrieve functions to ask questions of data using the program and facilitate the analysis phase of connecting themes or categories. NUD∗IST, ATLAS™, HyperRESEARCH®, QCA®, and AQUAD® have these capabilities. Various operators using a system of rules or formal logic are used in these programs to examine coded data for relationships, groupings, and proximity. These programs do not do the work for the research team, but they certainly make the organization and analysis of data more manageable. Finally, *conceptual network builders* add graphic network capabilities to theory building and testing, using not just drawings but semantic networks. Popular programs with graphics capabilities are Inspiration®, Decision Maker®, ATLAS™, MECA®, and the new NVIVO®.

Programs that exist for the analysis of qualitative data are in constant flux and development. Often, the companies with whom they originate closely monitor Internet chat groups and user groups to keep abreast of consumer and researcher requests. Revised versions of existing programs may incorporate popular features of other programs, and change is the rule, rather than the exception. The decision regarding what program to use for a project or a program of work is a challenging one, depending on the research team's computer literacy, the nature of the research, whether several people will be working on a project, what platform is most desired, available local or on-line support, and the nature of the derived texts. The organizing styles and interpretive approach being brought to bear in the project may also influence the choice of program—it may be felt that an immersion/crystallization style needs little more than a word processor, but a template style needs theory-testing capabilities. That said, most projects can usually use all the sophistication available, and oftentimes the research process and study findings cultivate increasing use of the fine points of a program.

` TO THE FIELD!

A recent discussion on the QSR Forum provides a powerful reminder that it is important to remember that programs for analyzing qualitative data are similar to those for quantitative data (i.e., SPSS®, SAS®) in that the program cannot do the analysis for the researcher. The program itself is a tool, analogous to earlier approaches using photocopies, colored highlighters, or simple sorting devices. A software program can be a powerful tool, but that is all that it is. Cries of, "I've coded all my data, now what do I do?" remind us that qualitative researchers are the brains behind the interpretations and in fact must actually do the analysis and interpretations themselves. The programs we discuss here can make that job much more manageable. However, in the end it is the researcher who decides on codes, devises searches for connections between themes or concepts, and interprets the findings.

Regardless of the approach to qualitative analysis that is being undertaken by the research team, in general, the aims of using a software program are to get the text into the program, use the program to create summaries of data or better organize it (organizing phase), and then proceed to making links and associations within the data that will satisfy the original research question and aid in interpretation (connecting phase). There are also two basic functions that a program needs to provide: a way to read the original text or documents, and a way to code or group pieces of data that represent concepts, themes, variables, or whatever categories are represented in the data. It is more convenient to have a way to move easily between these two groupings of data as the analysis proceeds, as this encourages the research team to stay close to the original data as the interpretation proceeds. Depending on the structure of the program, coded data may even become part of the data set, a feature known as *system closure.*

Research teams that decide to use immersion/crystallization as the primary organizing style need to be close to the data (see Chapter 10) to be able to work from the derived text in developing coding. Features that would be important for a software tool to have include quick access to the data and a way of writing memos about documents and thoughts about pieces of text to leave a paper trail that increases the credibility of the analysis process. Coding of the text would emerge as the analysts increase their familiarity with the data, so some flexibility in refining coding or adding to it is useful. As the interpretation proceeded, the ability to summarize coding and do comparisons among sets of coded text would prove useful. In a template style (Chapter 9), the analysis is guided by a basic pattern or template that is taken to the data as part of the process of identifying meaningful units in the text. The template may be developed from preexisting theory, research traditions, or knowledge the researcher had before working with the data, or it may be developed after a summary reading of the text. It is likely that for this type of organizing, the research team will develop a coding scheme either before using the analytic program or shortly after the team begins working with the data. The template style is iterative, with changes to the template likely and even desirable after work with the data has begun. A program that would be useful for a template organizing style needs to be flexible, possibly allowing an initial coding of the data as the meaningful units or parts of the data emerge. As the connecting phase progresses, the program will need to allow the coding scheme to be refined and begin to reflect the connections between and among units of meaning. The ability to search coding and explore hypotheses is also important to this approach to data analysis.

The editing organizing style (Chapter 8) is a more emergent method, yet it is one that also benefits from computer assistance. Coding of the data into meaningful units and grouping those units into patterns and themes is a key activity for this process, enhanced greatly by a program that encourages easy coding as well as simple revisions of codes and additional coding of new data as it becomes necessary. A second data collection from study participants or addition of cases may be part of this type of project; therefore the ability to smoothly add to both the project and the editing process is useful. Flexibility of the program is a key need, as approaches such as grounded theory (Glaser & Strauss, 1967) and long interview analysis (McCracken, 1988) often use an editing organizing style. Note that both the editing and template styles evolve in such a way that further data collection may be necessary, and there may often be a change in organizing style. A useful feature of a software program for these approaches would be the ability to track sampling and generate tables of key sample characteristics with the program. The import and export of tables, a relatively new feature of qualitative programs, is ideal for these needs.

A template style can also be applied with a stiffer structure. Content analysis is one example of this and is based on searching for words, terms, or semantic units of meaning. Once the basic units of analysis are identified, typically using a codebook, they are sorted into categories, at which time a statistical analysis of their relationship can be undertaken. Programs that would be useful for this type of analysis need features that allow quick and efficient searches of the derivative text, ways of organizing the results of these searches, and then a way to either export them to a quantitative statistical package or generate tables, vectors, and matrices. There is a lesser need to be able to interact with the data than in the other analytic approaches mentioned here; researchers using this style would likely be strongly attracted to programs that could automatically code data that answers questions, provides ratings, describes demographic characteristics, and the like. Command files would be an important feature of programs that would be useful to this more structured quasi-statistical-like template style.

It is important to realize that the goals and nature of the research, not the features of a software analytic package, should drive the research team's interpretive process. Some researchers will be more or less comfortable with the features of the software programs, and a few or many of the programs' functions may be used by the team. Doing the interpretation with the aid of the software program should enhance the process through saving time, presenting the data, coding, patterns, and meanings in a way that enhances the researcher's ability to practice her or his craft and see clearly what the texts are revealing about the topic under study. Many of the analytic approaches discussed in this section are based on the premise that the analysis and interpretation are done by a research team, sometimes with independent coding, even at remote sites. The ability to combine separate coding into one central project then becomes a consideration. Additionally, the ability to represent the project graphically, as opposed to in text alone, may be a feature that appeals to analysts.

In the following section, we briefly review two available programs, illustrating key features of them found useful in specific, current research endeavors. Folio Views illustrates a program that keeps the researchers very close to the text, organizes data well, and makes coding choices clear. NUD*IST, in the 4.0 revision, also allows the researcher to maintain close contact with the text and provides tools that can flow with the interpretive process, easily revise coding and patterns that emerge, and encourage the development of theory, should that be the goal.

EXAMINING WOMEN'S PERCEIVED
HEALTH ISSUES WITH QSR NUD*IST

Taking a new and somewhat rare perspective on midlife women's health is doubly interesting when the research team tells others that they are doing it with the help of NUD*IST! We really *can* find out a lot about the health of women 40 to 65 years old and their concerns surrounding it when both researchers and the women with whom they gather data have all their clothes on and use QSR NUD*IST as an aid to interpretation! In the WHEALTH study, texts are mostly derived from transcribed interviews and field notes, although as the analysis and interpretation proceeded the changed self was a constant; as issues emerged, concepts were articulated and connections in the data were explored. Data analysis began as soon as the first interview was transcribed and formatted as ASCII text so that it could be imported, or read into, the NUD*IST program. We (Meadows and Thurston) really wanted to listen to what women were sharing with us about their lives and health in our study and to get away from the view of midlife women as mainly concerned with reproductive issues and systems. We also wanted to be true to the process of qualitative inquiry as one in which sampling, data collection, and interpretation all occur at the same time.

NUD*IST is an acronym for non-numerical unstructured data indexing, searching, and theorizing. Just as an introductory sociology textbook tells most of what there is to know about sociology, so the name NUD*IST tells us all about what the program can do. NUD*IST provides the tools to index (or code) data, look through the results of that coding, and use those results to generate hypotheses and test them. NUD*IST 4.0 (N4), the most recent version of the program, is based on a document system and an indexing system.

The Program Basics

One phase of the WHEALTH study collected data from a sample of diverse midlife women, using semistructured interviews. The interviews were audiorecorded and transcribed verbatim. On the average, interviews lasted about an hour, but some were much shorter, and one marathon interview lasted 4 hours. Initial transcription of the interviews proceeded without formatting instructions, aside from noting with an asterisk when the person speaking changed and numbering questions sequentially from 1 onwards.

The NUD*IST coding and searching system uses user-designated segments of the data (e.g., words, lines, sentences, paragraphs) as the units of analysis in the project. These segments of data are the smallest pieces of data within that particular project that can be identified by the program and used in the analysis. These are called *text units* in the context of NUD*IST and are analogous to the unit of analysis in quantitative analysis. The text units are used by the program as the entity that is coded, searched, memoed, and questioned during the analysis. That unit can be a word, a line, a sentence, a paragraph, or a whole document.

In the WHEALTH study, women varied in the length of their answers to questions. Asking a woman to rate her health on a scale of 1 to 10 often resulted in a single number, but asking someone to describe a past illness could result in an answer that was a three-page paragraph. NUD*IST recognizes every hard return in the text as the end of a text unit. Larger pieces of text, known as sections, are delineated by asterisks (*) in the documents. Sections might be identified for individual questions and answers, by changing speakers in a focus group, or with changing dates on consecutive interviews. When using NUD*IST, it is always possible to extend the context of a text unit or chunk of data but impossible to make a text unit smaller. Therefore, users need to decide early on in the project what will constitute a segment of data.

In our case, we chose to have sentences be the unit of analysis. Although the person analyzing the data might clearly see new paragraphs emerging in the answer to a question, the transcriptionist might happily create page-long paragraphs, thus making the bounty of a text search more prolific than expected. Careful thought is important before designating text units—if they are too large, they will be cumbersome in later use.

A new NUD*IST project is simply started by going into the program, choosing "create new project," and entering in the information as requested. This will automatically create the four directories that are part of every NUD*IST project: raw files (where the ASCII files of text are introduced to the program), database (where all the components of the project file are stored), commands (where command files to automate functions of the program are stored), and reports (the default file for reports that you generate and wish to save). Once the new project has been created, documents for the project can be copied into the raw files directory of the project. It will be from that file that any on-line documents will be read into the program. These text files should be ASCII text files, appropriately formatted for the project (See Figure 11.1).

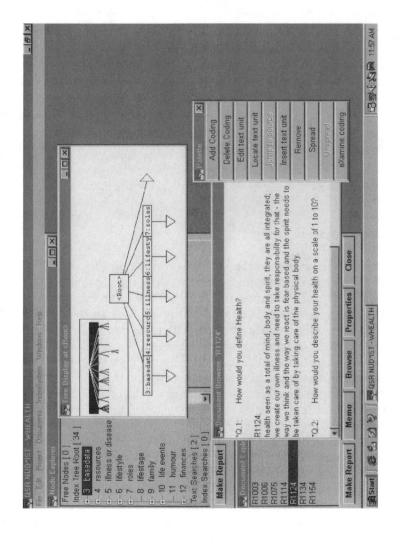

Figure 11.1. Creating Nodes in NUD*IST

203

The coding (or indexing) system in NUD*IST is based on *nodes.* In the program, nodes are locations within the project where references to coded texts are stored. In a project, one might have nodes for basic demographic data (gender, occupation, income, age) and also conceptual nodes such as health attitudes, family worries, and physician interactions. Nodes can be either free nodes, which are independent and unordered, or tree nodes, which are ordered hierarchically and organized in a tree diagram (see Figure 11.1). Tree nodes can be moved around the tree-like organizing structure through a system of cutting and pasting. Nodes that are either free nodes or tree nodes can be copied and placed in the other location if necessary or appropriate in later analysis. One advantage of this system is that as your analysis and understanding advance, your coding scheme, whether hierarchically ordered or not, can evolve and change. This invites early and enthusiastic exploration of the data—more than one avenue of thought regarding the data can be explored at the same time, and later these coding schemes can be revised, updated, or deleted as appropriate. Nodes of indexed or coded data provide the basis of the indexing system within NUD*IST.

The Document System

Textual documents provide the backbone to the operating system of NUD*IST. The NUD*IST document system works with documents that are introduced into the program from the raw files directory into the database directory. These derived texts can include references to whatever the research team is using as data sources: letters, reports, interview text, memos, photographs, artifacts, annotated bibliographies, or scanned written materials. When "import document" is selected under the document menu, the program automatically looks in the raw files directory for files. Although they can be in other locations (floppy disk, other directories), having the data files in the raw files directory allows execution of a quick command that will import, or introduce, all the data files into the project at one time. Files are then located in the database file, which is the essential file, along with reports and commands, to be a back-up for the security of the project. These actual data files are on-line documents—ones for which there is actual text in the project. In the WHEALTH study, the data files consist of numbered interviews, with the numbering differing according to the subpopulation sampled. Each file is the transcript of either a face-to-face or telephone interview. For example, local volunteer respondents are R1000s, immigrant women are R2000s, and ethnocultural minority women from another city are R3000s.

N4 also offers the option of cataloging off-line or supplementary documents into the project. These documents can be references to file folders in drawers, reports, newspaper reports, pictures, videotapes, or any other materials that are part of the project and need to be part of the analysis but are not available electronically. A newspaper series of articles on women's health could become part of the project, or pictures illustrating literacy or mobility barriers to health care access in a certain location could be an integral part of the project using off-line documents.

Memos are an integral part of the text of this project, as they are both a paper trail of our immersion/crystallization organizing and a way of talking with ourselves about emerging concepts, issues, and connections among women in their experience of health, work, and family in a broad environmental context. Memos can be generated through the document system, detailing thoughts about data analysis, instructions to other team members, and other information as it is important to link to the document. The *edit* menu of NUD*IST provides the option of inserting date and time so that the researcher can keep a chronology of the analysis process.

The Index System

The index system of NUD*IST is the heart and soul of the coding and organization of the project. As the research team goes through the derived text and begins identifying data to code, whether basic demographics and variablelike information or more conceptual or thematic information, references to those codes are placed in storage nodes. Coding is simple in N4. The analyst simply identifies the text that is to be coded (or indexed) to a node, uses the coding palette found within the document browser to "add coding," and verifies whether that piece of text is to be indexed at a coding node already in existence or a newly created one. If the project is based on a highly structured template organizing style, the index system is likely to be more structured, with, for example, coding nodes for sources of formal, informal, and indigenous sources of health information and care; numbers of visits to particular specialists; and a chronology of health issues and solutions. The coding nodes can be created first, then the text can be coded. On the other hand, if interpretation uses primarily an editing or even an immersion/crystallization style, conceptual nodes exploring relationships, abuse issues, effect of immigration, role of spirituality, meanings of energy, and other factors might emerge from the data, and the nodes can be created as the themes or meanings emerge. If a template style is used, the data may be best handled in organizing all answers to standard questions 1 through 10 as the past year's health is explored, along with family life stressors and formal health care encounters.

Once initial coding has been done by one or more of the research team, the results of that coding can then be used to continue the process. A series of logical operators will allow the index system to be searched to see if chronic headaches are mentioned near discussion of financial worries, if chronic illness and low self-rated health status occur together, or if women who talk about spirituality also speak of religion in their lives. Word and string searches can also be created that will ask questions of the document system; the questions can then be further explored using the index system. Memos about nodes or reflecting on the results of indexing can themselves become part of the document system and analyzed further, adding a system closure feature to the program.

Personal choice and the indexing system found to be appropriate for the project may play a part in whether quick reviews of the coding are made by viewing a summary of the nodes or by viewing the tree diagram. Either source will provide a way to do a quick check of how coding is progressing and, for some, provide a visual image of the progress of the project.

Our Project: Whealth Stage I

In our analysis of the first exciting data from the WHEALTH study, we wanted to quickly become familiar with the data to see how women were talking about their health, given that we wanted anything that they perceived as affecting their health as part of our data. We started with a very open-ended questionnaire and a sample of volunteer participants recruited through media attention. There was a need to track the characteristics of our sample (to make the best use of available resources), and see if our questionnaire was eliciting data that would allow us to interpret the text in a meaningful way. The ability to create demographic coding nodes to help track the sample characteristics and to then export this as a constantly updated table and to conversely quickly code data into initial categories with either apparent connections (gender role/traditional/finances) or information about emerging ideas (family physician interactions, abuse yes/no) were important functions. The practice of constantly adding memos to our coding nodes, containing both a paper trail of what we coded and when, along with our thoughts on the meanings of the coding categories, was an important part of the analytic process.

As the initial coding proceeded, it became apparent that, even at the pilot stage, our questionnaire was too open ended. Women were talking about their bodies, aches and pains, and current health status but not providing data that could help us "connect the dots" to better understand what it was about a husband's unemployment or a parent's dependence that was affecting health, and how. The demographic coding (ethnicity, income, education, immigration status, health status) quickly revealed that our sample was very homogeneous—White, middle-class, and healthy. It was also apparent that coding our data in NUD*IST and also using a spreadsheet program to track the sampling was repetitive and unnecessary.

As our data collection continued with a more heterogeneous sample and a revised questionnaire, more team members participated in the interpretative process. The *merge* feature of NUD*IST then became an important one, as it allows coding from more than one source to be combined with the core project. A sample of immigrant women was added to the project, and all project team members coded a number of interviews to search for emergent themes. At the same time, those interviews were searched for key words and phrases to see if the descriptions of health were similar or if the semantics were quite different. It became apparent that the nonimmigrant sample talked freely and openly about their bodies, their concerns for their own health, and contradictions in information and across sources. The immigrant women were more likely to speak of health in terms of providing for themselves and their families, security, and worries for those still in their homelands. This early analysis was invaluable in helping to move the project in a direction that more clearly spoke to our research interests and intentions in undertaking the research.

As work on the study continues and competitive funding proposals are generated, the ability to summarize coded data and export as tables, either as an actual table or to a spreadsheet or quantitative analysis program such as SPSS, is increasingly important. The ease of copying, cutting, and pasting nodes with their coded text is appreciated as new connections between themes emerge, meanings reveal themselves, and we move toward saturation of the sampling for this stage. The ability to make reports from the program that can be opened in a word processing program and to edit them within NUD*IST is also a useful feature. As promised, NUD*IST 4.0 isn't doing the analysis and interpretation but is providing valuable research assistance, going along with any proposed exploration of the data, working 24 hours a day, and spitting out the answers to our index searches and document searches as quickly as we ask the questions.

In later stages of the project, theory generation will be a goal. NUD*IST 4.0 allows the testing of hypotheses, exploring with great sophistication the connections between themes and categories, comparison of nodes of coded data, and questions exploring whether poor health rating is mentioned near or after discussion of chronic disease, only among those with dependents, or with financial constraints. The new function that allows the analyst to quickly move from text coded at a node to the derived text with its holistic context keeps the researcher closer to the data than in earlier versions and stimulates the process of iterative coding and connecting.

As we grow more sophisticated and refined in our analysis, we will explore more functions available to us. Users in other projects often present their wish list of features on the QSR Forum. These are as varied as the backgrounds and preferences of the users. Future versions will no doubt add more click-and-drop features, continue to supply basic command files to automate coding of data, and address other researcher-generated issues. The availability of training sessions through a number of venues, including instructors trained by QSR, distance training and consultation, and the forum are valuable aids to users. Courses for those who are assistants for the software operation, rather than experts on the program itself, are now being offered, as well as a support function for the program. In our experience, NUD*IST 4.0 has been a useful adjunct to our analysis and interpretation of the text of the WHEALTH pilot study. It has allowed us to remain close to the data, work as a team on the analysis and interpretation, and clearly track our work with the data and our sample of study participants. As other stages of the WHEALTH study are implemented, the program flexibility will aid other approaches and continue to be part of our menu of resources.

NUD*IST Alive: NVivo Is Here!

Early in 1999, QSR's newest software package was announced. NVivo® offers an upgrade route from NUD*IST 4.0. As this section is going to press before the software announcement, some details may differ (this quick introduction is based on test software), but we felt that readers who were making software decisions would find this information useful.

The differences between N4 and NVivo will be immediately apparent to users of N4—researchers can simply lift a project straight into NVivo. Once the project is inside NVivo, it comes alive—the desktop now appears in rich text, as will new documents that are added to the project. Font, color, and formatting now have a meaningful function in the project. Proxy documents can now be created, for example for summaries of videotapes. Links are a feature of NVivo and allow direct connections between your project and other text or files, documents, or nodes. These links may also include film clips, photos, or voices that are part of your project. Drag-and-drop features are part of NVivo, allowing researchers selected text for coding—now exactly the words or characters you wish—to a node.

Searches are performed differently in NVivo, allowing the researcher to refine searches and assay (or evaluate) them as the task progresses. A modeler is also incorporated in NVivo, allowing the research team to draw any number of models that illustrate how your project is being conceptualized, what relationships are emerging, and what is yet to be explored (see Figure 11.2). NVivo will no doubt add new steps to the dance of interpretation—making possible a change of rhythm as we work with our derivative texts.

No one approach to data management and interpretation can meet the requirements of all qualitative research teams. Earlier in the chapter, we saw that many qualitative analytic software programs are available. The

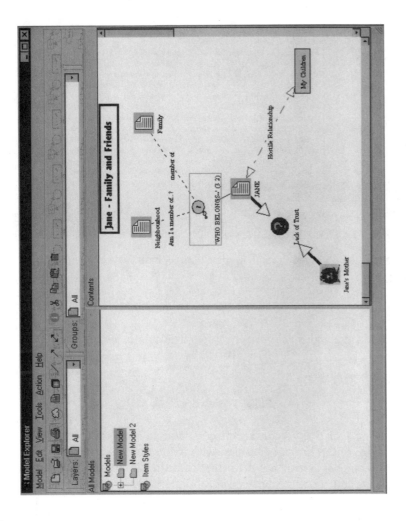

Figure 11.2. Example of NUD*IST Tree Node

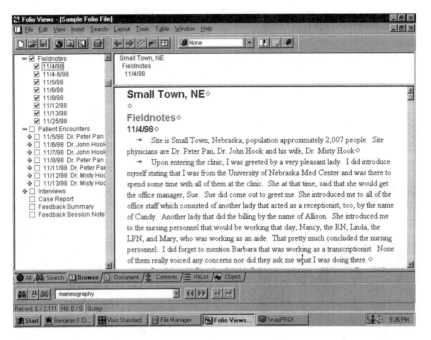

Figure 11.3. Folio Views Screen in "Browse" Mode, With Table of Contents and Text

next section highlights the many features available in Folio Views 4.11 (Figure 11.2).

Folio Views 4.11

Folio Views 4.11 is an infobase manager, that is, a freeform collection of information, both text and graphics, with a comprehensive index and a powerful retrieval system based on that index or an author-customized index (i.e., a code book). Folio Views is an international product available in English, French, German, Dutch, Spanish, and Portuguese. Folio Views includes a Windows-based word processor that allows formatting similar to most word processors, with fonts, paragraph styles, and other attributes. The Windows environment provides the usual features: title bar, menu bar, ribbon (editing features), ruler (tabs, indents, margins), document screen, vertical and horizontal scroll bars, and a status bar that indicates the cursor location by record number (see Figure 11.3).

Folio Views was originally developed for large businesses to manage complex data from multiple individuals and multiple locations. Therefore, it is highly developed for easy access to a "master file" by many users on a network (under the control of an administrator). It also has a feature whereby individuals can independently code the master file by using shadow files at their own workstation.

An Example of Folio Views in Action

The "Prevention and Competing Demands Study" is a large qualitative research project focusing on the delivery of preventive services in primary care practices in which research nurses dictate field notes and conduct interviews that are transcribed into MS Word files (for details of the project, refer to Chapter 16). A project coordinator imports these MS Word files directly into a Folio Views infobase to which all members of the team have access (refer ahead to Figure 16.1). An attractive feature of Folio Views is its ability to directly import word processor files, including both Word and WordPerfect. The infobase serves as the central repository for most of the data on each practice, including field notes of the practice, field notes on observed patient encounters, descriptions of patients' experiences in the practice, notes about charts and charting, audiotaped interviews, photographs (digital camera), and data tables.

Structure of the Project's Infobase

Folio Views 4.11 has a Word97® filter and an import function that brings in MS Word files cleanly. Folio has a number of filters that work with other word processing files as well as other formats. Folio will import the file wherever the cursor is when the file is named or selected with a mouse click. Each Folio infobase consists of an *info file*. Like most word-processing programs, the program has an "open" button in the file drop menu that opens current files, or the user can select "new" to create a new infobase. Under the File menu options, there is also an "information" option. Additional information regarding the new infobase can be entered in this dialogue box, which is useful for identification information. When a new infobase is created, it is considered a master file, that is, the original file (stored as *.nfo).

The preliminary formatting of the infobase includes several useful features. The infobase can be constructed with consistent fonts and margins, "levels" can be assigned to help organize the data (see next section), coloring of selected data can be done with "highlighters" (e.g., chart audit data), and coding is accomplished with "fields" (e.g., all references to prevention, such as tobacco or mammogram). Once the administrator or user has applied these features, a style file (*.sty) is created; this style file can be named and saved and subsequently applied to other infobases, which is very helpful if you will be setting up multiple files with similar formatting. For example, in the prevention study, we set up a separate infobase for each practice but only needed to set up the initial formatting once.

Levels

Folio *levels* establish an outline and some hierarchical order to the data, much like a book with chapters and sections. Levels can be thought of as the parts of an outline. The levels for the prevention case study infobase are (a) practice, (b) data type (field notes, patient encounters, patient pathways, interviews), (c) date (chronological ordering of dates within field notes and patient encounters), and (d) individual (individual patients per day as well as individual interviews). In addition, there is a default level of normal. To assign a level, the user blocks the text with the mouse and applies a particular level (that he or she had previously created) found under the Tools drop menu, similar to text formatting. The levels can be formatted with fonts and colors so that the outline is easily noted.

The application of levels to certain text creates a hierarchy of information and a Table of Contents (see left side of Figure 11.3) that is most useful. Level usage is a basic help with orientation while using the on-line document, particularly with large documents. A Reference Window feature, just above the text in Figure 11.3, shows the current levels only, allowing the user to recognize the current cursor location. For example, in Figure 11.3, the cursor is at the November 4 field notes in Small Town, NE. The visual hierarchical representation of the data in the contents pane can be visible while the document is open (browse mode) or hidden if the user chooses the "document" mode. The other use for the Table of Contents is data management, as it is a tool that can be used to monitor progress on data acquisition. The table can be printed as a separate document, and progress is noted as tapes are transcribed and entered into the infobase, as the preliminary coding is completed, and as sections are printed. If the user is able to plan the infobase with current as well as anticipated uses of the data, then levels can be created and applied to text that almost effortlessly organizes the data for increased ease in reading, analysis, and data management.

Coding and Organizing Data

"Highlighting" is just like using the old yellow highlighter marker in a book to label text that is considered important. The text in the infobase is blocked and a highlighter applied. The highlighters are created and named based on the qualitative analysis being conducted and formatted with fonts and colors to make them distinctive. For example, one of our highlighters is chart audit information; the highlighter is named "Chart Audit" and format-ted with a blue foreground; thus all text in the infobase containing information from the chart audit shows up as blue throughout the document.

Other selected text in the infobase is coded with a codebook in the form of *fields*. For example, in the prevention study, we developed a codebook that refers to different preventive services that can be coded. Fields are another way to organize and emphasize key data. Fields are similar to highlighters but are more powerful, in that fields can be defined as five types: text, date, time, integer, and real. Searching by field allows the user to add conditional operators ($<$, $>$, $=$, etc.) to refine the search and to test some hypotheses. One of the prevention fields is tobacco; any reference to tobacco is blocked with the mouse and the field applied using the layout drop menu. Terms such as smoking, chewing, quitting cigarettes, and pipe smoking are all marked as the field for tobacco (separate codes could also be developed). Another use of fields is to mark gender and birth dates of patients as fields. Then a search (query) of all women over the age of 50 years with another prevention field, such as mammogram, will produce all the records with just the focus needed for analysis.

This project also codes all text units in patient encounters using "group" according to the type of visit. Grouping is a tool used to organize informa-tion by topic. The advantage of grouping is that it allows the user to create a further refinement of a variable, for example, with "Office Visit Type" it is possible to specify acute, chronic, and health care maintenance visits. Unlike levels, highlighters, and fields, where the user can select colors and fonts that clearly identify coded data, a possible disadvantage of groups is that there is no visible indication that the data (records) have been assigned to a group. Nevertheless, grouping is useful for "query work" and with printing selected records.

The *Notes* feature is like putting a sticky note on the text. Readers can make notes to themselves while working in the infobase. These notes could be hunches or a hypothesis-generating statement. A small icon that looks like a sticky note appears at the beginning of the record in which the note was placed (simply double click on the note to read). Also, the note can be useful as a way for analysts to communicate with each other about the content and/or the analysis of the content without disturbing the form of the data. This project uses notes for a display of the timetable for each patient visit; this table provides data on the time spent during each of the various components of the doctor visit in units of minutes. The data is not in the document but can be accessed by a mouse click on the term *timetable*.

Object links can be created with files containing digital data (photos). In our study, we include a photograph of the clinic at the beginning of the file and photographs of individuals at the beginning of their respective interviews. To view the photo, the user simply clicks on the "hot spot," just as with the hypertext on web pages.

Because a lot of our coding takes advantage of the color formatting possible, the project uses a color printer to print the document. All the color coding is visible on the hard copy for reading and analysis if the analyst chooses to work on paper rather than on screen.

Security/Access

The nature of confidential data and the advantages of group analysis naturally lead to concerns about security. The program's security system allows the Rights Administrator to control the features for each of three user types: owner, administrator, and guest or specific individual user(s). The administrator may add other users to defined licenses that have various access and limit features to an infobase. Encryption and passwords are other security devices used to protect the data.

Shadow Files

With Folio, users have the option of creating several independent "shadow" files that refer to but do not change the master file. Shadow files are named by the user and end with *.sdw. A Shadow file is created by selecting "New" under the File Menu while in the original file and then choosing "Folio Shadow File" from the list of file types. Each shadow file can be personalized in the sense that the various coding tools and the toolbar can be modified and saved by each user. This feature is quite useful when there are several people working on the qualitative analysis. As the master file is updated (e.g., as new text is added), the shadow files will subsequently be reconciled for each user. Any previous independent coding by that team member is maintained; each user has the option of printing his or her version of the infobase as well. The work on the shadow files does not change the master file; it remains the "untouched" and protected file. Shadow files can be thought of as plastic overheads or filters on the computer screen. Each analyst can code the text in an independent manner without disturbing the original, master file.

Personalizing the Infobase For Analysis

The View tabs or mode (bottom of screen in Figure 11.3) can be selected, and each tab creates a different environment in which the researcher can work, thus personalizing the environment. There are seven different views that create a single pane in the window or some combination of panes. For example, a user may wish to have only the document open (document mode) or have three panes that include the document, reference window, and the Table of Contents (browse mode) open in the window at the same time. The toolbar (top of Figure 11.3) provides shortcut buttons for features available through the menu bar. Each user can personalize the toolbar to include the buttons that that user would most commonly use.

Analysis Work

There are several qualitative data analysis tools that the user will find quite useful and adaptable to a number of different needs and constraints. *Bookmark* is a tool that functions the same way that a bookmark does when reading a book. The user can place a marker at a certain location, for instance where the user stopped working for a session, and name the Bookmark "Stopped Here." Later, the user simply clicks on Bookmark and selects "Stopped Here" to go to that location in the infobase.

As mentioned earlier, highlighters are wonderful ways to code text; the user can pick a number of colors to use for highlighting and the process is like using a pen marker on text that is on paper. *Tagging* and untagging records provides a way to mark (visible as a red vertical line) selected text, usually for some other action, such as printing all references to a concept or term on one document or viewing tagged records together for analysis purposes. A researcher may tag reconciled records, which means that all changes in the master file will appear tagged in the shadow file.

Folio has a powerful *indexing system*; each text unit that is separated by spaces is indexed in the infobase (e.g., every word and number is indexed). This indexing design allows searching on all text, with a rapid search time. In Folio, the user can search the infobase for terms related to concepts or themes that are being developed or are already refined. The user can search for "hits" using the "Query" tool. A hit is an occurrence of a successful query. The user starts this tool by clicking on the Query button on the toolbar. After the user types in the text to search for, Folio shows the hits in a diagram form called a "Results Map" (see Figure 11.4). There are four different Query types available in Folio. The *simple query* finds the number of records in which the search text (natural language) appears. Putting the search term in quotes ("search term") will find text in exactly that form in the text, including capital letters and spaces. Clicking on the "Next" and "Previous" buttons on the toolbar takes the user through every hit identified in the infobase.

In a *combination query*, the user would use one of four conjunctive terms (and, or, exclusive or, not) to conduct a more refined search. An example would be a query for the terms *money* and *time*. The number of hits would be the number of records that contain both the word *money* and the word

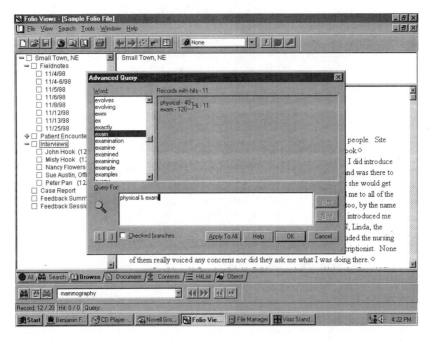

Figure 11.4. Results Map From a Search in Folio Views for the Occurrence of the Terms *Physical* and *Exam* in the Same Record

time. The use of "or" produces a search for all records that have either word in them. With the use of "exclusive or," the hits are records that contain one of the two words but not both words. "Not" is used to separate words that are commonly together, such as "Portland not Maine." The hits with this search would be records that contain the search word and do not contain the "not" word.

Proximity searches include the search term (exact order or any order) and possibly a number; the number indicates the number of intervening words that the user considers acceptable in searching for hits. For example, in a search for content related to "work force," the user may type "work force/4"; this would find all records with both words in it, in that exact order, separated by zero to four words.

A *pattern* or *meaning* query uses certain characters (? and *) as wild cards to search for text. A query for "r?n" will find hits for "run," "ran," "ron," and so on. Other patterns, such as a search for synonyms ($) and word forms (%) are possible with queries in Folio.

These four query types can be limited or refined in another way: by *scope.* If a user has applied grouping to certain text, such as "acute office visit" (visit type), then a search for a term "By Group" will find all records grouped as acute with that term. If a query for the term "Pap" limited the scope to text grouped as acute office visit, then the number of hits would reflect the number of records in which Pap smears were discussed in acute office visits versus chronic visits or health care maintenance visits.

Results of queries can be viewed in the infobase itself or in the Table of Contents view. In the infobase, hits can be followed with the Next button throughout the text; the search term is highlighted for easy viewing. If the hits are viewed in the Table of Contents, the number of hits is indicated to the left of the level.

When the analysis team meets for discussion, each member has the latest version available on his or her computer at the same time, has the advantage of the preliminary coding being completed, and has the individual analysis completed on shadow files; the team can then focus on relevant concepts or sections for analysis. It is not necessary to rely on hard copies of the text to be delivered to team members.

Advanced Features

Folio Views has a set of *links* that allows the user to connect to other locations, objects, or programs. By double clicking on a *Jump Link*, the user will be taken to another location in the infobase; thus double clicking on a Jump Link can reference many points in the infobase referenced to one theme or concept. An *Object Link* establishes a link in the text to an object, such as a photograph. A *Program Link* can take the user to another program, such as Excel® or Access®, for a review of related data.

Some of the advanced features of Folio allow for the importing and exporting of files from other file formats, such as word processing files, flat files, and tables. There is a procedure for enhancing the quality of the files; a user, usually the system administrator, can do a validation check on the integrity of the infobase. There are two processes for reconciling all shadow files with the master file.

The latest substantive versions of Folio Views (4.0 and 4.1) have a number of new features; one of the most appreciated is visual searching and narrowing (checkboxes), which eliminates the need to look up record numbers to print or export. Two new links were added: a *Web Link* type to connect to Web sites via the URL and a *Command Link,* which allows the user to create links within the infobase as well as linking to objects in another infobase. Another release (4.12) was out late in 1998. The exciting new feature in 4.11 is the "Undo" option; other new features are multico-lumn printing, better Query Template support, and an improved installation process.

The ease of use for beginners and the multiple features for sophisticated queries and linking makes Folio Views an asset for qualitative data management and analysis. With each new release adding more features, and now program and Web links, the versatility for analysts in local, regional, national, and international projects is tremendous. There is a time lag involved with new user training and with the facile use of the program; however, it is a tool that can allow the researcher to focus primarily on the task at hand—qualitative analysis—rather than data formats and management.

CONCLUSION

When research teams consider the use of computer programs to assist in data management and interpretation, and certainly when they decide to use a program, particular features of programs will be identified as of greater or lesser importance for their needs. In the preceding pages, we have discussed many currently available tools for the research team. Folio Views currently provides strong organizational and management functions, including features that allow the data to come alive through form and color, as well as links. NUD*IST 4.0 manages data well and supports data interpretation and theory generation at intriguing levels of complexity. NVivo provides many new features in NUD*IST development, and Folio Views is also always under development.

Users of software are constantly asking developers for more—as a result, our data management and interpretation can grow as quickly as our methodological approaches and our expertise will support. As always, the experience and expertise of the research team remains paramount in good qualitative research—but why not try out a new pair of dancing shoes once in a while?

PART
IV

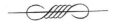

Special Designs

12

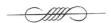

Narrative Approaches
to Qualitative Research
in Primary Care

Jessica H. Muller

N arratives, most simply put, are stories that relate the unfolding of events, human action, or human suffering from the perspective of an individual's lived experience. Stories, although varying in form, are ubiquitous, and storytelling, or narration, is one of the oldest and most significant of human activities (Rubenstein, 1995). It is in the telling and hearing of stories that people disclose, arrange, and make sense of their own experience as well as that of others (Churchill & Churchill, 1982; Gee, 1985). Nowhere is this more apparent than in the world of sickness and clinical practice, where the currency of communication is often the story. Patients tell stories of their illness and how they live with illness over time. Physicians and other health professionals relate stories to each other of patients, their diseases and treatments, and lessons learned. Patients and clinicians together negotiate therapeutic narratives, the stories of treatment. The story of the individual patient—"the case"—is still, despite the reliance of the medicine on scientific theory and generalizable results, an important mechanism for understanding how general scientific knowledge is applied to particular individuals (Brody, 1987; Hunter, 1991).

AUTHOR'S NOTE: I wish to thank Peter Sommers and George Saba for their insights and support, and Robert Bartz, Gay Becker, Molly Cooke, John Mergendoller, and William Miller for their critical comments on earlier drafts of this chapter.

In recent years, more formal study of narrative in medical domains has begun to attract the attention of researchers, teachers, and clinicians. Narrative analysis is an approach to research that takes as its focus narratives—or stories—as a means of representing and interpreting human action and individuals' lived experience. In the last two decades, scholars in various disciplines, finding the assumptions and methods of the scientific paradigm inadequate for explaining much of what goes on in individual or social life, have turned to narrative. Thus narrative studies have emerged in such diverse fields as anthropology, psychology, sociology, education, literary studies, and history[1] and are now beginning to appear in health research (Beeson, 1997). The purpose of this chapter is to introduce narrative study as a research activity, to provide examples of narrative investigations carried out with patients or in clinical and medical education settings, and to discuss the relevance of a narrative approach to qualitative research in primary care.

In this chapter, I use the term *narrative* as both text and method. First, it is employed interchangeably with *story* to refer to the process of storytelling as well as the product—the story itself. Second, I use the term *narrative* to refer to a method of inquiry—a qualitative research approach that solicits and analyzes personal accounts as stories and allows participants to use their own words and categories to describe their life experiences (Gordon & Paci, 1995). Taking the shape of an hourglass, this chapter begins by considering narrative generally as a form of inquiry with its particular theoretical groundings and assumptions. I then address, through examples from published research reports, the kinds of research questions that lend themselves to narrative research, how investigators go about carrying out the research, and how they begin to make sense of the data. Following, I examine in greater depth two narrative studies: a study of women's subjective experience of living with AIDS (Stevens & Tighe Doerr, 1997) and my own study of the construction of clinical stories. I end by discussing some of the benefits of narrative research in primary care.

In taking this approach, this chapter does not consider the use of literature in medical school classes to teach empathy, to raise questions of ethics, or to sensitize students to the patient's perspectives (e.g., Charon, 1994; Charon et al., 1995; Jones, 1997; Trautmann, 1982). Nor does it dwell on the healing function of storytelling (e.g., Brody, 1987; Kleinman, 1988; Remen, 1996; Shapiro, 1993). It also does not discuss the plethora of first-person accounts of illness that have been published in the last decade or so. These autobiographies have become so numerous that they have been given their own name—"pathographies"—and are being studied by literature scholars as a literary genre in their own right (e.g., Couser, 1997; Hawkins, 1993). Although these topics fall into the broad realm of narrative, this chapter focuses specifically on narrative as a research tool.

DIMENSIONS OF NARRATIVE

An underlying premise of narrative thinking is that it provides a way of understanding the world and ordering experience that contrasts with the prevalent positivist scientific paradigm that has characterized so much of modern research and thought (Bruner, 1986; Gordon, 1988). This paradigm, which underlies what we typically refer to as "good science," emphasizes the scientific method, hypothesis testing, quantitative measurement, and the search for objective "truths" with generalizable, predictable, and controllable outcomes (also see Chapter 1). A narrative approach, on the other hand, is firmly grounded in qualitative traditions and stresses the "lived experience" of individuals, the importance of multiple perspectives, the existence of context-bound, constructed social realities, and the impact of the researcher on the research process. The primary dimensions of a narrative approach are delineated in brief below.

First, a narrative approach assumes that people like to storytell, that they organize their significant experiences in terms of stories, and that the telling of stories is a way, perhaps the most basic way, for humans to make meaning of events in their lives. Stories are used to define who we are, to claim an identity. A story reflects individuals' experience as they see it and wish to present it to others (Becker, 1997). It is constructed in that it reflects a person's attempt to revise, select, and order biographical details to give meaning to their life experience (White, 1987). In Brock's (1995) view, we see ourselves as "storied:" "our 'life-narrative' is the story we tell ourselves that knits together our recollected past with a wished-for future, thereby influencing our sense of self in the present" (p. 152). Therefore, its "truth" may be selective in that it does not attempt to represent objective reality; rather, a narrative gives a rich understanding of an individual's sense of his or her reality. A researcher seeks the meaning an individual gives to life events in and through the story being told.

Second, narratives have structural properties of time and plot. Events unfold, following a sequence that is typically, although not always, chronological, in that it has a start, a development, and a "sense of an ending" (Bruner, 1986, p. 21). The story is made up of events that take place sequentially; it is assumed to go somewhere, to have some point or conclusion, even if that point has not yet been reached. People want to know how the story will "turn out." This unfolding of a story over time, in what Ricoeur (1991) calls "narrative time," is a compelling characteristic of storytelling. Moreover, events in a narrative are configured in certain patterns. They are perceived as connected and can only be fully understood as part of the ongoing narrative, not as discrete events occurring in isolation. Events are linked together by the *plot*: "the plot construes significant wholes out of scattered events" (Ricoeur, 1991, p. 106). Thus, actions, events, motives, desires are *emplotted* to make the story (Good, Munakata, Kobayashi, Mattingly, & Good, 1994; Mattingly, 1994), and the plot is developed, embellished, and communicated to the listener through core metaphors, imagery, and rhetorical devices. To understand the meaning of a narrative, a researcher may pay as much attention to these structural aspects of a narrative as to the content itself.

A third dimension of narrative concerns its power to actually shape human conduct as well as to reflect an individual's life experience. The stories Ilongit hunters in the Philippines tell about their hunts not only reflect what actually happened but also depict what the hunters plan to do in future hunts (Rosaldo, 1989). Stories may also be used to produce a moral narrative—how people are supposed to act. Among the Western Apache in the United States, for example, oral narratives are told about the land and events that took place on the land. Although these stories are "about" historical events and their geographical locations, they are also "about" systems of rules and values, about "what it means to *be* an Apache—what it is that being an Apache should normally and properly entail" (Basso, 1984, p. 36). In other words, the stories that are told produce moral narratives about how individuals within that culture are supposed to act. These stories are told, in effect, to edify and alarm social delinquents and, in so doing, to promote compliance with standards for acceptable social behavior. Closer to home, the stories told during hospitals' morbidity and mortality conferences could equally be analyzed for their moral messages about what it means to *be* a doctor.

A fourth characteristic of narrative is its contextual focus. Narratives do not arise by themselves; rather, they are nested within a cultural context. Although narratives are particularistic in that they are the stories of individuals, they also transmit or reflect cultural messages about the nature of reality. For example, they show us how cultural values shape our perceptions of our bodies, how we interpret symptoms, or how to act when we are sick. Moreover, culture influences not only which stories *can* be told but *how* they are told. The presentation and interpretation of experience is guided and shaped by shared cultural understandings. Storytellers learn from popular culture, friends, or family about the structure of narrative, its conventional metaphors and imagery, and standards of what is appropriate and not appropriate to tell. Thus, people tell their own unique stories, but they compose them by adapting the narrative types that a culture makes available. Frank (1995) argues, for example, that three general types of illness narratives are told in American culture, each containing its own plot structure: the *restitution* narrative ("yesterday I was healthy, today I am sick, but tomorrow I will be healthy again"); the *chaos* narrative ("life is never getting any better"); and the *quest* narrative ("illness is the occasion of a journey . . . something is to be gained through this experience"). Although Frank suggests that the restitution narrative is the preferred way of seeing illness among Americans, individuals often use a combination or adaptation of all of the narrative types to tell their particular illness story.

Finally, narratives are relational. Stories are told to others, whether or not the other is actually present (Rubenstein, 1995). Frank (1995) suggests that individuals recount illness narratives as much for their listeners as for themselves because the stories act as "a guide" to others who are ill. Narratives are also frequently produced in conversation: they are not simply "told" by teller to listener but take shape in the interaction between teller and listener. In research interviews, for example, the interviewer is often an active participant in the story-making process through the questions he or she asks and the interpretations made. These are, in turn, responded to and reinterpreted by the narrator. The answers continually inform the evolving conversation; thus, in a reciprocally interpretive process, the narrator and the listener develop the meaning of the story together (Riessman, 1993).

THE NARRATIVE RESEARCH
LANDSCAPE IN MEDICINE

What kinds of questions might be pursued by a primary care researcher interested in narrative? What methods of data collection are used in narrative research? How do narrative researchers analyze their data? This section considers these questions by examining, through illustrative examples drawn from published research accounts, how researchers interested in illness and medical care have engaged in three central research activities—choosing a research question, carrying out the research, and making sense of the research.

Choosing a Research Question

Certain questions or concerns in primary care research lend themselves to a narrative approach. It is especially fruitful if researchers are interested in how people give meaning to events and activities in their lives, how individual stories intersect with larger cultural or political narratives, and how stories are constructed in interactions between individuals. Research questions that have been investigated using a narrative frame fall into two general areas: individuals' illness narratives and clinical stories and interactions.

Much of narrative research in the medical arena focuses on the eliciting and analysis of stories of illness—in particular, the stories of patients with serious illness, chronic disease, or long-term suffering, or what Arthur

Frank (1998) calls the "deeply ill." The researchers carrying out these studies take as their premise that a narrative of sickness or disability is not simply the story of an illness but also the story of a life that is in some way altered by illness (Garro, 1994). A serious illness may represent a disruption in the story we are telling ourselves of our future; it becomes, as Howard Brody (1987) has observed, "a gap in the manuscript" of one's life story. Individuals attempt to make sense of that disruption or "to construct a new map" (Frank, 1995) in the telling of the story of their illness. Thus, the illness narrative, claims Kleinman (1988), is the "story the patient tells, and significant others retell, to give coherence to the distinctive events and long-term course of suffering" (p. 49). It becomes the task of the narrative researcher to examine the "distinctive events" that contribute to individuals' suffering, to see how they manage or make sense of their suffering, or to understand how broader cultural narratives of illness, recovery, or death are interwoven in individual narratives.

Scholars interested in this subjective experience of illness have used narrative methods to explore such questions as, How do people make sense of living daily with severe chronic pain? (e.g., Good, 1994; Kleinman, 1988); How do HIV-infected women respond to the discovery of their disease? (Stevens & Tighe Doerr, 1997); Why do some southern Black women delay treatment for advanced breast cancer? (Mathews, Lannin, & Mitchell, 1994); What are the individual explanatory models of persons who suffer from chronic pain attributed to the temporomandibular joint (TMJ), as well the broader cultural models that shape how they think about their illness? (Garro, 1994); What types of life disruption accompany infertility? (Becker, 1997); How do women live with breast cancer and its treatment through narrative? (Gordon & Paci, 1995); How do elderly patients find meaning after hip fractures? (Borkan, Quirk, & Sullivan, 1991); and How are new practices of genetic testing integrated into narratives of self and family life? (Brock, 1995).

The second area in which scholars have focused their research questions concerns clinical stories and interactions. A few investigators have taken a life history approach, as did Kaufman (1993) in her study of seven elderly physicians, in which she traced transformations spanning the 20th century in medicine, in American society, and in their personal lives. Others have examined clinicians' stories about their practices as narratives. The studies have focused on the construction of treatment plans as narratives (Good, 1995), cross-cultural narratives in the practice of oncology (Good et al., 1994; Gordon & Paci, 1995; Hunt, 1994), the ethical dilemmas faced by primary care physicians in the care of their elderly patients (Kaufman, 1997), or the narrative accounts of practitioners who care for the chronically ill (Kleinman, 1988). Still others have examined the narrative attributes of the case presentation or medical interview. For example, Kathryn

Montgomery Hunter (1991) studied physicians' use of narrative in the rituals of medical practice and in medical education, Cheryl Mattingly (1998) investigated what constitutes narrative talk among occupational therapists, and Manning and Cullum-Swan (1994) compared the formal "externally formatted" narrative of the medical interview or the case presentation to the wandering, expressive "self-formatted" personal narratives of patients.

Taking a different perspective, some researchers have formulated their research questions to focus on clinician-patient or clinician-clinician encounters. At issue here is the process by which stories are produced and negotiated in interactions between individuals, where together teller and listener create a "text." For example, interactions between oncologists and their patients have been analyzed in narrative form (Good, 1995; Good et al., 1994; Hunt, 1994), as have the interactions between brain-damaged patients and their occupational therapists (Mattingly, 1994). In the area of medical education, Ventres (1994) used narrative case reports of residents' interviews with patients to ascertain differences between patients' and physicians' perspectives; Shafer and Fish (1994) sought patients' stories in writing as a means of exploring how narratives could be used "to glimpse the world of the patient" for physicians in training.

Carrying Out the Research

To carry out their investigations, narrative researchers use many of the same sampling procedures and data collection techniques as other qualitative researchers. The research question is the primary guide to sample selection. To carry out a narrative research project, investigators may select a sample from clinical settings (e.g., Mattingly, 1994; Stevens & Tighe Doerr, 1997), from their own practices or teaching settings (e.g., Ventres, 1994), or from the community (e.g., Garro, 1994; Kaufman, 1997). Alternatively, they may choose to focus on a subset of subjects from a larger qualitative study or a study that is epidemiological in focus (e.g., Good, 1994; Gordon & Paci, 1995). Sometimes researchers may reanalyze existing data using a narrative frame. Becker (1997), for instance, did not initially set out to do a narrative study but later reexamined her interviews for their narrative content and structure. Sample sizes tend to be small: for example, 35 participants solicited from chronic disease support groups (Garro, 1994); 50 primary care physicians, selected by a snowball sampling technique from the community (Kaufman, 1997); or 38 low-income HIV-infected women, obtained through community-based purposive sampling (Stevens & Tighe-Doerr, 1997).

Although narrative research employs many of the same data collection strategies that are found in other qualitative research, the most common is probably the audiotaped and transcribed in-depth interview (see Chapter 5), a method that works particularly well for exploring individuals' subjective experience of illness. It is appropriate because the elicitation of individuals' stories takes time; stories usually do not emerge all at once in a linear, chronological order but meander, backtrack, jump ahead, or digress. Interviews, either one of substantial length or several interviews over time, allow the researcher to follow this meandering path of the story. These interviews may be either semistructured or unstructured, although many narrative researchers prefer an open-ended conversational style— starting with an open-ended question followed by probes—that allows the narrator ample opportunity to speak with his or her own voice.

Some researchers use a combination of written personal accounts and interviews as data collection strategies. For example, written accounts were collected by researchers in two clinical education studies. Interested in clarifying differences in the perspectives of house staff and their hospitalized patients, Ventres (1994) had residents talk to patients with whom they had problems communicating and write a narrative account of what they found. Using an open-ended interview format, he also interviewed residents about why they believed the problems existed. He then compared the two accounts and concluded that analysis of narrative case reports can be used to improve relationships with patients and to facilitate student and resident recognition of physician-patient communication issues. Shafer and Fish (1994) also elicited patients' stories in writing so that residents could read about their patients' experiences in the hospital. Their purpose was twofold: to analyze generated texts for content and themes that could provide insight into the phenomenon of hospitalization for surgery and to evaluate the pedagogical use of narrative for encouraging self-reflection and empathy in the hospital setting.

Making Sense of the Research

To analyze narratives, researchers treat the told stories, dialogues, or interactions as a type of text that can be interpreted and analyzed (Ricoeur, 1984). Once the data are in text form, they can be analyzed with various qualitative analysis schemes, depending on the goal of the analysis and the personal preferences of the researcher. Generally, the process of analysis includes the following steps. The first step is *entering the text,* either through the application of a preestablished coding scheme or by sifting and sorting the text to identify categories most pertinent to the research question. Once the researcher has entered the text, the process of *sense-making,* or finding connections and relationships in the data, begins. These links are not made through statistical manipulation of variables but from successive readings, critical reflection, and persistent immersion in the text.

The emphasis here is on discovery of themes and patterns in the texts. The third step consists of *verifying* or *confirming*, to achieve internal consistency of interpretation and to search for alternative explanations, disconfirming evidence, or negative cases. Finally, the researcher *represents an account* of what has been learned in the researching process. Although this process sounds linear, it is in reality more spiral in shape, as the researcher repeatedly immerses him- or herself in, and then steps back from, the data at various points in the research process (for a fuller account of the analysis process, see Chapter 7).

What distinguishes narrative analysis is its focus on the broad contours of a story. This contrasts with other types of qualitative research that may fracture the text by generalizing from pieces of data taken out of context (Riessman, 1993). Narrative researchers are, as I indicated earlier, not only interested in the content of a narrative but in its structure as well. They examine the informant's story to see how it is put together and what linguistic and cultural resources it draws on. Analysis includes different readings of the texts. First, each story is read for its content and underlying structural properties. Second, each story is read for its movement and plot development over time—its beginning, its middle, and its resolution (or lack thereof). Third, all stories are compared to find commonalities and differences in experience across individuals and to identify patterns in story plots. The goal is to keep intact, as much as possible, the context of each story, its sequential and structural features, and the consequences of events for each individual. Throughout, the process is an interpretive one—the narrators interpret or reconstruct events or their illness experience; the researcher interprets the narrators' stories and then reinterprets the stories in a text generated for a broader audience.

TWO NARRATIVE STUDIES

I turn now to an in-depth discussion of two research reports to examine in more detail how different narrative studies are carried out. One is a study of HIV-infected women by P. E. Stevens and B. Tighe Doerr, and the other is a study I carried out of the co-construction of student and teacher narratives in an ambulatory care clinic. Each study is examined in light of the research question, carrying out the research, and making sense of the research.

The Trauma of Discovery

The Research Question. As part of a larger investigation of women's experiences living with HIV, the study reported by Stevens and Tighe Doerr (1997) was informed by three research questions: What are women's

theorists on the workings of plot, Mattingly (1994) describes a process by which clinicians, in her case occupational therapists, "actively struggle to shape therapeutic events into a coherent form organized by a plot" (p. 811). She claims that these therapists create, out of the ordinary actions and interactions in therapy sessions, meaningful treatment stories for their brain-damaged patients. Through these therapeutic narratives—of hard work, rehabilitation, a sense of future—therapists solicit patients' participation in the therapy. In other words, clinicians "emplot" their actions, as well as the actions of patients, by seeing those actions as part of a larger therapeutic story they are attempting to carry out. I wanted to see if similar social processes occurred in teaching settings. Was there a process of story construction, and if so, what form did it take?

Carrying Out the Research. Research was conducted in a family practice center in an inner city public general hospital, one of the primary teaching sites for third- and fourth-year medical students participating in an 8-week required family medicine clerkship. A "consultation" model of one-to-one teaching is employed in this setting, where the medical student, who has the primary relationship with the patient, first sees the patient and then "presents" patient data to the attending physician, or consultant, while the patient is waiting. The student then completes the patient care visit.

An opportunistic sampling strategy was used to recruit six fourth-year students (three men and three women) for the study, all of whom participated in the fall clerkships at the family practice center in 1992 and 1993. Six physicians who attended in the center were also recruited according to the following criteria: a minimum of 5 years' teaching experience in this setting, consistently positive evaluations of their teaching from medical students, and a demonstrated commitment to ambulatory care teaching. Of the six teachers (five men and one woman), four were family physicians and two were internists, and all were core teaching faculty in the medical school's department of family and community medicine. Each attending physician was paired with a student with whom he or she had had at least one prior teaching encounter.

The methodology used for data collection consisted of videotaped observations and interviews. First, one teaching consultation for each of the six student-physician pairs was videotaped. I then interviewed each teacher and student individually while watching the videotape, as soon as possible after the consultation. Using an adaptation of the "stimulated recall" method (Calderhead, 1981), I encouraged each participant to stop the tape at any point to reflect on his or her observations. I also asked open-ended questions to solicit participants' comments on the consultation, their recollections of their thought processes and actions during the consultation, and their general beliefs, goals, and practices regarding one-to-one clinical teaching. These interviews were also videotaped, and both sets of videotapes were transcribed.

Making Sense of the Research. The data were analyzed according to two analytic schemes. Analysis was first conducted in an iterative process using the "grounded theory" method (Strauss & Corbin, 1990). After initially viewing the videotapes of both the consultation and the interviews for each student-physician pair, the researchers coded the transcripts and formed a preliminary set of thematic categories involving student and teacher beliefs, thought processes, and practices. As the analysis progressed, these categories were revised and refined until a final coding scheme was established. The data for each student and each physician were then analyzed; in addition, a cross-set analysis was completed to identify the beliefs and practices common to the group of students and the group of teachers. At each step of this process, agreement was reached among the researchers regarding the definition of the coding categories and their applications to the data under consideration.

The data were then reanalyzed using a multistaged narrative analysis procedure. First, I read through the transcripts of the interviews and teaching consultation of each student-physician pair for general content, with these initial questions being asked of the data: What are the stories being told here? How are they created and negotiated in the interaction between medical student and teacher? Second, the stories generated from the student's presentation and ensuing interactions between student and teacher were marked in each transcript and analyzed for their structural elements. I then analyzed the stories for their plot development over time and identified themes that could provide insight into the process of story construction. Finally, the stories and the process of story construction were interpreted within the larger cultural framework of medical training.

I illustrate this process with a discussion of one case taken from the research.

Case Presentation[2]

Nancy, a fourth-year student, comes into the consultation room and sits down across from the attending physician, Dr. Howard, who begins the teaching encounter with, "OK, what you got?" With these familiar words he invites the student to be the teller of the patient's tale. Well-rehearsed in her student role, Nancy slips easily into the opening words of the presentation: "This is a 65-year-old Filipino woman who . . . comes into

Acute Care with a complaint of left-sided chest pain and epigastric pain for about a week." [this patient is coming into the clinic for an acute problem; because this is an unscheduled visit, she cannot see her regular doctor].

Moving quickly through the history of the patient's present illness, Nancy explains that the woman's pain is always associated with activity, such as lifting heavy boxes, doing housework, or dancing, and that it goes away with rest. The woman was seen a few months earlier for low abdominal pain but has not experienced chest pain before. Nancy then notes that the woman's husband had died a few years earlier, and since then she seems to have had multiple somatic complaints, as well as a diagnosis of depression, noted in her chart. She adds that the woman appears lonely and is worried that her new pain will keep her from her only pleasure—dancing at the senior center.

After asking a few questions about the patient's depression, Dr. Howard reminds the student that this is an acute care visit and asks her what she thinks she needs to focus on today. Nancy replies that she doesn't think there is anything acute to worry about. The results of her physical exam were unremarkable, and the patient's EKG, which Nancy had reviewed earlier with the attending, was normal. She concludes that the woman probably strained a muscle but adds that there is definitely a psychosocial component as well. "She, you know, has a lot of sadness in her life, and I think that we need to address that at some point." She goes on to say that she will write a note for the woman's primary doctor to "consider antidepressants and definitely some counseling." For the immediate pain, she will recommend Tylenol, relaxing, and maybe some ice or heat.

Dr. Howard quickly asks Nancy if she has any other thoughts about what might be going on before she gets to her plan for treatment. In one form or another, he repeats this question three times in the next few minutes. In turn, she mentions the possibilities of an ulcer, a gastric cancer, or a pelvic cancer. Finally, the attending asks her more pointedly if she would think about anything vascular. She acknowledges cardiac pain should be considered, but that it is lower on her list of differential diagnoses.

When Dr. Howard asks Nancy for the first diagnosis in her differential, she returns to the subject of psychosocial causes and depression:

> I think it's more psychosocial than anything. I think she's depressed and she has somatic complaints. . . . I don't want to say they are not real. They're there, but I think they're intensified because she's worried. . . . I think that's number one. And the other thing, I think, is that she might have strained it, her abdominal muscles.

At this point Dr. Howard suggests another reading of the patient's story:

But pain with activity that goes away with rest in a 65-year-old woman, the first thing that I would be concerned about in terms of serious things that you don't want to overlook would be atypical angina or some kind of cardiovascular issue, even though her EKG is normal. . . So all these other things are going on, but that would be the thing I'd be most concerned about.

In the final few moments of the consultation, Dr. Howard and the student devise a plan of action that the student will then take back to the patient. Dr. Howard summarizes:

I think that's what you can tell her. I think what you can say is that you think it's mostly strain. Maybe it started from lifting these heavy boxes and then it's exacerbated by this dancing. . . . I think that's the trick—helping her find the things she can do without getting the symptoms. But if they do recur, especially with any frequency, she should not wait for this appointment. She should come in sooner. I think that's the overall message you want to give without terrifying her.

Case Discussion

Analysis of this teaching encounter shows that the initial narrative produced in this interaction is the student's construction of the patient's story. In her opening sentence, Nancy introduces the main character, the setting, and the beginnings of a plot. Elaborating a particular diagnostic story, she dwells on the patient's social history and uses this information to construct a narrative of depression, with a subplot of muscle strain, for which she suggests a treatment of antidepressants, counseling, and Tylenol.

The attending, however, hints that the student's effort at story making is not particularly persuasive. He continues to ask her, "Is there anything else to think about?" This repeated verbal intervention suggests that he thinks the student may be missing the main plot of the story completely. When he finally tells Nancy, "this is what I would be concerned about," Dr. Howard invites her to emplot a different story, to move from the portrayal of a patient afflicted with depression and muscle strain to an alternative narrative—one with a cardiac etiology.

At this point, the teacher and student have created during the interaction two competing plots to explain the patient's symptoms—two side-by-side texts. So what happens at this juncture? Dr. Howard assumes the role of conarrator of the patient's narrative. Building on the student's story, he emplots a sequence of actions for the patient to follow, into which are interwoven two subplots. The first—a plot of muscle pain—proposes a hopeful ending: If it is muscle pain, the patient will rest and do muscle strengthening exercises until the pain gets better. The second plot, however, is potentially more sobering. If the pain continues, it may, in fact, be atypical angina, and the patient needs to return to the clinic soon for further tests and medication. The attending does not include depression in this reconstructed narrative; apparently it is not enough of a concern for him to warrant its inclusion as a third plot.

As the narrative of the whole teaching encounter unfolds, the attending physician is seen to make a number of narrative turns that are directed to set two concurrent stories in motion. The first, as we have seen earlier, revolves around the "right" therapeutic story for this patient. He apparently does not believe the woman to be in imminent danger, as he does not simply reject the student's story outright and replace it with another, more emergent one—that of a potentially serious cardiovascular problem that demands immediate medical attention. Rather, he "emplots" future actions over time and structures multiple endings into the treatment story, giving the narrative a direction but leaving the outcomes open.

The second story set in motion encompasses a story of teaching. The attending physicians who work in this environment are teachers, as well as physicians. One of their tasks is to assess not only the content of the patient's story as it is told by students, but also how students construct the story itself. They listen to students' presentations for structure and plot as well as for coherency, comprehensiveness, and completeness. In the postconsultation interview, Dr. Howard reveals his concern that this student "gets stuck in psychosocial data" rather than dealing with medical issues and in this case had prematurely arrived at a diagnosis of depression. Thus interwoven with the treatment story for the patient is a teaching story for the student. Through the process of narrativization, he demonstrates how to produce a story that puts disease into the foreground and that classifies patients and their illnesses so that they become the appropriate focus of medical attention. At the same time, he illustrates the very process of story construction in medical culture—how to make sense of a patient's symptoms, how to devise an appropriate plot, how to think about a sequence of future actions, and how to direct a treatment toward "a sense of ending" without prematurely cutting off other possible outcomes.

This example illustrates how teaching encounters of this nature are narratively organized. Indeed, they embody multiple narrative processes. Students build a story from a patient's words and body, shape it into the standardized categories of the medical account, and then present—and represent—the patient's initiating presentation of body and self (Hunter, 1991). Together, attending physicians and students revise and reshape a patient's therapeutic narrative in an attempt to give coherence to a succession of clinical data. At the same time, teachers use these narratives to facilitate instruction in the very process of narrative construction. In much the same way as the Apache narratives dictate a course of action, the teachers' narratives set out a particular path for students to follow in how to think about patients, how to create a clinical story, and how to emplot a patient's therapeutic future. The analysis of unfolding narratives in clinical teaching allows us to examine what is highlighted and diminished in teacher-student talk. Employing a narrative frame reveals how stories about patients are culturally shaped and given particular meanings between clinicians and how they are packaged and presented back to patients.

CONCLUSION

The study of narratives can be an informative and valuable approach in primary care research. As demonstrated above, narrative research is a useful way of examining clinical encounters. Investigating the process of story construction in interactions gives us information about how medical knowledge is produced and reproduced in clinical situations. It can also illustrate the multiple perspectives involved in patient care and facilitate recognition of physician-patient communication issues.

Moreover, narrative analysis offers one response to the mandate set by Miller and Crabtree (1994a) for clinical qualitative researchers: "to join, listen to and speak what Mishler (1984) calls the 'voice of the lifeworld' " (p. 342). The biomedical model is built on a framework of positivism, therapeutic imperative, technological interventions, and explicit informa- tion gathering/decision making, but the realities of patient care reveal uncertainty and particularity. Eliciting illness stories is one way to grasp the nature of these realities. Patients' narrative accounts teach powerful lessons about the lives of sick people: narratives disclose how individuals restruc- ture and make sense of their lives as they struggle to meet the challenges brought on by chronic illness; they show how patients weave the story of their sickness into their larger, ongoing life story; they provide metaphors for understanding the experience of illness. Narratives also do more than simply convey the effect of illness on individuals' lives. By focusing on shared cultural understandings, researchers can transcend particular life histories to represent cultural models that give us information about groups of people and how they respond to illness and treatment.

Finally, narrative analysis provides a way of thinking about patients. What kind of story is the patient telling? What is its plot line? What metaphors do patients use to describe their illness? Where do patients place themselves in their story? Stories need a listener. Attending to the stories patients use to reveal the meanings they attach to their own suffering becomes a critical part of the clinical task. Telling and listening to stories can help in the process of healing, thereby complementing the biomedical emphasis on curing (Brody, 1987; Kleinman, 1988). It is the work of physicians not only to restore patients' health but to help patients "restory" their illness. Narrative research is a compelling way to capture the understanding and practices of physicians and patients.

NOTES

1. See, for example, Becker (1997), Good (1994), Gordon and Paci (1995), Kleinman (1988), Mattingly (1994, 1998), and Rosaldo (1989) in anthropology; Riessman (1993) in sociology; Bruner (1986) in psychology; Clandinin and Connelly (1995) in education; Couser (1997) and Ricoeur (1984, 1991) in literary studies; and White (1987) in history.

2. All names are pseudonyms.

13

Using Videotapes in Qualitative Research

Virginia Elderkin-Thompson
Howard Waitzkin

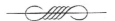

In the 1960s, recording technology made its debut as a research method in a clinical setting. Korsch and colleagues recorded the interaction between pediatricians, children, and their families in an emergency clinic (Freemon, Negrete, Davis, & Korsch, 1971; Korsch, Freemon, & Negrete, 1971; Korsch, Gozzi, & Francis, 1968). Korsch appreciated the importance of skillful communication, and she saw the potential in recordings for examining the quality of that communication. Today, conventional videotaping has become an important tool in nondiagnostic situations such as collecting data for analysis of interpersonal communication, providing the delivery vehicle for an intervention, or creating a permanent record for the evaluation of a program. After giving a quick overview of some research in these three areas, we will offer both precautions about pitfalls to be avoided and suggestions for procedures to increase the reliability and validity of videotaping projects. Because our experience lies in research of the personal interaction during physician-patient communication, we will focus on videotaping the medical encounter, but the ideas also have relevance for any videotaping project in a clinical setting.

Videotaped Data in Communication Research

Following the pattern set by earlier researchers using audiotaped encounters, many videotaped studies use a content analysis of the verbal

239

interaction between physicians and patients. The Roter Interaction Analysis System (RIAS) is a well-known method of content analysis (Roter, 1977) that has been used to investigate the relationship between clinical communication and such outcomes as ratings of satisfaction (Roter, Stewart, et al., 1997), malpractice suits (Levinson, Roter, Mullooly, Dull, & Frankel, 1997), patient health (Hall, Roter, Milburn, & Daltroy, 1996; Wissow, Roter, & Wilson, 1994), prescribing of psychotropic medications (Sleath, Svarstad, & Roter, 1997), and the association between gender and length of encounter (Roter, Lipkin, & Korsgaard, 1991). The scale has also pointed toward an interesting contradiction. Primary care physicians who use education and humor have fewer malpractice suits than physicians who do not, but the situation is reversed among surgeons (Levinson, Roter, et al., 1997).

The primary advantage of videotapes over audiotapes is the availability of nonverbal behavior for additional analysis. Nonverbal behaviors that indicate openness and interpersonal concern—head nods, open posture, or eye contact—have correlated with patient satisfaction in a number of studies (Bensing & Dronkers, 1992; DiMatteo, Prince & Hays, 1986a, 1986b; DiMatteo, Taranta, Friedman & Prince, 1980; Harrigan & Rosenthal, 1986). Despite the early expectations that physicians' nonverbal behavior might predict patients' satisfaction, correlational studies continued to produce disappointingly low results. Sociolinguists suggested that establishing the function of an utterance or behavior within the social context in which it occurs (as well as its meaning) might produce more significant results (Bruner, 1990; Edwards, 1997; Potter, 1996). Thus a behavior might have little predictive power individually, but it could operate within a more powerful constellation of behaviors that accomplishes a specific interactional function, such as the creation of affiliation, intimacy, or dominance (Patterson, 1983; Street, 1990; Street & Buller, 1987; Street, Mulack, & Weimann, 1988). If both physician and patient draw on the same constellation of behaviors to convey a function—affiliation, for example—their nonverbal styles are considered congruent, or in interactional *synchrony* (Koss & Rosenthal, 1997; Street, 1990; Tickle-Degnen & Rosenthal, 1990). Unfortunately, synchrony alone has not proven to be a reliable predictor of patient satisfaction either (Koss & Rosenthal, 1997). Nonverbal communication may function primarily as a modulator of other dimensions of the communication, such as the perception of technical competence or concern, with an indirect influence on satisfaction or compliance.

Recent research is integrating both verbal and nonverbal behaviors of patients to determine how they might influence the physicians' perceptions of the patients' illness narratives or the development of affective functions. The combined verbal-nonverbal message is referred to as the *metamessage,* and it represents a more powerful communicative channel than the additive value of its components would suggest. Unexpectedly, Girón and colleagues discovered that only a combination of verbal and nonverbal behaviors on the part of the *physicians* predicted their ability to identify emotional disorders in primary care patients (Girón, Manjón-Arce, Puerto-Barber, Sánches-García & Gómez-Beneyto, 1998). Identifying the relationship between nonverbal behaviors and diagnostic outcomes is not a straightforward problem.

The American Medical Association Task Force of the Council on Ethical and Judicial Affairs (1991) reported in the *Journal of the American Medical Association* that women are more often misdisagnosed and have less access to aggressive treatment than men. The most common reason cited by the task force for the errors was the attribution of women's symptoms to "overanxiousness." Clinical reviews and experimental studies also show women with higher rates of misdiagnoses for mental health problems than men after controlling for the higher epidemiological rates of emotional disorders among women (Badger et al., 1994; Bernstein, 1981; Redman, Webb, Hennrikus, Gordon, & Sanson-Fisher, 1991). The problem may corroborate feminist interpretations of the corrosive effect of an unequal power relationship on communication during encounters (Davis, 1988; Foster, 1989; Henley, 1977; Irish & Hall, 1995; Nathanson, 1975; West, 1984).

We suggest an alternative explanation for future research: physicians may have more difficulty determining the role of affect in women's symptom presentations than in men's, particularly in the early stages of patient management (Elderkin-Thompson & Waitzkin, 1999). In an experimental study, two groups of randomly assigned internists were shown one of two silent videotapes with identically scripted dialogue of cardiac symptoms in subtitles. One videotape featured the actress as a businesswoman and the other as an affectively expressive ("histrionic") woman. After viewing the videotapes, the physicians differed widely in their assessment of the problem. After viewing the patients' positive laboratory results, the physicians still differed markedly in their decisions to pursue a cardiac work-up: 93% who saw the videotape of the business-woman recommended a cardiac work-up, but only 53% who saw the emotional woman's videotape recommended a work-up (Birdwell, Herbers, & Kroenke, 1993). It appears that the emotional woman's manner of communicating was more germane to the diagnosis by a significant proportion of the internists than her symptomatology. If this interpretation is corroborated with replicated research, then the differing decisions regarding cardiac work-ups could be better explained with the well-established social psychological theory of attribution, which focuses on interpreting behavior

(Kelley, 1967), than with medical decision-making theories of probabilistic inference. What behaviors are associated with physicians' perceptions of "overanxiousness" and whether the behaviors represent a stable gender difference in communicative behaviors, an accurate indicator of anxiousness, or an inaccurate perception on the part of physicians is unknown.

Videotapes as Interventions

Nielsen and Sheppard (1988) reviewed the use of videotapes for delivering an intervention and found videotapes to be as effective as other presentational methods and more effective than the print medium. For example, clinicians applied Bandura's (1977) social learning theory to a videotaped preparation for children awaiting surgery. Puppets or peers modeled ways that the children could react to the situation to minimize their anxiety and pain (Faust & Melamed, 1984; McCue, 1980; Melamed & Siegel, 1975; Melamed, Yurcheson, Fleece, Hutcherson, & Hawes, 1978; Padilla et al., 1981; Peterson, Schultheis, Ridley-Johnson, Miller, & Tracy, 1984; Vernon, 1974; Vernon & Bailey, 1974). Although children still needed additional personal instruction and reinforcement from caregivers (Twardosz, Weddle, Borden, & Stevens, 1986), the information in the videotapes was sufficient to alleviate parents' concerns (Plavin, 1988).

Again using social learning theory, adults with chronic diseases were taught how to increase their daily functioning by watching similarly diagnosed patients who modeled ways to control their diseases (Marshall, Rothenberger, & Bunnell, 1984; Moldofsky, Broder, Davies, & Leznoff, 1979; Pace et al., 1983; Ward, Garlant, Paterson, Bone, & Hicks, 1984). A side effect of increased control can be an improvement in physiological indicators. In two groups of diabetic patients, one that received an intervention using videotapes and one whose members received usual patient care from their physicians, significantly greater improvement was seen in the intervention group in dietary behavior and serum cholesterol levels after 6 months, although glucose levels remained similar (Glasgow, Lachance, et al., 1997; Glasgow, Toobert, & Hampson, 1996). However, when longer time frames are included, intervention groups do not maintain their original advantage. For example, asthma patients who viewed an educational videotape lost their initial advantage by the 16-month follow-up evaluation (Moldofsky et al., 1979). If reinforcements and individualized instruction are incorporated into the intervention protocol, the advantage appears more likely to be retained (Greenfield, Kaplan, Ware, Yano, & Frank, 1988; Parrish & Babbitt, 1991). Possibly, clinical or quality of life outcomes could be improved among chronic care patients if a series of videotapes was developed in which the material increased gradually or provided sequential milestones for self-reinforcement.

Community health interventions have had some success with videotaped material (Klafta & Roizen, 1996; Rigg, 1979), but the context of the intervention should be considered. For example, two groups of mothers of young children were instructed via an educational videotape on the recognition of acute respiratory distress, a major killer of children under 5 years old. One group observed the videotape in a pediatrician's office and one group in a community setting. Mothers in the two settings remembered different aspects of the intervention, indicating that the setting in which a videotape is observed modulates the information that becomes salient to the observer (Ryan, Martinez, & Pelto, 1996).

Videotapes as an Evaluation Method

Occasionally, video recordings are used to evaluate the delivery of health care services. Videotapes of patients being managed for airway obstruction uncovered numerous performance deficiencies that decreased patient safety, and the videotapes informed the staff as to the contexts in which the deficiencies occurred (Mackenzie, Jefferies, Hunter, Bernhard, & Xiao, 1996). A similar videotaping project identified the reasons and contexts for nonusage of barriers for blood-borne pathogens (DiGiacomo et al., 1997). A videotaped study of children undergoing oncology treatments found nonpharmacologic ways in which parents and nurses can decrease the children's pain by increasing emotional support (Naber, Halstead, Broome, & Rehwaldt, 1995). One of our recent studies involved determining under what conditions bilingual nurses acting as translators make translation errors that are not rectified, and, on the other hand, how some nurse-physician teams avoid translation errors (Elderkin-Thompson, Silver, & Waitzkin, 1998c).

The most long-standing and common evaluative use of videotaping occurs in physician training programs, where the tapes provide real-time data for monitoring the acquisition of technical and interviewing skills by medical students, interns, and residents (Cassata, Conroy, & Clements, 1977; Enelow, Adler, & Wexler, 1970; Fuller & Manning, 1973; Gordon, Saunders, Hennrikus, & Sanson-Fisher, 1992; Ivey, 1971; Junek, Burra, & Leichner, 1979; Kahn, Cohen, & Jason, 1979; Pangaro, Worth-Dickstein, Macmillan, Klass, & Shatzer, 1997; Roter, Cole, Kern, Barker, & Grayson, 1990; Roter, Hall, & Katz, 1987). In addition to studying dialogue, medical students and residents can improve their ability to decipher simulated patients' nonverbal affect and formulate questions to address that affect (Doblin & Klamen, 1997). An evaluation of three training techniques for residents—observing attendings during encounters but no formal training, reading about interviewing, or receiving feedback from videotapes of their own encounters—found that residents who were provided with critical feedback on their own videotaped encounters improved in interviewing skills more than did the other groups (Quirk & Babineau, 1982). However, to overcome residents' hesitancy about being video recorded, a program that is nonthreatening, nonjudgmental, and learner oriented is less stressful for the residents and more likely to enlist their participation (Cassata et al., 1977; Edwards et al., 1996).

As with what has been demonstrated in interventions for patients, residents show enhanced short-term skill development if exposed to video-tapes of mentors (Adler, Ware, & Enelow, 1970; Branch, 1990). Also, as with patients, the degree of improvement increases if the videotapes are augmented with individualized instruction and role playing to provide additional reinforcement and modeling (Curry & Makoul, 1996; Roter, Stewart, et al., 1997). This combination has been successfully used to increase residents' confidence and to develop skill levels for psychosocial counseling (Gordon et al., 1992; Roter, Cole, et al., 1990; Wagstaff, Schreier, Shuenyane, & Ahmed, 1990), diagnostic ability (Del Mar & Isaacs, 1992), and breaking bad news to patients or their families (Cushing & Jones, 1995; Faulkner, Argent, Jones, & O'Keeffe, 1995).

Despite the widespread acceptance and agreement that videotaped reviews increase effective use of targeted communication skills, there is little data available to determine the degree to which acquisition of these skills makes long-term changes in the residents' communication with patients or in patient outcomes. An evaluation of videotapes of residents who had undergone training in giving distressing news found that residents warned patients and gave information at the patient's pace, but only 5% of the residents were able to pull the pieces together at the end of the discussion (Faulkner et al., 1995). On the other hand, in a controlled field trial, Roter and colleagues evaluated physicians' ability to address patients' emotional distress. The video-trained physicians used more emotion-handling skills, elicited more psychosocial problems, and engaged in more strategies for managing emotional problems with actual patients than did untrained physicians (Roter, Cole, et al., 1990; Roter, Hall, et al., 1995). Rigorous independent follow-up evaluations of videotaped training programs remain scarce, however, because videotaping is so widely accepted that control groups who are exposed to other training procedures are difficult to assemble. Generally, residents support the use of videotaping, particularly when feedback is combined with mentor modeling and peer discussions (Del Mar & Isaacs, 1992; Edwards et al., 1996; Wagstaff et al., 1990).

Physicians' impressions are that the changes in their interviewing and inter-personal skills are maintained over the long term (Edwards et al., 1996).

VIDEOTAPING PROJECTS

During our recent National Institute of Mental Health study (Waitzkin & Silver, 1992), we examined somatization among primary care patients. Somatizing patients repeatedly present physicians with symptoms for which no organic etiology can be found (*DSM-IV,* 1994). According to the psychodynamic theory, somatization is a defense mechanism for the release of suppressed emotional conflict that is outside of patients' awareness. The release then manifests as a disturbance in the functioning of one or more physiological systems (Barker, Burton, & Zieve, 1991; Berry & Penne-baker, 1993; Kiecolt-Glaser & Glaser, 1985; Malatesta & Culver, 1992; National Advisory Mental Health Council, 1985; Pennebaker & Traue, 1992). The main channel for communicating affect is the nonverbal, so we reasoned that if somatizers are suppressing emotion, they would be likely to show a general inhibition of nonverbal behavior. If somatizers do inhibit nonverbal behavior, the inhibition could be used diagnostically as a "marker" of possible somatization. Furthermore, we suspected that the emotional origin of the symptoms would disrupt somatizing patients' organization of their illness narratives because the symptoms would not have a clear onset or context (Elderkin-Thompson, 1996). Our methodology required all patients to complete a structured interview prior to their encounters to determine if they met criteria for somatization (Escobar, Rubio-Stipec, Canino, & Karno, 1989). Next, we videotaped the patients during their medical encounters so that we could examine whether the verbal and nonver-bal behaviors differed between somatizing and nonsomatizing patients.

The results showed that somatizing patients were more nonverbally inhibited than nonsomatizing patients, and the effect was large enough to be noticeable to a knowledgeable observer (Elderkin-Thompson, Silver, & Waitzkin, 1998b). Additionally, the affective suppression appeared to compromise the patients' ability to organize their narratives in cause-and-effect sequences, to establish time frames around their symptoms, and to communicate affect in a credible fashion (Elderkin-Thompson, Silver, & Waitzkin, 1998a). Affect was typically communicated with an incongruent combination of lexical hyperbole and prosodic or gestural inhibition; for example, an extreme description of pain might be spoken in a hushed voice without accompanying gestures. The incongruency of the two channels (i.e., verbal and nonverbal) suggested that patients who were unable to express their affect nonverbally attempted to use verbal hyperbole to compensate for their deficit.

Initiating Your Own Videotaping Project

As a first step in undertaking a videotaping project, we recommend assembling a physician panel to oversee the project's implementation and to lend scientific credibility to the research. Senior physicians and residents are more likely to participate in projects that are being monitored by a respected physician panel (Levinson, Dull, Roter, Chaumeton, & Frankel, 1998). If a panel has been created, residents have some confidence that their supervisory personnel will not be reviewing the videotaped encounters without their awareness and permission. Third, sampling strategies that require the selection of "typical" encounters are problematic for all researchers, but particularly for nonphysicians. If there is no supervisory relationship between panel members and participating physicians, the physician panel can help select the "typical" encounters or determine if randomly selected tapes contain relevant material. Mishler, Clark, Ingelfinger, and Simon (1989) used an independent physician panel to select those encounters that represented typical primary care encounters even though the researchers were themselves physicians. If one disease is being focused on, such as diabetes or coronary artery disease, an expert in that disorder would be an asset to the panel. Finally, the physician panel can help the recruitment effort by anticipating potential barriers to participation (Levinson, Dull, et al., 1998).

Some type of screen for mental health disorders is advisable. We discovered that depressed, dysthymic, or traumatized women were more likely to participate in a videotaping project than were nondepressed, nondysthymic, or nontraumatized women. Among men, no difference was found. We administered the Comprehensive International Diagnostic Interview, a long, structured questionnaire, before the encounters that we videotaped to identify the most common emotional disorders in primary care populations. We could then control for them in our analyses. Shorter but less reliable measures such as the Medical Outcome Study (MOS) Short-Form General Health Survey or the Primary Care Evaluation of Mental Disorders (PRIME-MD) allow assessment of physical and social functioning and mental health status in approximately 10 minutes, but they must be administered by the attending physician (Spitzer et al., 1994; Stewart, Hays, & Ware, 1988).

After methodological issues have been decided, it is time to approach the staff to gain their cooperation. Despite support by senior staff, we found physicians to be the most reluctant of all staff members to participate (Baird & Gillies, 1993; Del Mar & Isaacs, 1992; Edwards et al., 1996). Clinicians are aware of the importance of communication in securing complete data and cooperation from the patient, yet many have reservations about their communication skills and fear that the videotapes will reflect unfavorably on their skill level (Alexander, Knox, & Morrison, 1977; Edwards et al., 1996). Physicians are scientists, so their reluctance to being video recorded suggests that they fear the empirical paradox: in the pursuit of science, observers assume that seeing the encounters can lead to scientific understanding of the encounters. On the other hand, the "empirical" findings are inherently biased because they are controlled by the expectations or biases of the viewer/researcher (Potter, 1996). A collegial atmosphere of trust must be established so that physicians are assured that they will not be professionally embarrassed or made unduly vulnerable to researcher biases.

Some More Suggestions

We gathered permission from others who might be on the tape, such as nurses and translators. Our project entailed extra work for the nurses in the form of new routines that needed to be followed and additional paperwork that had to be completed, so we compensated the receptionist who was to act as a gatekeeper for potential participants. We had a short training session for the nurses so that they could understand the logic of our system and question our motives. The nurses became supportive and well informed (although blind to the research hypothesis) and were excellent sources of information and reassurance for patients. On the other hand, if any nurse perceives that videotaped patients are subject to any disadvantage by virtue of participation, he or she can sabotage the project by routing consenting patients away from the consenting physicians or by suggesting that patients change their consent.

More effort is required to protect patients' personal privacy during videotaping than during audiotaping. Our camera was focused on chairs where the patient and physician sat during the history taking, and the camera was angled so that it did not include the examining table. Signs in the examining room reminded patients where to stand when they disrobed, and physicians were instructed on procedures for maintaining privacy. We did not take further precautions for women who were using gynecological services, although it might be advisable. Some gynecological patients requested that only the history taking and conclusion be videotaped, and one changed her mind after the encounter, so the tape was destroyed. If the physician is supportive, she or he may be willing to turn the camera off at the time requested or cover the lens with a cap during the physical examination. Before any tapes were analyzed in our study, a senior researcher edited them to ensure the privacy of everyone.

Maintaining a steady flow of patients in a busy primary clinic with multiple doctors, some of whom are participating and some of whom are not, can be challenging. Whether in resident training facilities or offices of established doctors, the clinicians move from room to room. We had only one room equipped with a videocamera, so potential participants were occasionally lost because the room was not immediately available. We had a clear rule that patients could not be forced to wait longer than would have occurred without the video recording. Some clinics associated with medical centers are equipped with cameras in every examining room, and video recording is done routinely for training purposes. The ideal situation is to have the camera built into the wall or ceiling so that it is available, yet invisible, save for the opening for the lens. The added logistical burden of using video recordings rather than portable audio recordings is a methodological as well as conceptual or theoretical decision.

Whether encounters with first-time patients or long-term patients are selected is another methodological, as well as conceptual, issue. We selected first-time encounters because we wanted to hear illness narratives. Encounters between physicians and their familiar patients are more likely to be maintenance encounters than are first-time encounters, so there may be limited history taking. On the other hand, physicians feel more free to use humor with patients with whom they are acquainted, and they may be cognizant of emotional or psychological disturbances of the patient that would be unknown to physicians in first-time encounters. When the type of encounter has been selected, it should be compared to other similar but nonrecorded encounters to determine if video recording is prolonging the length of the encounters.

Reliability and Validity Concerns

The presence of a video camera may affect the communication between physicians and patients, but there was no indication in our study that the participating physicians or patients were reacting to the camera. Physicians had the choice of whether or not to participate, and those who did appeared primarily concerned with the comfort of and acceptance by patients. When the physicians were assured of this, they tried to ignore the logistics of the study. The participating patients did not appear to restrain their comments. As an additional precaution, we provided physicians with a small remote control for the camera, the size of a credit card, that could be carried in a shirt or coat pocket. If the physician feared that the camera was intimidating the patient or compromising his or her frankness, the physician could stop the recording. Other researchers have concluded that the presence of the camera had little impact on patients' behavior (Pringle

& Stewart-Evans, 1990; Redman, Dickinson, Cockburn, Hennrikus, & Sanson-Fisher, 1989; Wilson, 1991).

The number of residents who were reluctant to participate (approximately one third) did cause some concern on our part. Arborelius and Timpka (1990, 1991) asked patients and physicians to review their medical encounters and make comments about what they observed and whether they felt that the camera had changed their behavior. Ninety percent of the patients said that they felt only slightly or not at all influenced by the video recording of the consultation. However, the physicians felt significantly more influenced. They said that they felt more tense than usual or that they conducted a more thorough examination than they would normally. Physicians who strongly oppose the presence of video cameras do so on the grounds that patients feel intimidated and are reluctant to refuse participation (Bain & Mackay, 1993). Some evidence suggests that this is true: patients may feel obliged to participate in any research approved by their physicians despite reassurances from the research assistant (Lavelle-Jones, Byrne, Rice, & Cushieri, 1993). However, the bulk of the evidence suggests that physicians are the more intimidated because they can be evaluated unfavorably.

Tapes should be transcribed according to predetermined and accepted methods of transcription. The social sciences have developed sophisticated and precise methods of transcribing material, although professional transcription can be costly for large data sets. If less precise transcription than that used for sociolinguistic studies is sufficient, a standardized transcription technique developed in earlier sociolinguistic studies has been adapted to medical encounters, and it can be done by research assistants without special equipment (Fisher, 1984; Frankel, 1984; Mishler et al., 1989; Waitzkin, 1991; West, 1984). Either method will capture the flow of the conversation by including speech hitches, pauses, simultaneous speech, fluctuations in volume, and disjunctures of speech.

Selection of data for presentation should be made under some process that is made clear to the readers. Sometimes random sampling may be possible (Waitzkin, 1990) if all encounters provide material relevant to the research questions, but random sampling does not ensure the absence of interpretive bias. If multiple excerpts from a number of encounters are used to demonstrate the breadth of the result, the distinction between the data and its interpretation can become blurred. The analyst might use the quotations from patients as illustrations of the analyst's opinions or generalizations. The analyst's authorial voice and interpretative commentary, which knit the disparate elements together, will determine how the reader comes to understand the excerpts (Edwards, 1997; Mishler, 1990). Consequently, both the selection of data and the manner of presentation of the excerpts is vulnerable to biases of the author, and the conclusions can be shaped by the same biases (Waitzkin, 1990).

If, on the other hand, the researcher wants to do an in-depth interactional interpretation of only a few encounters, perhaps two or three, focused purposive sampling may be substituted for random sampling. An expert panel is particularly helpful for selecting these few representative encounters, or a research team could select them by consensus and in response to articulated selection criteria. The use of an independent panel is advised if the clinicians are to be scrutinized for interpersonal skills or interviewing techniques. Whichever method is selected, it is helpful if it is driven by theoretical considerations that can be justified to readers. To "deepen" the observations and clarify the context under which the phenomenon in question emerges, disconfirming evidence can also be presented with explanations as to why the encounters differed (Huberman & Miles, 1994; Kuzel, 1992; Waitzkin, 1990).

The authorial voice can be made more credible if multiple observers analyze the material independently (Waitzkin, 1990). Analysis of videotapes for personal interaction is considerably more complex than analyzing audiotapes when only discrete behaviors or utterances are the focus of the research. Even if the focus is the verbal message, what the researcher "hears" in a videotaped encounter depends as much on what the participants do as what they say, that is, the "metamessage" can interfere with the "message." From our own experience, we found that some patients can be perceived sympathetically when only the audio portion is used but considered irritating and uncooperative when the videotape is shown. Similarly, a physician's line of inquiry might sound reasonable when listened to, but when the complete metamessage is reviewed and the social dynamics between patient and physician become apparent, the same inquiry can appear domineering. Epstein and colleagues (1998) used this problem imaginatively by having physicians review their own videotapes of HIV-related discussion for errors in handling sensitive and awkward moments in the discussion. The awkwardness might not be discernible from audiotaped dialogue, but it was apparent in the videotaped interaction, and the physicians readily recognized it.

If analysts arrive at their interpretation of the material independently and then begin the collaborative effort, the likelihood of biasing the interpretation decreases. The videotape may need to be replayed many times during the collaboration so that the multiple actions (e.g., verbal and nonverbal behaviors of both physician and patient) can be reexamined by all analysts. If possible, both men and women should be included in the analysis team, as markedly different interpretations of nonverbal behavior can occur according to gender, and these differences affect interpretation of the accompanying verbal behavior (Kendall & Tannen, 1997; Tannen, 1990). Consensual conclusions emerge from a willingness to reenter

"Shiva's Circle" (see Chapter 1) whenever disagreements appear, until consensus is reached.

Ethical Issues

Issues of patient confidentiality, autonomy, and respect must be addressed, especially as they relate to shame and humiliation. Despite the precautions that are taken, video recording a medical encounter must be seen as a challenge to the confidentiality of the physician-patient relationship (Butler, 1996). The interaction is legally recognized as privileged, and the capturing of images during that encounter for view by noninvolved personnel is always assumed to be a breach of that confidentiality. Audiotapes can be made anonymous by deleting proper names. Controlling confidentiality of videotaped participants is more difficult because both the person's image and words can be made public. Consequently, videotapes cannot be as readily provided for review by other researchers to satisfy questions concerning validity, although transcripts can be provided. The importance of the research must be secondary to the protection of the patients' words and images and of the physicians' professional standing and respect.

Obtaining consent can not be considered sufficient grounds for waiving the challenge to confidentiality. Instead, informed consent is required. Patients must be assured that nonparticipation will not affect their care and that they have the authority to stop the camera at any time if they so choose. If patients are told that the tape is for scientific analysis only and that their confidentiality will be protected, then public viewings of the recordings are precluded. If they are told that the tapes may be used for educational purposes, then some potential participants might decline participation. They must be told the extent of the anticipated public exposure and the target audiences. If some patients are not fluent in English, then bilingual and bicultural research assistants are needed to ensure that these patients understand and participate voluntarily.

CONCLUSION

In conclusion, videotaping projects have the potential of providing a rich source of data, and the effects of the observer are somewhat minimized. However, the decision to use videotaping methodology must be based on the research questions and the clinical context (Miller & Crabtree, 1994b). Only if the research questions or hypotheses require videotaping is this methodology likely to be worth the added logistical and ethical concerns.

Audiotapes are less invasive, more easily monitored, more portable, and more acceptable to patients and physicians. On the other hand, if the research is going to focus on qualitative and quantitative data from the encounters, or post hoc analyses are planned, then videotaping may be the better technique, although any subsequent analyses should indicate that they are based on a convenience sample. The current research trend is toward examining the metamessage during communication or analyzing how constellations of behaviors fulfill communicative functions. For these purposes, as well as some intervention and evaluation purposes, the drawbacks of using videotape technology are outweighed by the richness of the data available.

14

An Armchair Adventure
in Case Study Research

Virginia A. Aita
Helen E. McIlvain

E very clinician has at some time in their practice puzzled over the
mysterious black box of practice and considered changes that might
make it more efficient and/or fulfilling. Taking care of patients involves
much more than the doctor-patient interaction in the examination room.
It is a complex process involving personnel with different roles and
responsibilities, patients with different needs and expectations, and external systems with competing requirements and recommendations. Although
generally seen as negative, these circumstances also create opportunities
for creative problem identification and resolution.

In this chapter, we invite you to imagine yourself involved in an armchair
adventure, journeying into case study research to discover how this method
may be useful in answering some of the mystifying questions about practice.
As guides on your journey, we explain some of the practical issues that
might be encountered in designing a project, identifying the field of study,
choosing tools, and making sense of what is learned along the way. To do
this, we refer to a number of authors whose insights into case study research
have helped inform our process and to a case study that Helen and her
small team completed. So . . . settle into a comfortable chair where you can

consider the process from beginning to end, for there is much to think about and appreciate on this journey.

HISTORICAL BACKGROUND

The case study approach to research has a long history. Hamel, Dufour, and Fortin (1993) trace the traditions of case study to Bronislaw Malinowski's field work in the Tobriand Islands during the early twentieth century and to Frédéric Le Play, founder of French sociological field work and developer of the case study method of inquiry. In the early to mid-19th century, Le Play was involved in the social, political, and scientific currents of societal change. His close ties to familial and religious traditions, however, influenced his decision to study working class populations and the family as a unit of social organization. By comparing the various organizations of family units and the societies of which they were a part, he developed the comparative methods that we are familiar with today (Hamel et al., 1993).

The case study method became an important tool of sociologists in the Chicago School during the late 19th and early 20th centuries. Faced with enormous urban problems related to industrialization and the influx of immigrants that resulted in subsequent urban crowding, poverty, illness, and violence, sociologists adapted case study methods to explore these problems from an impersonal perspective. It was Robert Parks of the Chicago School who encouraged the use of the case study as a means to gain subjective insight into problems by going into the "field." Parks documented life in these neighborhoods by going into the streets and homes of the poor and displaced to obtain face-to-face interviews, letters, on-site personal observations of immigrant experience, and other evidence (Hamel et al., 1993). The approaches used in each of these historical examples were all largely descriptive or documentary in nature, with the motive in each situation being to better understand the complex dynamics of the field in question.

Similar methods have been used in medicine. Physicians will be familiar with the case report, a study of one patient's illness or experience. The case study methods we describe are not unlike the strategies used in the case report and the historical examples described above; they draw together many elements needed to understand the complex nature of a problem. Examples of case studies in the medical literature are abundant. One of the best known situational case studies in the medical literature is Becker's *Boys in White: Student Culture in Medical School* (Becker et al., 1961). A more recent example would be Miller's (1992) "Routine, Ceremony, or Drama: An Exploratory Field Study of the Primary Care Clinical Encounter."

PREPARING FOR THE JOURNEY, OR
"DO I REALLY WANT TO DO THIS?"

So where does one begin to prepare for such a project? A good place to start is with the questions that provoke one's curiosity in the first place, prompting one to consider venturing into research. We may wonder why something happens or doesn't happen or why events unfold in one way rather than in another. The stimulus for research manifests itself in these early stirrings when we begin to question, "Why?" This questioning process stimulated Helen to conduct the project that serves as our example.

A few years prior to doing this case study project, Helen had completed a study that looked at residents' smoking counseling rates. She found that physicians' self-reported estimates of counseling were considerably higher than reports from their patients after their appointments. Residents were then given counseling training, and although counseling rates subsequently increased, they returned to baseline after only 6 months. Given this minimal effect of training, Helen began to wonder what physicians in practice were actually doing in terms of smoking cessation counseling. Most physicians were aware of the importance of tobacco counseling and its effectiveness through professional literature, but most had received no formal training in cessation techniques. Additionally, most existing research concerning physician tobacco counseling patterns had been conducted by focusing on resident behaviors or using self-report data from practicing physicians. Having serious doubts about the representativeness of the former and the validity of the latter, Helen was intrigued by the question, "What are physicians really doing out there regarding smoking cessation counseling?" The goal of this chapter (and this adventure) is to figure out how to approach this kind of question.

It is important to remember that case study research is iterative in nature (see Chapter 7). Although our discussion of methodology may appear to be linear, it is indeed a circular adventure of wondering, inquiry, insight, hypothesis formulation, discovery, and renewed inquiry. To enhance your understanding, we recommend several authors who have helped explain the process to us. They provide a wealth of valuable insights into case study research, as do authors who have written chapters in this book about different aspects of qualitative research.

Robert K. Yin (1993) has detailed some of the earlier applications of case study research and provides some of the basic nuts and bolts needed to engage in the process. Robert E. Stake (1995) provides a very readable and concise text on case study methods, and Sharan B. Merriam (1998) contributes a solid philosophical treatise on the applications of case study approaches in the field of education. John W. Creswell's (1998) excellent comparative survey of five qualitative research traditions includes case study as one approach. Finally, we refer to Czarniawska (1998), who writes so eloquently on the role of storytelling in case study research.

Decisions, Decisions!

Once the researcher has decided to use the case study method to help answer his or her questions, one of the first decisions to be made concerns the type of case study to do. Robert Stake (1995) differentiates between quantitative and qualitative case studies. He argues that one must first identify the goal of the research. If the research goal is to generalize across cases to explain phenomena, a quantitative design should be used. The qualitative design is better suited for looking at the interrelationship of variables to understand phenomena within a case (p. 36). We would counter Stake's recommendation of choosing either a quantitative or qualitative case study design by suggesting that the circumstances of the case(s) and the unanswered questions of the researcher determine the methods for data collection, which may include both quantitative and qualitative sources. The researcher may simultaneously seek not only explanations of questions but insights generalizable across cases. Being a novice, Helen designed her study not by asking whether or not to use quantitative or qualitative approaches but by determining what types of data would help to answer her research question. She decided that multiple data sources, both quantitative and qualitative, were needed.

Types of Case Studies, or
"Could Someone Please Explain This to Me?"

As Helen thought about trying to find out "What are they doing out there?" she decided to write a tobacco grant to obtain state health department funding to look at the question. She wasn't sure what kind of design to use, but she knew that she wanted to actually go into the practices to see what was being done rather than using physicians' self-reports. She had done quantitative research in the past but knew nothing about case studies. Ben Crabtree, the research director in her department, suggested that because this type of project had not been done previously, Helen would probably need to develop her own instruments, based on her prior experience with tobacco research, the current literature on behavior change and smoking cessation, and current guidelines on "best practice."

Ben also suggested that it would be helpful in developing these instruments if Helen did a few in-depth case studies to get an idea of the potential range of behaviors she might expect to see. With this direction, Helen began to see that there were really two studies that she needed to do. The goal of the first case study was essentially to discover what was going on "out there" in a qualitative sense, to discover the range of variables that were important in practice around tobacco cessation. The second part of the project would be a later, larger quantitative study to identify the prevalence of key variables within a random sample of Nebraska family physicians. The first case study is the project we will continue to report on in this chapter.

Putting Helen's study into a theoretical context, let's consider the differences among types of case studies. Stake (1995) differentiates three types. In the "intrinsic" case study, the motive is to learn about a particular case for its own sake. In the "instrumental" case study, the desire is to understand a particular case as an instrument for understanding something else. Finally, in the "collective case study," several cases are selected for the purpose of comparison (see Chapter 16). Yin (1993) categorizes six basic categories of case study: single or multiple case studies that are exploratory, descriptive, or explanatory by design. An exploratory case study is one that defines questions or hypotheses, a descriptive case study depicts a "phenomenon within its context," and an explanatory study identifies cause and effect relationships among variables in a particular case (p. 5). Similarly, Merriam (1998, pp. 27-34) describes categories of case study as particularistic (focused on a given situation), descriptive (where the goal is a "thick and rich" description of the case), and heuristic (where the goal is to enlighten the reader about the case situation).

Stake (1995) would classify the first of Helen's studies as an intrinsic study with instrumental overtones. Yin (1993) would categorize the project as a multiple exploratory study, and Merriam (1998) would classify the study as heuristic. The next question Helen had to think through was, Who would she study?

Sampling, or "What Is My Destination and Whom Will I Study?"

Helen believed the study needed to include a range of the different types of practices across the state, as different practices might have different resources available or demands made on them that could affect what they chose to do regarding tobacco counseling. By identifying her unit of analysis, the practice, she had a starting point for her sampling strategy. She decided to do purposeful sampling of practices based on their location by the population each served (urban, rural, frontier), by the gender (male or female) of the practice physician, and by the practice configuration (solo or group practice). The funding and time line were limited, so Helen decided to study only one established Nebraska practice in each of the possible 12 categories. Having made this decision, she had to figure out how to identify those 12 practices.

Yin (1993) argues that no decision in research design is more important than defining the unit of analysis, for the definition of the object of study determines the boundaries within which research is done. The unit under study, what some refer to as a "bounded system" (Creswell, 1998; Merriam, 1998), can be either a single person engaged in a particular situation or activity of interest or a larger organization, such as a hospital unit or a practice, where a group is engaged in a common activity. Whatever the unit of analysis turns out to be, the decision is critical because it guides the process of picking or "sampling" the study cases.

Sampling strategies differ in quantitative and qualitative approaches because the goal of each is different. In quantitative research, the goal is to obtain a small probability sample that is representative of the larger population, minimizing cost and effort while maintaining a large enough sample to ensure that the results will be generalizable to the larger population. Sample size determination and randomization of subjects are the primary tools used.

In qualitative case study research, the goal is to achieve exploration, description, or explanation of a particular situation. Cases are chosen "to maximize what we can learn" (Stake, 1995, p. 4). Sampling is purposeful to obtain rich information. As Merriam (1998) explains, purposeful sampling may choose to represent the "typical," the "unique," or the "maximum variation." Creswell (1998) prefers "to select unusual cases in collective case studies and employ 'maximum variation' as a strategy to represent diverse cases to fully display multiple perspectives about the cases" (p. 120).

Yin (1993), on the other hand, separates "sampling logic" from "replication logic." Sampling logic refers to representation of the larger universe. Using this approach, the researcher selects cases based on representative a priori criteria. Replication logic refers to two or more cases in the same study where the investigator is looking for congruence that indicates increased confidence in the overall findings. Yin does not think that using sampling logic works well with multiple case studies and may detract from the rationale for applying the case study approach in the first place. In case study research, and especially in multiple case studies, he believes that cases should be selected using a "replication logic" that will either confirm or disconfirm expected findings based on what has been learned from prior cases. Therefore, the investigator may use sampling logic to select the initial case(s) but use replication logic as a strategy for building the sample in an iterative process one case at a time. Sampling decisions will help determine the number of cases desired. As Merriam (1998, p. 64) states, sample size depends on "the questions being asked, the data being gathered, the analysis in progress, [and] the resources you have to support the study." Sampling should conclude shortly after saturation occurs, that is, when fewer and fewer new insights occur during data analysis. For a more in-depth discussion of sampling, see Chapter 2.

As good luck would have it, one of Helen's colleagues helped her begin recruiting her sample by granting her permission to use the mailing list of the Nebraska Academy of Family Physicians. After getting the membership list, Helen broke the list down by county population so that she could begin to identify the practices according to their urban, rural, or frontier status. Then she went through the three lists and picked out the names of males and females in both group and solo practices, looking for physicians that she did not know personally. Once she had identified a group of eligible physician practices, Helen sent a letter to each physician briefly describing the study and indicating that she would be calling a week later to talk with the physician personally about participation. Expecting some refusals, Helen mailed 20 to 30 letters in all, contacting several practices in each of the 12 categories she wished to study. A week later, she telephoned the physicians asking for their participation. The only category she was not able to fill was the male, frontier, solo physician practice. As Helen discovered during the recruiting process, solo frontier practices were fast becoming a thing of the past, so she didn't worry about not having a practice in that category.

Helen's a priori approach to sampling was not as ideal, methodologi-cally, as an iterative process working toward saturation might have been. She decided ahead of time what practice features—gender, county popu-lation, and practice type—would determine her sample. This method had the time advantage of allowing her to recruit practices before data collec-tion began and to standardize her approach to the practices. However, the approach also had the disadvantage of ruling out the possibility of Helen adjusting her selection criteria as she gleaned insights from the first practices as to what other kinds of selection criteria might have been important to include in the selection of later practices.

Theoretical Frameworks, or "Do We Need a Map for This Trip?"

Merriam (1998) views theory as a map, helping to define the research problem. Because "explorers" like Helen are discovering and describing new ground, they may not have a map, or at best they may have only a crude map. But where better developed "maps" (theory) exist, they can help determine the research problem, research questions, data collection strategies, and analysis techniques as Helen's study did for our later research projects. Merriam (1998, p. 45) speaks of the theoretical frame-work as the "structure, the scaffolding, the frame of your study." Some people erroneously believe that because qualitative research is inductive, theory is unnecessary. Merriam argues that theory is indeed important because it can frame the orientation, or "the lens through which you view the world." She believes the easiest way to identify a theoretical framework concerning a given question or set of questions is to do a thoughtful and careful review of the literature, which should uncover a number of possible theoretical perspectives from which to view the issues under study. Helen's review of the literature served as the foundation for the interpretive part of her project. With an awareness that theoretical concepts are, if not in the forefront of the research design, at least a subtle influence on the researcher's approach to data collection, we move now to the more active phase of preparing to enter the field.

Strategies for Data Collection, or "What Gear (Tools) Will I Need in the Field?"

After reviewing the literature and consulting with Ben, Helen decided that she was most interested in obtaining information on the following variables: practice demographics, environmental cues, patient education, methods of identifying and documenting tobacco use and cessation efforts, physician behavior in patient encounters, and perceptions of the target physician and office manager about the role of tobacco prevention and cessation in practice activities. Consequently, she developed a chart audit checklist looking for documentation of tobacco use and counseling, a patient encounter form looking for tobacco history taking and counseling, a revision of a practice environment checklist that had been used in another study of practice behavior (Stange, Zyzanski, Jaen, et al., 1998), and in-depth interview guides for physicians and office managers. Additionally, she would have the field worker dictate field notes at the end of each day regarding his impressions of the physician and practice activities that centered around tobacco prevention and cessation. Having made these decisions, and after gathering and developing needed data collection tools, Helen was ready to move this project into the field.

Stake (1995) points out that data collection does not really have a formal initiation. He maintains that data collection begins even before the researcher has decided to do a study, when observations and experiences are informing the preliminary understanding that brings the investigator to the point of wanting to know more about a certain phenomenon. Another important idea that Stake discusses is the difference in perspective between quantitative and qualitative observational data. The approach taken depends on the relevance of data type to research questions. For example, when describing observational data, Stake describes a quantitative approach as a "tally" of "categories or key events." He differentiates this approach from the qualitative approach in which observational data, gathered during a specific time and place, tells its own story. In the former situation, data must be categorized and sorted to derive meaning. In the latter situation, the story itself is an interpretation of meaning.

Merriam (1998) has made other important observations about data collection. She thinks that notions of data collection can be deceiving, as data are not objective things awaiting collection. Instead, our ideas about what comprise "data" are determined by the meanings that are attributed to particular types of information, be they observations of activities or environmental contexts, conversations (interviews), relevant documents, or other quantitative or qualitative elements. This insight leads Merriam to conclude that decisions about questions for research, the sample selected for study, and the theoretical framework, as discussed above, all determine what become "data" and how it will be collected.

Yin (1993) approaches data collection in a manner similar to Merriam's but places more emphasis on the importance of the project's overall theoretical perspective as the determinant of data collection methods. Discussing the dichotomy between quantitative and qualitative research, he dispels the notion that one is built on hard data and the other on soft. He shows how case study, ethnography, grounded theory, and quasiexperimental study each call for different types of data. He concludes that the case study, by its theoretical nature, calls for multiple data collection strategies, incorporating both quantitative and qualitative elements.

Preparing to Enter the Field, or
"What Else Do I Need to Do Before I Get There?"

While planning to begin data collection, Helen found that she could get a first-year medical student to assist her during the summer as a field worker. Later she found that having a medical student do the research was an asset because it enhanced physicians' receptivity to the study. Physicians seem to enjoy opportunities to interact with medical students because they become potential partners after graduation. This was really the only participation benefit for the practices.

The student's limited availability helped Helen decide that he would spend only 2 to 3 days in each practice. He was given brief training in the overall goals of the study, the use of the specific data-gathering instruments, observational techniques, taking field notes, and interviewing, and he proved to be a very reliable and conscientious researcher. The biggest difficulty in setting up the field work schedule was to coordinate the timetable of 2- to 3-day site visits so that the time frames corresponded with physicians' preferences but did not require the medical student to constantly backtrack to and fro across Nebraska.

Entering the field begins with gaining access to the site(s) and setting up the schedule as Helen did. To understand what is involved in this process and in field work in general, it is important to grasp the research roles of the principal investigator and the field worker, although these roles may be assumed by one person. The *principal investigator* (PI), as the overall administrator of the project, is responsible and instrumental in recruiting the "case" sites for the study. Case recruitment is a time-consuming job. Once the first case is identified, initial contact is made with the site.

Stake (1995, p. 57) discusses the process of gaining access and permissions. He suggests that a brief written description of the study be offered to case candidates for their review, along with other specific information that individuals from the site might request. Stake points out that obtaining written permission from formal authorities to enter the site for the collection of data is essential. Personnel at the site should also be informed. Consulting with the "informal authorities" at the site can also smooth the field worker's entry into the study. These informal authorities may include the office manager or other professionally or highly skilled people within the setting who are recognized for their leadership ability. The principal investigator needs to communicate with them about what is going to happen and how long the data collection phase will last. It is important to acknowledge that having a field worker in their midst is a burden, but it is just as important to ask for their cooperation and that of the other staff. This information, along with the answers to specific questions that site personnel have, should be given freely and early in the process to maximize cooperation and make the entry process as quiet and organized as possible.

The *field worker,* who may also be the primary investigator, is the most important person on the research team at this point because she or he has a direct connection to the case; everything understood about the case will come through his or her senses during the process of data collection. We have chosen to use health professionals to fill the field worker positions on our projects because of their interpersonal skills and familiarity with health care situations. Even though our field workers are highly skilled when hired, they need to be trained in the use of all the assessment tools they will use on site and how these tools will be used in the analysis. We make every effort to prepare our field workers for some of the challenges they will face by having them read Bernard (1994) and Bogdewic (1992) on participant observation during their training period. We also have them practice doing observation in our clinics and with our physicians during encounters. After they practice their observational skills, we have them dictate field notes and encounter notes. Members of our research faculty then review and discuss the dictated data, giving feedback to the field worker on the high and low inference of observations, giving him or her the opportunity to discuss problems, personal feelings about the process, and other concerns. A similar process is involved in their training to do interviews. Field workers also need to understand the goals of each facet of data collection (what we are trying to find out and why). Because field workers provide the direct contact with the on-site research process, their deep understanding of project goals and methods is essential if they are to know if something is not working or if there is a problem that needs to be addressed. In this way, the field worker is an extension of the primary investigator and is able to troubleshoot on site if something is amiss.

Collecting the Data, or Discovering What's Going on Out There

Once the medical student started his field work in the tobacco study practices, he completed all the data-gathering instruments, dictated his field notes, and then brought the information back to the office when he returned to Omaha. Toward the end of field work, he was spending only 2 days in the practice rather than 3 because he was more accomplished in gathering the necessary information. In the office, the dictated audiotapes, with field notes and interviews, were transcribed and put into Folio Views® (Weitzman & Miles, 1995; see also Chapter 11). The medical student seldom had more than 5 to 10 pages of dictated field notes. In addition to the data in Folio Views, paper files were made that contained the data related to chart audits, practice encounters, practice environment checklists, collected documents, and hard copies of field notes and interviews. The medical student field worker was able to complete all data collection within the summer time frame.

Because of the time limitations in this data collection phase, all data were collected before the interpretive phase of the study began. In many qualitative studies, however, analysis is ongoing throughout the data collection process. When the interpretive process coincides with data collection, the process takes on a more iterative nature, and corrections and refinements are possible that can enhance the quality and overall outcomes of the study. For example, it may become apparent that a data collection strategy is not working and that some other type of data, or a more specific type of data, is needed. If interpretation is ongoing, the investigator can alter the data collection process in midstream to take a different approach. This is an advantage qualitative researchers have that quantitative researchers must resist.

Another thing to consider during data collection concerns the interaction between the field worker and the environment. Manners, consideration, and unobtrusiveness are essential characteristics of the field worker assuming a "fly on the wall" perspective during periods of observation. In the beginning, the field worker will be treated like "company" because of being a new person in the site. In our experience, it takes several days, depending on the situation, before the field worker will begin to "blend into the crowd" and others on the site will be less self-conscious about the field worker's presence. It is at this point that the field worker's observations take on more validity, as people are less guarded in their interactions with one another. We have found, in general, that doing the interviews after completing other data collection is usually a good idea because by that time, people in the practice have become a little more comfortable with the researcher. Our field workers often do less sensitive tasks in the first days, such as making a map of the office layout or identifying all the staff and their job responsibilities. The time involved in data collection varies depending on the size and complexity of the project, its goals, and the site being explored.

The field worker needs to be both organized and flexible in his or her approach to data collection. Time demands may be uncertain; the organization's needs and the personal schedules of those being observed may disrupt the best-laid plans. It is important for the quality of the data that dictation be done soon after observations are made, so field workers may find they are working long days. In extended data collection, there is the tension between the demands on the field worker, perhaps away from home and living in a hotel, and the intrusion into and disruption of normal schedules in a research site where the generation of quality data demands time.

Success in data collection depends on the field worker's ability to affiliate with others while maintaining a "mental separateness." Rapport and a sense of trust must be established with others who are asked to share thoughts, beliefs, and feelings on a personal level. The field worker must then be able to report or describe this information from an objective perspective. Difficulty may arise, as it did in one of our projects, if a field worker feels that reporting such sensitive data subverts the trust of the informant. This may present a moral dilemma for the field worker.

There are also moral dilemmas involved in taking the intrusive stance that is required in field work. Stake (1995) discusses this and points out the unnatural sense of intimacy involved in hearing and knowing about the personal situations of others, which one would not encounter in normal circumstances. Anticipation and discussion of moral issues involved in field relationships are prudent and wise during field worker training.

As data collection nears completion, the field worker needs to begin the process of withdrawing from the site. Stake (1995) reminds researchers to leave the site as it was when the field worker entered and to remember and keep promises made during the process. The longer the field worker has been in the field, the more difficult this becomes and the more necessary it is that some formal closure take place. Finally, as the field worker is winding down work on site, she or he will probably be spending more time assisting with the analysis process.

Data Management and Analysis, or "How Do I Make Sense of All This Stuff?

Deciding whom to include in the interpretive phase is important, and the primary investigator may decide to form a team, involving one or two others in addition to the field worker in the analysis of data. We believe that the application of many different professional perspectives to data analysis increases the validity of findings by increasing the likelihood of maintaining objectivity. Helen's team included a physician colleague because she felt it essential to have a physician's interpretive "voice" familiar with the day-to-day demands of practice. It is helpful if participants possess good interpersonal skills and the ability to tolerate ambiguity and conflict, as different "voices" often present different points of view and analysis can be prolonged.

By this point, the reader as well as the PI may be wondering, "What should I do with all this data? How do I store it? How do I access it? How do I work with it?" There is just a lot to manage. Case studies do accumulate a lot of data, and its management can be made easier by having a data management program such as NUD*IST® or Folio Views (see Chapter 11). Such a program has many advantages, not the least of which is just getting the data organized so that it is easily accessed. These programs allow the data to be organized as if it is a book with a table of contents and many chapters. By going to the table of contents, the researcher can go to the specific piece of data of interest and can maneuver through the text with relative ease. This technology allows data to be added as it is transcribed and imported into the database. It also allows the researcher to code data easily and to search and manipulate coded terms, themes, and patterns with ease. Data management by computer program does require a moderate level of technical proficiency, and there are courses available to assist researchers in learning these skills if necessary. It is also possible to manage the data entirely using paper files, if that is preferred.

The interpretive process in the tobacco study did not start until all of the site visits had been completed. Helen was not initially familiar with data management computer programs, so she began to interpret the data by taking the 11 practice site files home and spending a day with a yellow pad and a pen collating the information from the chart audits, practice, encounters, and the practice environment checklists. First she tabulated the quantitative data for each site, looking for the presence or absence of materials, such as patient education brochures and office systems used to identify and record patients' tobacco usage. Then she tabulated scores across sites because she was looking for the variety of activities and totals for each. Meanwhile, Ben entered the qualitative data, including the transcribed field notes and interviews into Folio Views and gave Helen and her physician colleague a brief training session. They then coded the text, identifying the following variables: intensity, confidence, skills, outcome expectations, and locus of control.

There are many simple ways to code data, such as highlighting text with colored markers where each color represents a different concept, theme, or pattern, to using the editing, organizing approach that Helen used (see Chapters 7 and 8). Preferring the latter style, we make notes on the margins of our paper files as we read through the data. We find we feel more relaxed when thinking about, making notes, and coding data at ease in a comfortable chair, or in bed with a cup of coffee, than when we sit before a computer screen. But whether coding on paper files or on computer, the researcher's initial ideas about what may or may not be important in early stages of the process may change by the end of the process, especially when there are large amounts of data. When coding categories seem to change, it is usually because the researcher has learned and understands more about the case through the analysis process.

Because there are different types of data, there are also different ways of doing interpretation. For example, field notes may be coded or notated as to patterns and themes that emerge as described above. Interviews may be coded similarly to field notes, but in analyzing interviews, the researcher takes a slightly different perspective, interpreting what the interviewee is saying given an understanding of the context of the situation that is usually gained from insight gleaned from the field notes. But there are other types of data as well, such as the practice environment checklist and chart audit data forms as from the tobacco study, which are more concrete forms of data that may be evaluated quantitatively. In the case of quantitative data, the interpretation process is more comparative in nature, looking at what exists compared to other comparable data sets or, possibly, a priori standards or guidelines. Once each type of data is analyzed independently, it is "triangulated," a term used by qualitative researchers to see if data sources are internally consistent and supportive of larger ideas arising in the analysis process (Creswell, 1998). For more discussion of analysis techniques and issues, see Creswell (1998, pp. 139-165), Merriam (1998, pp. 155-197), Stake (1995, pp. 107-120), and Chapters 7 through 10 in this book. What seems most cogent is that sensitivity to the data will guide the process, and the most important ideas will rise to the top in the minds of those doing the interpretation. How the data are coded does not matter; of more importance is the inductive process of determining what ideas, patterns, and themes are important. When "saturation" is reached, the important ideas keep coming up repeatedly, and little new information arises. When the main ideas, patterns, and themes have been established, the process can move into higher levels of interpretation, synthesizing what has been learned with theoretical perspectives that may have guided the case study from its inception. Where theory has been incorporated, we witness the closing of the inquiry circle, as theoretical concepts are brought to bear on the analysis and interpretation of data.

Writing The Case Report, or "How Do I Wrap This Up?"

Many think that analysis precedes the actual writing of the case report, but that is not necessarily the case. The interpretation team working on the tobacco study met every week or two for a number of months. In each of these meetings, writing was an important part of the interpretive process, from the initial summarization of each practice to the final draft of the paper submitted for publication, "Current Trends in Tobacco Prevention and Cessation in Nebraska Physicians' Offices" (McIlvain, Crabtree, Gilbert, Havranek, & Backer, 1997). We have found this to be true in our experiences doing other case study projects, and we think that writing helps the researcher grasp the story.

Czarniawska (1998) has argued that storytelling is an important facet of pulling the research puzzle together. She believes that stories contain metaphors, which are "condensed stories" that can help us to understand and interpret the meanings that lie underneath the larger story that the data have to tell. Czarniawska (pp. 29-31) states that in narrative interviews, the interviewee reveals the plot (structure) and main concepts (metaphors) of the story. As an example, the metaphor "research is an adventure" provides the structure and concepts of the methodological story that we are trying to tell. The use of metaphor potentially helps make sense of the relationships of actors and other variables that may lead to theoretical or hypothetical prediction. By writing the case report as Helen's interpretation team did, the story becomes a collage, constructed not just by one perspective but by a number of voices, incorporating multiple viewpoints over time while the interpretive process is under way.

Czarniawska's (1998) way of approaching writing is different from methods suggested by others such as Lincoln and Guba (1985) and Stake (1995). The latter suggest a "substantive case report" or a template format consisting of several different sections, including a description of the problem; development of the situational context and associated observations; a thorough discussion of important actions, processes, or relationships; triangulation confirming or disconfirming data; and the authors' assertions about the case. Stake suggests beginning and ending the report with a vignette taken from the data. The report culminates in the identification of themes and, finally, "lessons to be learned" from the situation (Lincoln & Guba, 1985; Stake, 1995).

By contrast, our approach is more like Czarniawska's in that we try to tell the story from "the inside out." We think that such a perspective allows for a richer narrative, which weaves together discrepant findings, inconsistencies, and contradictions that generally arise from triangulation of multiple data sources. All of the elements of the "substantive case report" can be found in our "inside-out story," but the perspective is subtly different, and we believe that validity is enhanced. If multiple case studies are conducted, as in Helen's study, each case must be analyzed independently before a cross-case comparison can be started for the purposes of comparing and contrasting cases.

If this were the end of an adventure short story, you might be left feeling that adventure only happens to other people, but in this case the end is only the beginning. Case study research offers a real-life adventure in your own practice, a nearby community, or any place your questions and curiosity may lead. We hope that you feel better prepared to address some of those intriguing questions and begin to dream about how you might study them using the case study method. Like any adventure, a case study research project takes some time to plan. One must define the goals of the journey, identify the field or destination of the study, bring along the right gear—maybe a map or two and tools for data collection—and, in the process of doing field work, try to make sense of what is going on out there. But what is most important, your curiosity, is already inside of you. This is an adventure that you can experience by yourself, or you can take some of your friends and associates with you. In either case, we encourage you to participate, for you will end up in a different place than you started.

15

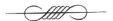

Participatory Inquiry

Janecke Thesen
Anton J. Kuzel

Research that produces nothing but books will not suffice.

Kurt Lewin, 1948

PARTICIPATORY INQUIRY:
TYPICAL FORMS, ASSUMPTIONS, AND ISSUES

Participatory inquiry is a general term for several academic traditions. Reason (1994) has reviewed three of these: cooperative inquiry, participatory action research (PAR), and action science. Cooperative inquiry, according to Reason, is rooted in humanistic psychology (e.g., Maslow, 1968; Rogers, 1961) and focuses on personal and group development. The cooperative inquiry cycle involves group processes of (a) defining an area of inquiry, (b) implementing action steps, (c) experiencing the consequences, and (d) learning from the experience. PAR is more explicitly focused on liberating oppressed peoples (Fals-Borda & Rahman, 1991). Reason (1994) says PAR has two objectives:

> One aim is to produce knowledge and action directly useful to a group of people—through research, adult education, and sociopolitical action. The second aim is to empower people at a second and deeper level through the process of constructing and using their own knowledge: They "see through"

269

the ways in which the establishment monopolizes the production and use of knowledge for the benefit of its members. (p. 328)

The third form of inquiry, action science, is the most recently developed and is based on the work of Argyris and Schön (1974). Here the emphasis is on intensive personal development with the goal of participating in the improvement of organizational function. In action science, organizations bring the assumptions (theories) behind their actions to the surface so that these can be challenged and modified, thereby promoting greater effectiveness and greater justice (Reason, 1994). They pay full attention to their mission, strategy, operations, and outcomes and seek to bring these four "territories of human experience" into harmony (Torbert, 1991).

The three traditions have different emphases. Cooperative inquiry explores experience to promote development, PAR challenges and recreates power to liberate oppressed communities, and action science seeks better theories of action. The traditions also have obvious similarities. They are all oriented toward reform rather than simply toward description or meaning and so are examples of a *critical/ecological* paradigm (Chapter 1). Each is a kind of "disciplined inquiry (research) which seeks focused efforts to improve the quality of people's organizational, community and family lives" (Calhoun, 1993, p. 62). Finally, all three approaches use an iterative cycle of inquiry that Stringer (1996) has captured with simple language: *look*—defining and describing the problem, *think*—analyzing and interpreting the problem, and *act*—formulating and implementing solutions to the problem.

> As participants work through each of the major stages, they will explore the details of their activities through a constant process of observation, reflection, and action. At the completion of each set of activities, they will review (look again), reflect (reanalyze), and re-act (modify their actions). (Stringer, 1996, p. 17)

These research traditions are sensitive to the role of participants. McTaggart (1997) brings into focus the obligations of academics who wish to do participatory research:

> Other kinds of research . . . typically involve researchers from the academy doing research *on* people, making the people objects of the research. . . . The knowledge produced from such research can be used in coercive kinds of ways, but somewhat contradictorily can create the *illusion* of participation. People can be required to work out ways of implementing policy developed on the basis of knowledge produced by research *on* them rather than *by* them. . . . To counter this expectation of the academic role,

considerable energy must be directed at ensuring reciprocity and symmetry of relations in the participatory action research group, and at maintaining community control of the project (and its staff). (pp. 29, 33; italics in original)

Participatory inquiry has deep roots in the field of education. In the first third of this century, curriculum theorist and philosopher John Dewey (1929) called for an educational system in which teachers and learners collaborate as coinvestigators. Dewey's ideas were echoed and developed by Hilda Taba, who coordinated an effort to improve relations between majority-minority groups through curriculum development (Taba, Brady, & Robinson, 1952). More recent champions of participatory inquiry in education include the British curricularist John Elliott (1991) and the Australian critical educational action researchers at Deakin University (Kemmis & McTaggart, 1988). These authors believe that "education is a 'contested terrain' in which contrasting conceptions of what should be taught and how are struggled over, with some conceptions becoming dominant and other suppressed" (Hursh, 1997, p. 124). They see social efficiency (education in the service of capital) as the dominant approach in this decade, resisted by social meliorism or social reconstruction, which focuses on education "as a means of achieving democracy, justice, and equality" (Hursh, 1997, p. 124).

The ideals and methods of participatory inquiry are finding expression in a wide variety of other disciplines and traditions. Feminism's activist approach to redress the oppression of women is particularly resonant with PAR (e.g., Fine, 1992; Lather, 1991). Evaluation specialists are adopting emancipatory principles and tactics and calling it "empowerment evaluation" (Fetterman, 1994). Analysts of organizational function advocate for worker participation under the names of "continuous quality improvement" (e.g., Deming, 1986) or "the learning organization" (e.g., Senge, 1990), both of which are essentially forms of participatory inquiry in the workplace. Anthropology has developed a strand—action anthropology—that is not content with the description and interpretation of culture but rather is oriented to "intensive intervention in the problems and requirements of local communities" (Bennet, 1996). Another strand is critical medical anthropology, which examines how social issues of class, race, gender, and sexual orientation interact with dominant models of disease and health care to create oppression in marginalized groups (e.g., Singer, 1990, 1994).

Participatory Inquiry in Health Care

There are many examples of participatory inquiry in the health professions literature. They all pay attention to individual and group development, to relationships and power, and to environmental and structural determinants of behavior and experience. They differ in the relative emphasis on each of these aspects of participatory inquiry. Those studies that focus on professional development include Malterud's (1995a) use of action research to improve the quality of consultations (see also Chapter 17). In this "patient-centered clinical method," she shows how

> improvements in practice and increased knowledge and understanding are linked together in an integrated and dynamic cycle of activities, in which each phase learns from the previous one and in turn shapes the next. The stages of research involve problem identification, planning, action and evaluation. (Malterud, 1995a, p. 476)

Balint groups (Balint, 1957) are a kind of action research whereby practitioners come together to reflect on their relationships with patients and the meaning of their work. Brigley, Young, Littlejohns, and McEwen (1997) describe a "reflective model" of continuing education in which practitioners widen their accountability to patients, the community, managers, and policy makers. They seek collaboration with these stakeholders and with other providers to develop ways of learning that address the needs of those serving and those served. Other professional development inquiries emphasize historical and structural reasons for the dominance of some provider groups, such as medicine, and the subordinate position of other groups, such as nursing (Henderson, 1995; Street, 1995). These studies adopt a critical theory or explicitly feminist approach (Lather, 1991) to promote more evenly shared power among the health professions.

Other participatory inquiries emphasize the environmental context of health and illness. Schurman (1996) reports on a longitudinal project that reduced stress-related illness and disability in a U.S. automobile parts factory. The Motala, Sweden Injury Prevention Program employed a participatory research model that led to the establishment of a safety board for the municipality. The project created new prevention activities that continued after the initial study was completed (Lindqvist, Timpka, & Schelp, 1996).

Many participatory projects are set in underserved areas in both the developed and the developing world. Canadian family physician Carol Herbert (1996) and colleagues collaborated with Aboriginal communities in British Columbia to improve the health of local residents. Herbert describes how the community leaders chose the focus of the work (diabetes), designed culturally appropriate interventions, and controlled both the use of resources and the content of resulting publications. Rains and Ray (1995) report on the "Healthy Cities" initiative in rural Indiana. Here, public health nurses collaborated with community representatives to identify priority health problems—in this case, cancer and heart disease—and devise community-level interventions on specific issues. These issues included smoking, exercise, alcohol use/abuse, mental health, and dietary choices. The group eventually decided to focus their efforts on one issue—smoking—and implemented both policy and prevention actions. Urban U.S. examples include Detroit's East Side Village Health Worker Partnership, in which lay health advisors assist the local community while following PAR principles (Parker, Schultz, Israel, & Hollis, 1998), and a collaborative community intervention to improve breast and cervical cancer screening behavior among Korean women in Oakland, California (Chen et al., 1997). From South Africa, Hildebrandt (1994) describes "community involvement in health" in a Black township whereby community groups and individuals identified the health needs of the elderly and the capacity of the current system to meet them. They implemented, evaluated, and maintained four new programs to improve services. From India comes Emmel and O'Keefe's (1996) report of how slum dwellers in Bombay, through dialogue with investigators, exposed "the differences in perceptions between professional health deliverers and the women of Budh Mandir . . . [that] have important implications in redefining health delivery." The authors argue that "participatory methods can act as a process through which slum dwellers can demand appropriate health care for themselves and their families." Numerous other examples are cited by Macaulay and colleagues in their 1998 report to the North American Primary Care Research Group on participatory research with communities.

Challenges

It is apparent that participatory inquiry differs from other kinds of qualitative research in the degree of emphasis on participant control and on personal and political reform. Other qualitative research might ask questions like, "What is going on in life?" and use participant observation (Chapter 3) or "What is the meaning of life?" and use various kinds of interviews (Chapters 4 through 6). Participatory inquiry asks, "How can life be better?" and will seek both the "reconstructed logic" found in interviews as well as the "logic in use" found through participant observation. The methods are the same as other qualitative work, but the purposes and players are different.

The ideals and forms of participatory inquiry also create unique issues and tensions for the team. This kind of research is often in and for the *community.* Yet the investigator must deal with the expectations of *academe* to conform to acceptable structures and publish in scholarly journals

Ethical issues must be included in all steps.

Preparing. Don't do it alone! Find allies. This step includes:

- Focusing on the question/issue
- Focusing on the need for special requirements (especially because one of the goals is transformation—not everyone wants that or is ready for that)
- Doing a stakeholder analysis
- Deciding who needs to be on the team, both from a stakeholder perspective and from a methods perspective: Who has the necessary competence?

Gathering. This step includes:

- Group dynamics, negotiation skills, conflict resolution
- Stages and process of community development
- Acknowledging and addressing tension (academe versus street, powerful versus oppressed, agenda of principal investigator versus agendas of coresearchers [the community, etc.], agenda of funder versus agenda of researchers, etc.)

Working/reflecting. This step includes:

- Sampling issues (because the sampled are the researchers, or at least some of them are)
- Working up from down (doing research as a resident alien or doing research to change those who might lose power as a result of the change)
- Creating reflective positions from which to analyse and synthesize the data and experiences

Transferring. This step includes:

- Creating an account of the research (in a form that speaks to the people who want and need these insights and is congruent with the research aim and the project phase)
- Entering a new cycle of preparing, gathering, working, and transferring

Final transferring step, when one chooses to leave the process:

- Creating an overall account of the research (in a form that speaks to the people who want and need these insights and is congruent with the research aim)
- Leaving the research process

Figure 15.1. The Steps of Doing Participatory Inquiry

and guided by "the user perspective" and implemented through "user involvement." No one really knew what user perspective and user involvement meant. In explaining the term "users," the authors of the background paper said: "those who themselves have serious psychiatric illness, with or without serious addiction to drugs or alcohol (dual diagnosis) in addition" (SME, 1990).

The objective was very broad: "To elicit knowledge concerning what kind of collaboration and what kind of help is relevant for people with serious mental illness, and those who care about them." This was based in the evidence that services for users with mental illness were inadequate, often nonexisting, and sometimes even harmful. These are problems Norway shares with most other countries in the Western world, especially after implementation of deinstitutionalisation. TCP had a broad focus and was organizationally complicated. This presentation focuses only on those parts of the story that are relevant to this chapter.

The project initiators made contact with seven different potential project leaders from different sectors of the services and in different parts of the country—in psychiatric specialist services as well as in primary care, in rural and urban, southern and northern parts of the country. They all accepted the challenge of designing, applying for funding, implementing, and reporting the experiences over a 3- to 4-year time span. I (Janecke Thesen—JT) was the only primary care physician invited. I had worked in the project area for more than 15 years.

Preparing

The first task was to analyze who the actors in this field were, who would be most in power, who would be most positive, who would be most opposed, and so forth, to the ideas embedded in the project objective and background paper—in short, doing a stakeholder analysis. Did we have enough allies to make this happen at all? Were those opposed to ideas of user perspective and user involvement so powerful that we would be opposed or sabotaged? Were those in favor of these new ideas powerful enough to support the work, take part in it, make it happen? Did I really believe in these ideas myself? Crucial to me at that point was the opportunity to pose these questions as we-questions so I would not feel alone through this process. I carefully chose a small number of people with whom I could discuss these questions at great length, feeling safe and supported while at the same time being tenderly confronted with my own inadequacies and prejudices and all the challenges that would come up. I call these good people my personal advisors. Two of them (Kirsti Malterud—KM, and Unni Kristiansen—UK) have stayed with me through the whole process and have secured my ability to stick with it. These two advisors also had important competence that the project needed: Although I had extensive inside knowledge about the local culture and sufficient authority and skills to shoulder the leadership role, I lacked the research experience. KM (a GP/family doctor and researcher) had competence in qualitative, statistical, and action research methods, and UK (a psychiatrist) brought us the skills of systemic family therapy and group processes. Besides, we were close friends, all women, and we did not have to spend time on creating a mutually trusting and safe environment. What we did not have was inside knowledge about what it is like to have serious mental illness in this part of Norway.

We organized the project by establishing a multitude of groups and key people, of which the most important were

- a planning committee of 20 people, in which I served as the secretary;
- a smaller advisory group especially designed to give me ideas and constructive critique in a safer, more informal, and more supportive climate; and
- a research and internal evaluation supervisor from the nearest University—6 hours away by car and ferry.

The basic idea of involving an evaluation supervisor was to help establish and implement an internal evaluation process that would both deliver data and establish metapositions that would facilitate the review and reflection processes so crucial for driving the cycle of action in this action research project (Malterud, 1995a; Malterud & Kristiansen, 1995; Stringer, 1996). I later came to learn that these principles were in agreement with "empowerment evaluation," defined as "a method for using evaluation concepts, techniques and findings to foster improvement and self-determination. It is designed to help people help themselves and improve their programs using a form of self-evaluation and reflection" (Fetterman, Kaftarian, & Wandersman, 1996, p. 4).

Within these structures and by the help of my personal advisors, we developed a project plan where the time span was 3 years. The overarching objective was broken down into 14 more specific objectives. The means for achieving these objectives were user involvement and establishing multidisciplinary teams with a team case-management approach in every municipality. The project plan was applauded and the project successfully financed. The planning committee was transformed into a steering committee (one user representative, one mother of a user representing family members), and we established a project committee to follow the daily work more closely and decide on day-to-day finances (no user representatives). I left my main job as a family doctor for 3 years to lead the project.

Gathering and Working/Reflecting

So there we were, a lot of people, a lot of money, 3 years in front of us and a well-intended commitment to user involvement. We had no ideas on how to do it, and no local user organizations to lean on. The process of trial and error that followed was a long and complicated one.

We contacted the geographically closest user organization, requesting help. This was the county chapter of Mental Helse Norge (MHN = Mental Health Norway), the largest user/survivor organization in Norway. They allowed us to have one day at one of their conferences to present thoughts on TCP and organized a group process to answer the question: How can TCP achieve user involvement? They gave us some very clear guiding principles: (a) the users must be in the majority to be able to voice thoughts and ideas and to be heard and (b) the users need local groups that are their own.

What the users had told us was validated quite soon from our own experiences in the project structure, particularly the steering committee. We were proud of having representatives from users and their families in the committee, as most projects had none; however, it soon became painful to watch the hostage position we had put these representatives in. They were present in a democratic process, being held responsible for the decisions made. At the same time, the power imbalances, the language used, the speed of the decision process, and a myriad of unspoken rules made it quite impossible for them to have any but window-dressing influence on what was going on. As a country doctor without a hospital-based specialty, and as a woman, I was able to recognize the double catch that often had made me despair in influential committees of professors and high-powered managers, where I was the only one representing the three following groups: women, family doctors, and rural populations.

We arranged an evaluation workshop and invited all the professionals from the local multidisciplinary groups, in addition to other people involved locally—except the users. From this experience, we learned that people working locally, without research experience or familiarity with research language, can deliver very useful material for evaluation processes and cycle-of-action processes. When enough attention is spent on careful planning of the process, it is possible to create group processes that feel safe enough to enable people to voice not only good, but also bad, experiences (Malterud & Thesen, 1994). The hypothesis emerged: if this is the case when we invite local professionals, it may also be the case if we invite users and their family members.

On the basis of these three main experiences, we designed what became the turning point for user participation in TCP: the "Knowledge Workshop."

The Knowledge Workshop

What Is a Knowledge Workshop?

A Knowledge Workshop is a meeting between two or more groups with the clear goal of producing or eliciting new knowledge. The meeting is directed in such a way that inequalities (in status, meeting competence, argumentation skills, and power) are addressed and minimized. The main objective is to bring forth experiences and knowledge from people who are usually not heard or allowed to exert their influence.

We planned and implemented the first Knowledge Workshop with two groups, users, and professionals. The workshop itself was divided into four steps (or phases) of different duration: preparing, gathering, working/reflecting, and transferring. The aim was to generate/elicit/produce knowledge based on the user's experience with the services for people with psychiatric illness in the project area.

Preparing

We formulated and circulated six specific questions (only one question on each sheet of paper) 1 month before the workshop, asking users to discuss them (see Figure 15.2). By then, we had a network of user groups and connections through the project organization, so we did not have to recruit from patient-provider relationships.

We asked the users to discuss the questions—in organizations, with their friends and lovers, with their psychiatrist or social worker, or think about them privately—in whatever way they thought helpful to them. We asked them to mail or bring the written answers to the second step: the gathering. One man, being too sick to attend any meeting or write anything, called me on the phone and contributed by discussing the themes focused by the questions.

Gathering

We used the conference hotel where the professionals usually have their seminars and meetings and made sure that the meals were just as good as usual. We had hired four leaders from MHN to function as observers for the whole workshop. Unfortunately, only two showed up, so we had to use any nonprofessionals at hand that very morning—two social anthropologists working in the project field. A main point was that the meeting should not be "contaminated" by any typical healthcare professionals. Thus even I, as a project leader but still a physician, had to withdraw, apart from

1. What are the main problems for people with serious mental illness in this region? (Think about your own situation or someone you know quite well. Use examples you have experienced yourself, not only heard about. Make a list, and feel free to use extra paper.)

2. What are the main problems for people (relatives, family members, friends) who care about persons with serious mental illness in this region? (Think about your own situation or someone you know quite well. Use examples you have experienced yourself, not only heard about. Make a list, and feel free to use extra paper.)

3. What difficulties do you experience with municipal services? (Health services, social services, housing authorities, schools, social insurance offices, vocational authorities, and so on. Use examples you have experienced yourself, not only heard about. Make a list, and feel free to use extra paper. What is needed to change the situation?)

4. What difficulties do you experience with county and specialist services? (Psychiatric clinics and hospitals, psychiatric centers, psychiatric nursing homes, psychiatric outpatient departments, county-level vocational offices, and so on. Use examples you have experienced yourself, not only heard about. Make a list, and feel free to use extra paper. What is needed to change the situation?)

5. Make a list of positive and good collaboration with the services, things you want to happen more often. (Use examples you have experienced yourself, not only heard about. Feel free to use extra paper.)

6. What important questions would you like to focus on, in addition to the other 5 questions? (Think about your own situation, both as individuals and as a group of people. Possible starting points could be: [here follows a list of materials produced by users in TCP and closely related projects and directions of how to get hold of the material]. Feel free to use extra paper.)

Figure 15.2. The Questions From the Knowledge Workshop

welcoming people to the workshop and having lunch with them. The 13 users and the four observers worked on the six questions the whole day, mostly in groups. I sat in my hotel room going through the written answers to the questions.

Working/Reflecting

Two system-oriented family therapists from outside the project area had arrived by plane by the next morning: one psychiatrist and one psychiatric

diagnosis, that happened in the context of diagnosis-as-label, diagnosis-as-doom, diagnosis-as-unappeasable-verdict, a context used by the local communities to discriminate against them, deem them incompetent, harass them. The local community also includes the managers, the professional helpers like the social workers and the doctors—in short, it also included me and the other professionals in the project. Even though I did not have any provider-patient relations to any users during the project phase, some were my previous patients, and the stories told were from periods when I had been their doctor. The users made me see things differently. For example, they taught me how my concept of poverty (perhaps meaning having to wait another year before I could buy a new pair of skis or having to refuse to allow one of my kids to go to a very attractive private school) was totally inadequate to describe their experience of poverty (e.g., not being able to join the user collective or visit your father because you never had money for the bus or not having a telephone because you could not afford the phone bills). In a similar way, I had to revise my perceptions of loneliness, isolation, lack of love, and so on. Another example is that the users did not restrict themselves to roles that I considered appropriate for them: when speaking of helping acts, they freely varied their examples, sometimes with themselves on the receiving end, sometimes in the helping role.

During the Knowledge Workshop, I was tempted to turn their intense plea for respect and deference around to justify a similar demand for respect and deference for myself. What I did not realize until much later was the huge power differential between me and the users, making such demands coming from me highly oppressive.

The learning process that I have described in the previous paragraphs is itself the result of a long process: listening to the tapes, production of the initial report, and an in-depth qualitative analysis of the transcribed tapes from the Knowledge Workshop. I handled the material as if it had been a focus group session, supplemented with the written material, the flip charts, and photographs of the whiteboard at different stages of the process. I used the modification of Giorgi's phenomenological method recommended by Malterud (1996). In the analysis, I tried to stay as close as possible to the concepts and words employed by the users. It required putting my worldviews and theoretical models as a general practitioner in the background. Thus, I could better grasp what I now define as the user perspective. It is not what I think the user really means when I use my theoretical background to interpret his words and actions, looking for some hidden intention or plot. This is the style of analysis that Kvale (1996) calls "meaning interpretation," inspired by hermeneutical philosophy (also see Chapter 8). Rather, the user perspective is what I as a human being see if I place myself in the shoes of the user and look at the world through his or her eyes (or glasses). As that is, of course, impossible, I strive for the closest I can get to that ideal. To do this, I used what Miller and Crabtree call an editing analysis style, trying to be more a person living in this region than a GP when I interpretively determined the connections between categories (see Chapter 7).

Changing My View as an Inquirer:
Pushing Me Against a More Participatory Research Style,
Learning About Model Monopoly,
and Developing New Instruments

Before the Knowledge Workshop, I tried to read texts produced by users—some in the research literature, some in more informal reports, some accounts and stories, and some in the world literature. They did not produce a great impact on me, nor did they change my perception of the people we call users. I mainly found the texts lengthy and often boring. After the Knowledge Workshop, I actively looked up this literature again. This time, it stirred my interest and captured my attention. I think this was because I recognized themes and phenomena from the data collected and lessons learned from the Knowledge Workshop. I think it no coincidence that the authors that stirred my newborn interest were people in the user movement who also are mental health professionals or researchers. I think it has to do with language and cultural similarity. As Blanch, Fisher, Tucker, Walsh, and Chassman (1993) state:

> a growing number of people with a psychiatric history are entering the mental health field, and some professionals have started to disclose their own psychiatric histories. As these "consumer-practitioners" openly discuss their own process of recovery, they express many of the ideas developed by the consumer/ex-patient movement in a context and a language that encourages professionals to listen. (p. 17)

Fossen (1994) states the phenomenon in a slightly different way:

> Luhman introduces the image of an aeroplane high above the sky to describe a self-referential system. To get information about the world outside, it must rely on its internal instruments. If something happens on the outside that cannot be attended to by one of the instruments, the aeroplane is blind to these phenomena. What is meaningful will always be internally decided. Social systems both within and outside the academic community can be modeled with this conceptual apparatus. Action research can then be modeled as a symmetrical process in which two self-referential systems encounter each other. Neither of the parties will be able to import meaning from the other system. (p. 3)

It is a fascinating hypothesis that I was in such an airplane high above the sky, with no instruments with which to pick up the signals from the user community. Being present at the Knowledge Workshop and working with the data had made me develop new instruments that increased my ability to pick up signals from "the translators" between the user and medical communities, the people with both user and mental health professional experience.

Being the pilot who suddenly became aware of the inadequacy of the airplane's instruments, I started to question the biomedical models and the focus of medical attention in mental illness. The inadequacy of these models was no news to me, but this fact had so far made little impact on me. Up to that point, I had used models in which we as service providers should "put the user at the center," make him the focus of our attention. The reciprocal effect of that is that the user must focus on us and make us the center of his attention. But we are not, and should not be! By following the leads from the literature and contacting authors from the user movement, I made contact with the National Empowerment Center (NEC) (specifically, with Fisher, Deegan, Chamberlin, and others), located in Boston, Massachusetts. I was able to visit the Center for Psychiatric Rehabilitation (CPR) at Boston University for 6 months. NEC and CPR collaborate closely, and I was able to work with both groups. I was introduced to user-led and user-assisted development of recovery-based models (Anthony, 1993; Deegan, 1996, 1997; Harding & Zahniser, 1994; Spaniol, Gagne, & Koehler, 1997). They have a different focus, namely the user's own project of hope and recovery. To remove the cause and alleviate symptoms of the illness—the focus of treatment—is but one of three important tasks. The other two are reconnecting with communities in acceptable social roles (mainly focused in rehabilitation) and action directed toward disempowerment and hopelessness (mainly alleviated through self-help and peer support and ensuring that treatment and rehabilitation do not function in a disempowering way).

Working with these alternative models made me acknowledge the concept of medical model monopoly. The concept of "model monopoly" was introduced by the Norwegian sociologist Stein Bråten in the early 1970s. It is defined as

> influence on others by virtue of a powerful model of reality that the others define as the source of the only valid answers to questions in the field. Model monopoly excludes the horizon of questioning from other perspectives and definitions of reality. As a consequence, what seems like a dialogue becomes a mock dialogue on the terms of the knowledgeable (model-strong) actors. (Bråten quoted in Korsnes, Andersen, & Brate, 1997, my translation)

Bråten (1988) states that there are at least four possible strategies for overcoming model monopoly:

1. Shifting the boundary of the universe of discourse or redefining the domain in a manner which reveals the limit of the monolithic perspective.
2. Opening up for rival knowledge sources and admitting propositions in alternative languages.
3. Developing knowledge on own premises. . . . canceling or escaping submittance to a mono-perspective, such as resorting to a meta level, entering a dialectic modus, stepping back for reflection! Or, just break off interaction while developing and consolidating your own perspective. (p. 214)
4. More generally, being aware of the kind of conditions that may promote model-monopoly and evoke psycho-logical tendencies toward cognitive consistency, monadic closing and conformity that prevent a creative horizon in the individual and in the community. (p. 215)

On afterthought, I think the Knowledge Workshop made use of several of these strategies, although I did not know about the concept of model monopoly at that time.

Transferring

When I entered TCP, I was skeptical about research and *happy about the fact* that my principals did not require any scientific publications from the project beyond extensive reports (e.g., Thesen, 1994, and several evaluation reports). My view has changed, however. When I realized how little emphasis the medical community gives to these kinds of reports, it made me determined to communicate the knowledge from TCP to fellow MDs in a scientific language. To challenge medical model monopoly, you must learn to play by the rules of the game. That brings me into the dilemma described in the first part of this chapter: "the investigator must deal with the implicit expectations of academe to conform to acceptable structures and publish in scholarly journals and books." This part of the project has so far been successfully financed as a grant for a medical dissertation, and the work is still in progress. Only time will show whether it will succeed.

FINAL REMARKS AND THE WAY BEYOND

On Participation

In almost all research there is participation. The ingenious lone researcher and thinker is becoming more and more rare. The news in participatory inquiry is that the people traditionally left out of the reflecting phases and merely studied as "things," as "rocks in the road," are invited into the processes as thinking and feeling human beings. They are expected to participate as human subjects with real influence in the processes, not only as objects to be studied.

Important checkpoints for whether or not the research is participatory are

- Who gets invited? Are all those affected, particularly at the bottom of the hierarchies, included?
- How are the power issues addressed and handled?
- Who formulates and refines the research question?
- Who has real influence on the processes?
- Who can allocate the resources when conflicts of interest arise between different stakeholders in a project?
- Who has the power to formulate and transfer the account of the process and outcomes of the project?

On Participatory Inquiry Versus Action Research

Because participatory research has developed in the context of action research/qualitative methods, there is a lot of confusion. But participatory inquiry and action research, although closely related, are not the same. We need to revise the models we use when designing participatory inquiry. Today, we usually adapt the models of action research, without changing them. A good model for participatory inquiry has yet to be developed. Changing the names and changing the grouping together of the different stages in the action research models is, however, a good start in developing a participatory inquiry model—emphasizing we-words like gathering, stakeholder analysis, team, community development, agenda, power, and so on (see Figure 15.1).

A participatory ideal should be used as a guiding star, not a compulsory straightjacket. In real life, the starting point is often a traditional and rigid research structure, at least for projects that get funded. It is possible to accept this as a fact and then consistently push in a more participatory direction. We know this to be true for action research projects and qualitative research methods, which allow for discovery and change during the research process. It may be much more difficult in more traditional medical experimental designs (see Chapter 1).

There may be reasons not to work in a participatory mode. In such a case, that should be justified based on the objective of the project. If the objective justifies a participatory mode (as with the objective "To elicit knowledge concerning what kind of collaboration and what kind of help is relevant for people with serious mental illness and those who care about them"), the potential benefits are at least two: (a) empowerment of disempowered groups and (b) production of better, more relevant research that is less dependent on the model monopoly of Western medical thinking.

On Empowerment

Empowerment is probably one of the most misused and coopted words in the English language. It may also have different meanings in different contexts. Numerous definitions exist, but for this chapter we will join Garcia (1997): "it is the ability to choose among alternatives, to act, to intervene and to change. It involves an appropriate use and sharing, and not the abnegation, of power" (p. 28).

There are hidden dangers in the good intentions of academics who do participatory inquiry. What if the ideals of advocacy for the oppressed, for empowerment, are really codes for investigator agendas and needs for control? Is Foucault correct when he argues that "humanistic values have become the ideological vessels through which the norms and expectations of a specific way of life are imposed upon individuals, thus reducing human freedom and eradicating human differences" (Fahy, 1997; Foucault, 1984)? How are we to resolve this tension?

Reason (1994, p. 335) suggests that this is a paradox of participatory research that must be acknowledged and lived with "to find creative resolution moment to moment." Heightened awareness of this potential ethical dilemma seems a necessary ingredient for creative resolution. This is why it is so crucial that ethical issues are included in all steps of the research process (see Figure 15.1). Another ingredient is the ideal of stewardship, the willingness to be accountable for the well-being of the larger community by operating in service to those around us (Block, 1993).

It is important that anyone wanting to do participatory inquiry in primary care keep the following points in mind:

- Empowerment is particularly important to the most disempowered patients (e.g., people who have been psychiatrically labeled) because perceived influence and control in their lives are central to the recovery processes.
- You cannot "empower" someone—but you can stop taking people's power away, and you can stop blocking empowerment and switch to facilitating the process of people regaining their own power.
- The people you want to "empower" possess important knowledge about their own situation. This is true even if that knowledge is not articulated in a language you are able to understand.

- You cannot control the direction of an empowerment process, or the process itself, if you succeed in stimulating such a process.
- Don't confuse *your* agenda with *their* agenda; focus on how to create *our agenda.*
- Don't introduce anything that induces dependency and is not available when the project ends—including yourself.

Ernest Stringer (1996) speaks of his work with Aboriginal populations in West Australia:

Professionals tend to approach Aboriginal people with the intent of "helping" them, or as people in need of "training." They talk in terms of the "cultural deficits" of Aboriginal children and the need for Aboriginal people to learn "social skills." Their ethnocentrism would be merely annoying if it were not for the fact that many of them are in positions of professional power that permit them to have significant impacts on the lives of people for whom they have so little regard. Aboriginal people often find their lives controlled by experts and public servants who have little understanding of their social and cultural realities and are apt to act in ways that are inappropriate or demeaning from an Aboriginal perspective.

I am once again reminded of the words of the Aboriginal social worker Lila Watson: "If you've come to help me, you're wasting your time. But if you've come because your liberation is bound up with mine, then let us work together." (p. 147)

PART
V

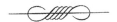

Putting It All Together

16

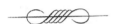

Researching
Practice Settings

A Case Study Approach

Benjamin F. Crabtree
William L. Miller

SETTING THE CONTEXT

The "Prevention and Competing Demands in Primary Care" study was a complicated project that evolved and matured over several years. Designing and conducting a research study of this magnitude and intricacy took more than a good research question and a desire to do research. There was, by necessity, a history of small studies that provided a conceptual foundation, contributed essential experience in the use of multiple methods, and produced a sufficient track record for a funding agency to believe it was worth investing their money in this project and not another. The focus of this chapter is on describing a comparative case study of family physicians' clinical practices. We begin with the historical context and our personal journeys, which made it possible to conceptualize the study, obtain funding, and eventually carry out the project. This is followed by a description of the research, including the ongoing modifications that occurred over time as the project was implemented. The chapter ends with a summary of some of the key learnings.

THE QUEST

By fall 1995, we were beginning to visualize the pieces of a very complex puzzle. Over the preceding 5 years, as part of our search for understanding of the variation in family physician practices, we had completed a series of depth interview studies that focused on physicians and their perceptions of what they do. These encompassed a wide range of topics that included pain and pain management (Miller, Yanoshik, et al., 1994), approaches to diabetes care (Helseth, Susman, Crabtree, & O'Connor, 1999), depression management (Susman et al., 1995), mammography and breast cancer screening (Smith et al., 1996), and tobacco cessation efforts (McIlvain, Crabtree, Gilbert, et al., 1997). In different ways, these studies had each challenged the assumption that it was possible to understand the variation in practice behavior described in the medical literature by focusing on individual physician perceptions or isolating specific health problems. Physicians were part of bigger systems, and specific health problems were not independent of the whole complex range of problems seen in primary care practices. We were also getting glimpses of the great diversity in the way practices organized their office systems, making it clear that we needed to better understand the contexts in which physicians worked and health problems presented.

We were also changing as researchers. We were becoming increasingly dissatisfied with the limitations of the research methods we were using, even some of the methods that we had personally committed a lot of effort to disseminate. After making a major commitment to developing our skills in qualitative methods, we were still concerned by our heavy reliance on interviews. We were finding that our interview-based studies were missing context at the very moment when context was increasingly seen as important. This was a time for much self-reflection, which resulted in greatly expanding our research scope.

Another important development was the start of a long research collaboration between the two of us, when we were both in the Department of Family Medicine at the University of Connecticut, and with investigators from Case Western Reserve University, particularly Kurt Stange and Stephen Zyzanski. Early in 1991, Kurt and Steve approached us about putting together an article that described ways of integrating qualitative and quantitative approaches. This article would eventually be published (Stange, Miller, et al., 1994), but our discussions pushed us to consider how qualitative research could be incorporated into a large descriptive study of family medicine practices that Kurt was preparing for submission to the Agency for Health Care Policy and Research (AHCPR) and the National Cancer Institute (NCI). When the proposal was finally submitted in February 1992, we had developed a strategy whereby research nurses would dictate qualitative field notes about their impressions of physicians and their practices while collecting a large volume of data that was otherwise quite structured. By the time the "Direct Observation of Primary Care" (DOPC) project was funded in May 1994, Ben had moved to the University of Nebraska Medical Center in Omaha and Will had moved to Lehigh Valley Hospital in Allentown, Pennsylvania. Nevertheless, the collaboration continued; now, however, with additional members from Nebraska and Pennsylvania.

The DOPC study got under way with great excitement early in summer 1994. As the group of collaborators on the project discussed the impressive array of data collection protocols for the study (see Stange, Zyzanski, Smith, et al., 1998, for details of the DOPC methods), we realized that this would be an incredibly rich data set, albeit primarily within the survey research tradition of epidemiology. The qualitative component appeared to be very limited, and we felt the need to have a richer source of text to really understand the intricacies of practices. It was during one of the DOPC planning meetings that summer that the idea of developing a follow-up study to the DOPC to better understand both successful and struggling practices was conceived. This was to be one of the first large-scale qualitative studies ever submitted to AHCPR and NCI, a challenge to them as funders and reviewers, as well as to us. Thus, the "Prevention and Competing Demands in Primary Care" study was born.

The task of putting together a proposal to conduct these comparative case studies of DOPC practices fell to Ben at the University of Nebraska. The "Prevention and Competing Demands in Primary Care" project was designed and written during an intense 2 months and submitted to AHCPR in October 1994. Although this was not known to us at the time, the November elections in 1994 would have a grave impact on our project and challenge our collaboration. The project received an outstanding score at the eighth percentile when reviewed the following February, but funding seemed remote as AHCPR's budget was drastically cut by the new Congress. By summer 1995, the project appeared doomed as AHCPR struggled just to survive, and the National Cancer Institute was not interested in funding a qualitative case study project.

Meanwhile, at the University of Nebraska, new colleagues Jeff Susman and Jim Medder, both family physicians, and Helen McIlvain, a behavioral scientist, were interested in pursuing an evaluation of the soon to be released Put Prevention Into Practice (PPIP) program that was to be distributed by the American Academy of Family Physicians (AAFP). The primary interest at the AAFP was an accounting of sales, but after we presented them with a proposal for a substantially scaled-down version of the AHCPR project, the AAFP was willing to fund some limited case studies of practices that had purchased the PPIP program (see Chapter 9 for a description of the project). In summer 1995, the PPIP study began as our first serious effort toward conducting case studies of practices and an opportunity to test some of the methods we would later use in the "Prevention and Competing Demands" study (see McVea et al., 1996).

The PPIP project was a real eye opener, both about the need to be multimethod and about the complexity of family practices as organizations. To capture this complexity, the concept of a "practice genogram" was created to provide a visual display of a practice's organization and the interrelationships of participants (see McIlvain, Crabtree, Medder, et al., 1998). This view of practices as complex systems was further reinforced as Ben, Will, and a new member of the team, Virginia Aita, began to work more intensely with the DOPC data and see linkages with chaos and complexity theory (see Chapter 9; Miller, Crabtree, et al., 1998). The data from both of these studies pointed toward new possibilities in understanding primary care practices as nonlinear complex systems (Miller, Crabtree, et al., 1998) and in the role for case study designs in providing the data necessary for capturing the complexity of practices.

During summer 1995, a third study, "A Study of Tobacco Use Prevention in Physicians' Offices," was just getting under way in Nebraska and would later prove to be instrumental in identifying practices for future studies (see Chapter 14 for a description of this project). Helen McIlvain and Ben began this two-phase State of Nebraska-funded project to study tobacco prevention and cessation efforts in family practices. The first phase (McIlvain, Crabtree, Gilbert, et al., 1997) used a brief case study design much like the PPIP project. The second phase, which becomes very important to this story, did very brief one day evaluations of tobacco and mammography in a random sample of 91 practices throughout Nebraska. A trained research nurse spent half a day observing clinical encounters of one physician and the remainder of the day filling out a practice-level observational checklist, conducting a depth interview with the physician, and performing chart audits. Data collection for the second phase began in fall 1995 and would last for 1 year.

By early 1996, things did not seem quite as dismal at AHCPR, and we once again began to get excited about pursuing funding for the "Prevention and Competing Demands" study. Initial inquiries at AHCPR seemed promising, but a complication had arisen at Case Western Reserve University. Kurt Stange had submitted a follow-up clinical trial, the "Study To Enhance Prevention through Understanding Practice" (STEP-UP), to NCI. This new study planned to randomize the practices participating in the DOPC into either a control or an intervention group based on our emerging work on practice organization, particularly from the PPIP study and the DOPC study itself. Members of the collaboration had anticipated that it would take several submissions to obtain funding; thus we were sure there would be ample time to complete the comparative case study before STEP-UP. To our surprise, STEP-UP received an outstanding priority score on the first submission. Much to our chagrin, it appeared that, somehow, the "Prevention and Competing Demands" project and STEP-UP needed to be done simultaneously in Cleveland and in the same practices.

Faced with this dilemma, we (Will and Ben) took several days after the spring 1996 Society of Teachers of Family Medicine (STFM) Conference in San Francisco, rented a car, and headed north to contemplate in the redwood forests of California. We had the forests and miles of rugged Pacific coast to ourselves, as the chill of early spring seemed to discourage others from sampling the incredible beauty of the area. With 2,000-year-old redwoods as our companions, we waited patiently for new insights to emerge. They did! It was going to require tremendous coordination between the University of Nebraska and Case Western, and a lot of personal give and take between Kurt and Ben as the two principal investigators, to make it possible.

In May 1996, Ben flew to Cleveland to work with Kurt on integrating these two large projects with combined budgets of well over $3 million. The proposal we developed seemed feasible, but Kurt was legitimately concerned about overwhelming the practices and contaminating the clinical trial. He was also concerned that having the staff required for two major R0-1 projects would be overpowering. The collaborators from Case Western suggested that the "Prevention and Competing Demands" study be conducted in Nebraska using the practices from Helen McIlvain's tobacco and mammography study instead of those from the DOPC. Ben saw little hope in this because the data available from the Nebraska study were just a drop in the bucket compared to that from the DOPC study, and this could represent a major weakness to AHCPR. Ben went home dejected and wondered whether the collaboration was sustainable.

In a series of e-mail communications, Ben presented the idea of the study location change to the project officer at AHCPR. He argued that it would be possible to greatly reduce the $1.2 million budget, which could be very attractive to a money-strapped AHCPR. After the initial e-mail negotiations, Helen McIlvain and Ben flew to Washington in mid-June for a face-to-face slide presentation and discussion with members of AHCPR. The day did not get off to a good start. The early direct Washington flight from Omaha was delayed by two hours, making it impossible for them to be at the scheduled 11:00 a.m. briefing. When they finally did arrive in Washington at noon, they logically decided to take a taxi to Rockville to save time, and again fate seemed to be against them. Despite the news program on the radio specifically saying to stay off the interstate, the taxi driver headed directly into the bumper-to-bumper crawl, and this on a 95° day without air conditioning. To make matters worse, the taxi driver did not have a clue where the building was located and began to drive in circles looking for the street. Hot, sweaty, and completely dejected, Helen and Ben jumped out of the taxi, looked at each other and said, "Guess this wasn't meant to happen." Helen called AHCPR, and the project officer came to pick them up. They eventually did present their ideas to two of the staff in an otherwise empty conference room.

By late July, it appeared that the efforts had not been in vain after all; we received word that the "Prevention and Competing Demands" study would be funded, with funding beginning in September 1996. This saga, from conceptualization through funding, taught us a lot about what it takes to get a major qualitative study funded. Persistence is essential. We could have given up at many points along the way. The collaboration and patience of many people were essential for this complex project but were constantly tested. We learned that maintaining a collaborative relationship requires going through ups and downs, doing a lot of listening and compromising, and making the adjustments. Equally important, during the 2 years of waiting, we had continued doing other smaller studies while the "Prevention and Competing Demands" project was being reviewed and put on hold by forces outside our control. These studies provided valuable experience in the methods and helped to coalesce our group into a working team.

DREAMING IT

The "Prevention and Competing Demands" study was conceptualized as an in-depth examination of family physician practices, with the goal of better understanding the organizational and office-system features that promote or inhibit preventive services delivery. A longer term goal was that of developing interventions to assist practices that are currently struggling to provide these services. A multimethod comparative case study design was conceived that combined prolonged direct observation of the practice and semistructured and key informant interviews with members of the practice. All data were to be collected by full-time field workers with a health care background, who would be provided with extensive training in field research methods. A planned feature was to have the field worker substitute for one of the office nursing staff for 2 of their 6 to 8 weeks at the practice—thus the project's nickname, "vacation study." Field notes were to be dictated daily and rapidly transcribed to preserve the iterative process. Ongoing analysis would take place by having the investigators at the medical center write summary case reports resulting from the triangulation of interpretation from an editing analysis of the individual depth interviews, coding of the field notes with an evolving code book, and summary statistics of the checklist and chart audit data. There would be continual feedback discussions with the field worker.

This comparative case study design would include an initial phase of purposefully selected practices that included both urban and rural practices and practices with different intensity of preventive services delivery; the second phase would search for confirming or challenging cases using replication logic (Yin, 1989). As mentioned earlier, cases were to be selected from the "Tobacco Use Prevention in Physicians' Offices" study, after it became impossible to use the DOPC practices. Although the initial plan was to conduct a total of 26 case studies, the reduction in funding changed the sample size to 18, 10 initial and eight confirming or challenging cases.

The overall plan for data gathering included pairing structured checklists with open-ended descriptive field notes; the checklists could also serve as loose templates for the field notes. The pairings included separate checklist/observation templates for clinical encounters and for the overall practice environment. Data from informal key informant interviews with the physicians and staff were also in the field notes, and a semistructured taped depth interview was scheduled with each physician and key staff members. Thus, the primary data for each practice were to include observational field notes (see Chapter 3), key informant interviews (see Chapter 4), and individual depth interviews (see Chapter 5). These were supplemented with the structured checklists; chart audits of all patients observed; patient exit cards; photographs of all personnel and the physical location; and samples of documents, chart materials, and patient education materials.

The nurse researcher's first goal when entering the practice was to try to gain an initial understanding of the practice. One of the early steps was to create a detailed map or floor plan of the practice and to begin identifying individuals and activities that occurred in different areas of the practice. Over the course of 6 to 8 weeks, the researcher was to learn about each practice setting by directly observing the activities at the practice, including observing 30 clinical encounters with each physician. They would also have numerous informal conversations or key informant interviews with office staff. Short reminders or jottings were to be noted throughout the day and then expanded into more formal field notes in the evening by dictating into a tape recorder. These field notes were to provide details on a wide range of topics, such as the different roles of staff, the various office systems, office politics, and interpersonal relationships.

During the observation of each patient encounter, the field workers were to complete a clinical encounter observation checklist that was used to record information on basic patient demographics, type of visit, and types of services provided. The checklist was also to include more than 75 of the preventive services recommended by the U.S. Preventive Services Task Force. Each evening, more detailed field notes were to be dictated for each encounter, based on field jottings written at the bottom of the encounter checklist during the visit. These expanded field notes would describe in some detail the chronology of the encounter, often resulting in two or more pages of notes per encounter.

After an initial 2 to 3 weeks in the practice, the field worker was to return to the medical center to meet with the rest of the team and to construct a practice genogram (McIlvain, Crabtree, Medder, et al., 1998). Over the course of 1 to 2 hours, the research team would interview the field worker and construct the genogram on a large whiteboard. The construction was to begin with an organizational chart based on the assumed hierarchy of authority and responsibility, with notation of important demographic information such as age and length of service. Once the basic genogram structure had been constructed, details on functional and emotional relationships would be added. In addition to constructing the genogram, these sessions would serve to perform some preliminary analyses, leading to additional questions and content areas for the field workers to explore when they returned to the practice.

With the genogram completed and a list of follow-up questions identified, the field worker was to return to the practice to complete data gathering. Only after the field worker was very familiar with the practice and the personnel were individual depth interviews of physicians and staff to be conducted. All office providers would be asked for verbal confirmation prior to scheduling an interview, with written informed consent to be obtained at the time of the interview. These were to consist of a 1- to 2½-hour depth interview, during which the respondent would be asked open-ended questions designed to elicit long, in-depth responses (see Chapter 5). As the focus of the study was to be on preventive services delivery, most of these grand tour questions would center on the physician's or staff's perception of prevention and their role in providing these services. The interview would be audiotaped and transcribed.

Chart audits would be conducted to provide an independent assessment of adherence to preventive guidelines and to identify office strategies for prevention. A chart audit form would be filled out and a brief verbal description of the chart dictated. These latter would include the overall organization of the chart and the ease with which the field worker was able to locate information.

Documents from the office would be collected whenever possible. These would include samples of patient education materials and any innovative practice enhancements, such as flow sheets and reminder cards. Photographs were to be taken of the physical location, including both the outside and the different areas within the practice, and of all the physicians and staff.

LIVING IT

The overall design of the study, as just described, proved to be well conceived; however, there were continual modifications and adjustments that needed to be made. We were surprised to find that it was possible for the researcher to become oriented to the practice quickly, in part because practices routinely have outside observers, particularly medical students and residents, and the field workers were health care professionals familiar with the clinical setting. On the other hand, we quickly discovered that we had underestimated the overwhelming volume of data and the enormity of managing and interpreting these data. In this section, we look at some of the details of implementing the project and the ongoing adjustments that were deemed necessary.

Before beginning data collection, we spent several weeks training the field workers in the use of the methods. This included having outside consultants providing hands-on training. John Creswell, a widely published educational psychologist from the University of Nebraska in Lincoln, and Kim Yanoshik, a very experienced interviewer from Case Western Reserve University, spent several days working with the field workers. In addition, we also had the field workers practice observing encounters and dictating field notes in residency training practices. These were then reviewed by project staff, who provided feedback to the field workers so they could enhance their skills.

Finding a Place

To recruit practices into the study, we began with the list of 91 practices that had participated in the earlier tobacco and mammography study. Based on the existing data, we had indicators of which practices performed well in these two areas of preventive services delivery and which practices struggled. Thus, we were able to rank the 91 practices in terms of their intensity of delivery of tobacco prevention and/or screening mammography performance. In addition, the previous data had information on the number and gender of physicians in the practice and its location. From these data, we were able to purposefully select large versus small practices, independent versus health system-affiliated practices, and rural versus urban practices.

To recruit practices, a letter was sent to the physicians in the practice that explained the overall design of the project and what participation would entail. A follow-up phone call was made, and, if the practices expressed an interest in participating, a visit was made to the office by the principal investigator (Ben Crabtree) and the project coordinator (Diane Dodendorf). During the office visit, the whole project was explained to the physicians and office manager and any additional staff they invited. After the physicians had all agreed to participate, a letter was drafted to provide written confirmation of willingness to participate. It was assumed that this implied that office staff had also consented to being observed, which, in retrospect, proved to be not always the case. All offices were provided with a copy of the study design.

Recruiting practices turned out to be a time-consuming process; however, most practices that were contacted did eventually agree to participate (it required contacting 24 practices to get the 18 that participated in the study). Among the practices that did not participate, we generally found that one or more of the physicians were willing to participate, but we could not get consensus of all the physicians. This was a practice-level study, so we decided to work only with practices in which all the physicians had consented.

The initial site was selected because we had a very positive relationship with the practice, and we anticipated having a large learning curve in the early data-gathering process (and were we right!). This was a three-physician, independently owned rural practice that was a 7-hour drive from our office in Omaha. We sent the letter to all three physicians in the practice and then made phone contact with one of the physicians with whom we had previously worked most closely. She readily agreed to participate and was looking forward to our coming. When we arrived, however, it was apparent that either this had not been passed on to the two partners or that they had forgotten completely about the study. They did agree, but this alerted us to the need for more direct communication. As the study progressed, we found that the recruitment process required the persistence of the project director, who had to make numerous phone calls and sometimes found it difficult even to talk to the physicians due to overly protective staff.

Gathering the Data

The actual data gathering proceeded much as anticipated in the research design. The one big exception was our immediate discovery that the "vacation" component, in which the research nurse was to take the place of an office nurse, needed to be scrapped. Neither the research nurse nor the practice were comfortable with this aspect of the study. Both expressed concerns about liability.

Additional changes were needed in the data-gathering protocol. After the first few practices, we began to realize we were missing the community's perspective on the practice and on prevention. We added the use of key informant trees (see Chapter 4) to get at the community perspective. Similarly, while we were getting the physician's perspective of the clinical encounter, we became disturbed by our lack of the patient's perspective and thus added patient paths (Pommerenke & Dietrich, 1992a, 1992b), in which the field worker followed the patient throughout his or her visit. This approach used yet another pairing of a semistructured checklist along with dictated field notes and also included informal interviews of the patients. Finally, we discovered digital camera technology, which was very useful but did require the addition of new software programs and learning how to incorporate the photographs into Folio Views.

We quickly found that the process of getting patient informed consent required custom tailoring for each practice. In addition to the practice-level consent, another whole strategy was used to inform patients of the study and provide them with an opportunity to participate—or not. A notice with a brief description of the project was posted in the waiting room of each practice, informing everybody that the practice was participating in the project. When recruiting patients to allow observation of their physician visit, the receptionist or the office nurse gave copies of the notice and an informed consent form to all patients and/or their parent/guardian. Each office had to find the least disruptive way to ask patients if they would be willing to have their encounter with the physician observed and to allow the research team access to their chart. Effort was made to ensure that patients understood that not participating in the study was acceptable and would not influence their care. In some practices, the receptionist would do the consent process; in others, it was done by the nursing staff. Often it took several days for the process to be worked out. For example, in one practice, the nurse was initially responsible, but it was found that she did not have time to get the consent forms signed, leading to our missing many opportunities. Eventually, the receptionist stepped in to get the consent forms signed and placed in the chart so the research nurse would know that the patient had consented to be observed.

Processing and Managing the Data

The project presented many data management challenges that were not anticipated when the study began. The volume of data was simply overwhelming. A complex system needed to be set up to catalog and track the numerous tapes that the field workers sent for transcription, and once these were transcribed, there needed to be a process to ensure that the data were correctly incorporated into the appropriate file, printed, and distributed to team members in a timely fashion. The enormity of this process became all too clear when the practices explicitly indicated that they wanted feedback from the study. Given the very large volume of data, this request created a major challenge for data management and interpretation if the feedback was to be given within a reasonable time after completion of data gathering. The dedication of a full-time project coordinator was essential, as was formulating the very detailed process shown in Figure 16.1.

Each practice generated 30 or more audiotapes, along with quantitative checklists, other forms, and photographs (Step 1 in Figure 16.1). Each of these needed to be labeled and logged in by the project coordinator (Step 2). As part of the logging-in process, every patient encounter and matching chart audit needed to be assigned a unique identification number by the coordinator. Audiotapes of practice-level field notes, encounter field notes, and interviews were given to a transcriptionist, who transcribed the tapes in the order suggested by the project coordinator (Step 3). Once transcribed, both the tapes and a diskette copy of the data were returned to the coordinator for importing into Folio Views (Step 6). The Folio Views file that was set up for each practice (see Chapter 11) contained all the transcribed field notes in chronological order, along with the transcriptions of the dictated observed encounters and associated chart audits and the transcribed interviews. Data from the checklists were entered into Access (Step 4) and chart audit information into Excel (Step 5). Throughout the project, the project coordinator also maintained a "blue binder" of written materials collected during the project and a file cabinet of signed informed consent forms (Step 7).

Once the data had undergone these preliminary data management steps, an iterative process of analysis and interpretation took place. The quantitative data that had been entered into Access and Excel were used to create tables that profiled the observed patients (Step 8) and to track the extent to which preventive service recommendations were being followed for more than 25 different preventive services. This latter was done in detailed "hit/miss" tables in which each individual patient was given a "hit" or "miss" for a list of services based on the chart audits, the encounter checklist, and the written description of the encounter (Step 9). To do this, the project coordinator began with the chart audit of each observed patient and then read the field notes for that same patient to determine what occurred in the encounter. A file was created for each practice in which each line represented a patient and included data on the date of visit, the type of visit, the number of visits in the prior 2 years, and a determination as to whether the patient was eligible or not for up to 25 different preventive services. If the patient was not eligible under current recommendations, he or she was simply given an "X." If the patient was eligible, then based on the chart audit and the encounter notes, each service was designated with an "H," indicating that the service was a hit during the observed encounter, an "h," indicating that it was not done during the

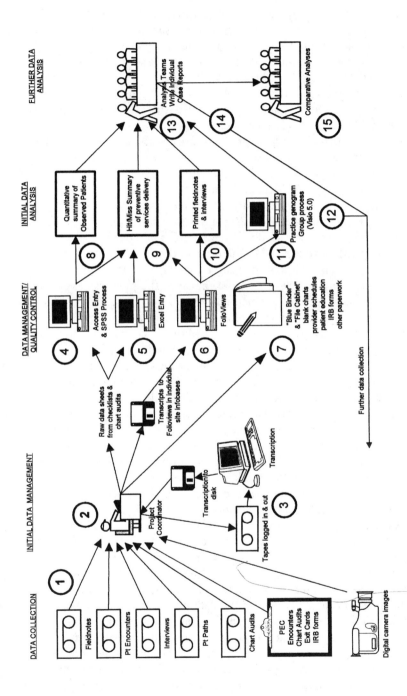

Figure 16.1. Data Management for Prevention and Competing Demands Case Study

encounter but was up to date according the chart, or an "M," indicating a miss. Once all encounters had been coded, a summary hit/miss table was constructed and printed for inclusion in the interpretation.

After reading the initial field notes from Folio Views (Step 10), the field worker worked with the larger team in a group process to construct a practice genogram (McIlvain, Crabtree, Medder, et al., 1998), with a computer-generated diagram being produced with a design program, Visio Standard 5.0 (Step 11). The practice genogram provided a visual picture of the practice that was very helpful in future discussions (see Figure 16.2). Based on the genogram session, additional areas of exploration were identified for the field worker to explore further (Step 12), and this cycled the process back into the data collection steps.

Throughout the study, the analysis team met to review the evolving data with the goal of writing a 10- to 20-page written case study report for each practice and producing a feedback report that could be used as a member check (Step 13). Beyond the data management challenges, this data analysis and interpretation also presented several major unanticipated challenges. As mentioned previously, right from the start, the practices expressed a desire to receive feedback, which put pressure on the team members to create timely descriptive case reports and then summarize these into feedback reports. Depending on the size of the practice, those working on the analysis were faced with reading several hundred single-spaced pages of field notes and interview transcripts, reviewing summary tables, deciding what was important, and writing a concise 10- to 20-page description of each practice site. These reports then needed to be summarized into a 4- to 5-page feedback report that could be presented to the practice along with the quantitative summary table. The process was relentless; no sooner had one practice been completed then another was waiting in the wings.

In addition to writing the two reports, during the analysis process, the analysis team provided feedback to the field worker on areas where clarification or further data were required (Step 14). Finally, once the final reports were written and data collection completed, comparative case analysis began (Step 15). At the time of the writing of this chapter, more than 70 separate analyses had been identified, and plans were made to revisit each of the practices for yet another iterative cycle of data collection.

There were real struggles to make the iterative process of collection and interpretation work (refer to Chapter 7). Initially, all five faculty and staff at the medical center worked on the data from each practice, but we just simply couldn't keep up. The grant funding cycle would not allow us to slow up the data-gathering process, so we divided our team members into two interpretation teams so the practices could be divided up. We "re-cruited" two additional physician faculty to work with us on interpretation so that each team had at least one family physician and a faculty member

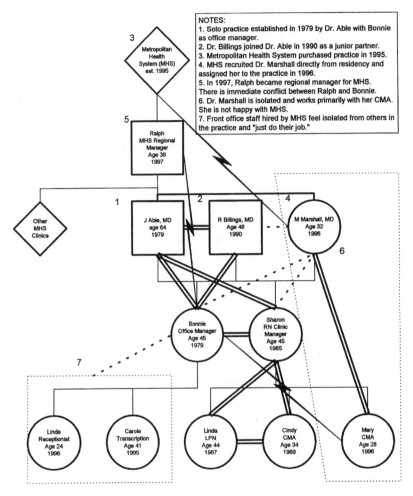

NOTES:
1. Solo practice established in 1979 by Dr. Able with Bonnie as office manager.
2. Dr. Billings joined Dr. Able in 1990 as a junior partner.
3. Metropolitan Health System purchased practice in 1995.
4. MHS recruited Dr. Marshall directly from residency and assigned her to the practice in 1996.
5. In 1997, Ralph became regional manager for MHS. There is immediate conflict between Ralph and Bonnie.
6. Dr. Marshall is isolated and works primarily with her CMA. She is not happy with MHS.
7. Front office staff hired by MHS feel isolated from others in the practice and "just do their job."

Figure 16.2. Example of a Genogram of a Three-Physician Family Practice (Not an Actual Practice)

with expertise in qualitative methods. Everybody still met for an hour or more each week as a larger group and participated in the genogram construction meetings; thus we were able to communicate enough to at least partially maintain the desired iterative process. This two-team approach did allow us the time to get the case report completed and the feedback presented to the practice in less than 6 months after data collection. Eighteen months and 14 practices into the study, attrition of team members to other positions and general burn-out necessitated a slow down and a return to a single team.

Becoming a single interpretive team had less impact than one might initially think because of data saturation. After preliminary analysis of 14 practices, both the field workers and the analysts were experiencing much redundancy. They weren't learning anything that was new except for specific details of the practice. Recently, one of the field workers even commented that she was really finished after only 2 weeks in the practice. Qualitative researchers refer to this as data saturation, and it is an indication that the sample size is sufficient.

The analysis/interpretation process just described included only the steps necessary to write the preliminary case reports and the feedback summaries; this was just the beginning of the interpretive process and one that would never be published. The study team needed to be cognizant of their progress in addressing the research questions outlined in the grant proposal. Comparative case study interpretation would be needed to address key study questions (Step 15 in Figure 16.1). What are the distinguishing features of high- and low-intensity prevention practices? What are the competing demands within daily family practice? What are the organizational structures that support preventive service delivery?

In addition to the primary research questions, a "consultant conference" was convened to explore other manuscript ideas that should be pursued with the more than 10,000 pages of field note data collected from 18 practices, which included data from about 50 family physicians and more than 1,500 observed patient encounters. Conference attendees (see acknowledgments for list of attendees) identified more than 60 such manuscripts, ranging from the use of patient education materials in physicians' offices to describing the metaphors that capture the essence of practices. Working on these manuscripts will require a completely new strategy of data management and interpretation.

Providing Feedback and Member Checking

Although not incorporated into the initial design, providing feedback to the practices provided a valuable member-checking function in addition to satisfying the wishes of the practices themselves. As the descriptive case reports were nearing completion, the practice was contacted and a time for the feedback session scheduled. These sessions were generally over the lunch hour, but several were scheduled for the evenings. We left it up to the practice to determine who should attend the sessions. In most cases, all the physicians attended, generally with the office manager. In two practices, all the office staff were also invited and attended; in another two, only one of the physicians from the large group attended.

In preparation for the session, the research team compiled a packet for each physician that included a 4- to 5-page written summary, the practice genogram, a quantitative summary of the observed patients, and a hit/miss summary of key preventive services. A plaque was also prepared for each physician and for the practice. The principal investigator attended all the sessions and initially did most of the presentations. In most cases, the field worker who collected the data also attended and used the opportunity to express appreciation and say good-bye to the friends she had made at the practice.

Initially, we dreaded going to these sessions, perhaps fearing that the practices would not agree with our assessment, but after experiencing the overwhelmingly positive responses and gratitude expressed, we came to look forward to these as reaffirming. Immediately after each session, those who attended debriefed and constructed field notes that were added to the database. In the feedback sessions, there were, occasionally, additional insights or interpretations provided, but usually the practices confirmed our interpretations with comments such as "this is just like looking in a mirror."

Spelunking: The Dark Side

From the preceding description, it must be evident that the project required a lot of hard work, but it was also repeatedly threatened by what Harry Wolcott (1995) would call the dark side. There were always self-reflective questions about how much data we should collect and who should have access to it. We were also continually plagued by not enough time and not enough money.

The experience of one of our field workers serves to illustrate one of the perils of digging too deeply and overidentifying with research participants (see Chapter 7). As we were completing data gathering in the first practice, we were able to hire a second nurse researcher. After several weeks of intense training, she began data gathering in an inner city practice. She provided excellent data, but as she began to develop rapport with the practice, more and more personal information was revealed to her. She began to question which part of this data should be included in the field notes and which she should "suppress." Despite long discussions acknowledging her concerns, she finally felt forced to resign after completing the data gathering at only this one practice. She was never able to resolve her role as a "spy," and her struggles with the data were too much to endure.

We have also had continuous concern with how to maintain confidentiality. Patient identifiers were never recorded, but the names of the practice, physicians, and staff were part of the dictation and thus part of the transcription. Initial attempts to create pseudonyms proved fruitless; there were just too many names and too few resources to make the changes. Protocols for ensuring that data are always securely locked were developed and regularly reviewed. In addition, discussions of confidentiality were regularly brought up at our weekly group sessions. Nevertheless, this was and is a continual concern.

A commensurate concern relates to who should have access to the data. It is obvious that the primary investigative team requires full access to the data, but what about others such as consultants, coauthors, and those wishing to do secondary analysis of the data with our team? The language of the informed consent certainly indicated that the data were to be used for research purposes by the research team, but did that include individuals who were not part of the original study? After considerable discussion and debate, we decided that the consultants and those working as coinvestigators on manuscripts should be granted access to the data. We developed a confidentiality agreement for them to sign that reinforced the need to be careful with the data. Nevertheless, this will always be a legitimate concern about the data; it is very different than anonymous quantitative data with numerical identifiers and a code book.

Crawling Toward Light:
Turns and Decisions

Having persevered through the arduous process of getting the grant funded, the challenges and struggles to gather the data, and the deep reflections of the dark side, it was the support, encouragement, and collaboration of an interdisciplinary group of investigators that made this study possible. Members of the team at the medical center in Nebraska gave a lot of themselves for the project (see acknowledgments). In each of the first 2 years, a 2-day "consultant conference" provided guidance at critical points. In the early phase of the project, the consultants helped to refine the tools and to focus the lens for producing the case reports and feedback summaries; midway through the study they provided reassurance and some new ideas for obtaining community-level data; and near the end of data collection, they provided the insights for moving the next stages of analysis forward. This was absolutely a collaborative effort.

The wonderfully rich data provide the potential to greatly enhance the knowledge base of current family practice well beyond the prevention focus. We are now faced with the task of being good stewards of the data and ensuring their appropriate use. The true test of this stewardship will be in our ability to produce evidence that matters to practicing clinicians, evidence that they can use to make a difference in their practices.

The journey has been long and sometimes perilous, but through perseverance and determination we did get the data. Our team has traveled many uncharted regions and completed the very first steps toward interpreting the tome. It is important that we were able to provide feedback to practices in a timely manner. The response of the practices has been reaffirming, and we feel reenergized as we take our next steps in our quest for understanding the "black box" of clinical practice.

LEARNINGS:
THE EMPEROR RECLOTHED

One of the principal lessons learned from this project is that data management and interpretation for a project of this scope take considerable time; it is easy to underestimate the resources required and the complexity of managing such a project. Over the course of 2 years, we tried different configurations of analysis teams and continually struggled to find sufficient time. Having a full-time faculty member dedicated to the project, Virginia Aita, was essential for our survival, as was the hard work and dedication of a full-time project manager, Diane Dodendorf. It is also easy to underestimate the amount of support staff time required. We required a full-time data manager and a full-time transcriptionist. When putting a grant proposal together, it may seem expedient to shave some of these costs, but in the long run it can potentially compromise the whole project.

Participation in this study has changed us all. We all grew as researchers, but most impressive was that the collaborative relationships that were repeatedly tested throughout the project have come out even stronger. New collaborations have also been discovered and been integrated into our group. The strength of this collaboration was demonstrated when, late in 1998, our group successfully applied for funding from the American Academy of Family Physicians to establish the Research Center for the Value of Family Practice. Funding from this 4-year grant will be used to move us to the next phases of our collaborative research effort.

ACKNOWLEDGMENTS

This project was supported by a grant from the Agency for Health Care Policy and Research (1 R01 HS08776). The project was only possible through the hard work and dedication of many individuals, particularly the two primary field workers, Connie Gibb, RN, and Jenine Rouse, MS. Additional data-gathering assistance was provided by medical students Julie Rothlisberger and family medicine resident Greg Nelson. Countless hours of reading and interpreting of data were contributed by Lisa Backer, MD; Helen McIlvain, PhD; Virginia Aita, PhD; William Minier, MD; and Paul Turner, PhD. Diane Dodendorf's work as project coordinator, Jason

Lebsack's role in data management, and Mary McAndrew's dedication to transcription were instrumental, as was the grants management assistance of Marlene Hawver and Joyce Juracek. Finally, outside consultations from William Miller, MD (Lehigh Valley Hospital); Kurt Stange, MD, PhD (Case Western Reserve University); Reuben McDaniel (University of Texas, Austin); Ruth Anderson, RN, PhD (Duke University); Valerie Gilchrist, MD (NEOUCOM); Carlos Jaen, MD, PhD (SUNY-Buffalo); and Paul Nutting, MD (Ambulatory Sentinel Practice Network) served to enrich both us and the project.

17

Making Changes
With Key Questions
in Medical Practices

Studying What Makes a Difference

Kirsti Malterud

Some years ago, as a practitioner I wanted to make some changes in my practice; however, I also wanted to know what was going on along the path of change. This latter aspiration turned my efforts into a research project. By sticking to the clinical problems I wanted to untangle, I found myself within a field where methodological challenges were abundant and ready-made solutions were scarce. In retrospect, I am happy that as a novice researcher I did not realize the magnitude of the challenge. Today, I appreciate how my professional identity as a practitioner reminded me to stick to the core of clinical knowledge while asking my research questions, even though this brought me to the margins of traditional medical research.

Turning my ideas of change into a qualitative research project provided a framework where practical knowledge could be developed in a systematic way, and strategies and experiences could be shared with others. In this chapter, I present my experiences as an example of how practical clinical knowledge can be approached and developed and how theory can support the translation through research design and method. I will discuss the potentials of this research strategy but also give some warnings to those who believe that it is possible to make every tiny step in clinical practice documented and evidence based. The field of research I present here inhabits the borderland between the art and the science of medicine. My presentation will argue that areas within the so-called art of medicine can be explored in a scientific way, although I do not endorse the view that science is the only valuable base of medical knowledge (Malterud, 1995b). My approach is also a deliberate attempt to upset the medical belief that subjective and objective matters are fundamentally different and should always be so. Qualitative research methods are my tools in these endeavors.

CLINICAL PROBLEM

After some years in clinical practice, I found myself repeatedly stuck with women patients presenting with medically unexplained problems—long-lasting, painful, and vague conditions where no objective findings could be demonstrated (Malterud, 1987). These disorders presented in various appearances, often as musculoskeletal complaints, fatigue, or mental problems. The patients suffered from pain syndromes related to various and multiple organ systems, concentration problems, sleep disorders, vaginal discharge, urination problems, dyspepsia, irritable bowel, or inner tension. Empirical evidence told me that these problems were seen not only in my practice but actually comprised a considerable proportion of women's health problems in general (van Wijk, Kolk, van den Bosch, & van den Hoogen, 1992). Medical textbooks offered no solutions for understanding and management except various psychiatric diagnoses, which most often were rejected by the women. For some years I felt awkward and incompetent as a physician, constantly reproaching myself for having forgotten or never having learned the essential facts of medicine that supposedly would have given me access to understanding and management. Feelings of helplessness provoked my professional identity of needing to be in charge, which unfortunately was sometimes transformed into more aggressive behavior. I shamefully realized that in my disapproving attitudes I had been blaming the patient.

The obvious suffering of the patients told me that the resolution was not to deny or discard their illness. As time passed in my practice, the ill-structured and unexplained problems gradually became more available for understanding and management. Experience gently taught me the art of recognizing patterns of symptom presentation, comparing these to the individual's particular needs and resources, and subsequently transferring this understanding into medical management, which sometimes seemed to work. Gradually I acquired various clinical strategies, and a more skillful feeling replaced my helplessness. My enthusiasm was triggered by events where something I said somehow seemed to make a major difference. I am talking not just about the emotional atmosphere but even more about the problem-solving part of the consultation. I felt that such incidents were about shared knowledge, perhaps made available by empowering the voice of the woman by means of something I did or said—a key to mutual understanding that served to unlock hitherto closed gateways (Malterud, 1993a).

I wanted to explore this hypothesis further by elaborating my communication style to expand the empowered space for the woman in a more conscious way, by turning intuitive talk to a key question. The aims of the research project were to describe how key questions for this purpose were worked out, what happened when the key questions were used in the consultation, and how I found a way to study and report my advances and experiences in a systematic way. My approach can be summarized as a research strategy based on action research (see Chapter 15) and qualitative evaluation that describes the development of a clinical approach on a process level (What is going on?) and an outcome level (What happens when this is done?). It is also an example of how to handle the dual roles of observing and participation (myself as the physician whose pursuit for change is the object of study and, at the same time, myself as the researcher studying this), assisted by metapositions.

Key Questions: Why and How?

In most cultures across the world, men still maintain more influence and power in society than women do. Throughout their lives, men and women encounter different expectations and experiences attributed to their gender. Overall gender differences such as these are most likely to have an impact on women's health (Craft, 1997). Health care may reinforce and reproduce disempowerment and lack of influence (Candib, 1995; Waitzkin, 1979). Even when the medical encounter seems to be an interaction between mutually understanding individuals, the doctor and patient in many regards belong to different lifeworlds—often without the doctor noticing this (Mishler, 1984). This is more often experienced by women patients than by men. Expressions from women patients are not assigned significance as adequate medical information (Armitage, Schneiderman, & Bass, 1979; Wallen, Waitzkin, & Stoeckle, 1979). Gender has a strong impact on medical communication and can partly explain why misunderstandings can occur between the woman patient and her physician (Hall, Irish, Roter, Ehrlich, & Miller, 1994; Roter, Lipkin, et al., 1991). However, power issues also have a strong impact on the diagnostic interaction, assigning power to the doctor to decide which information is valid and relevant (Candib, 1995; Mishler, 1984). Communication is a strong agent for gendered interaction, and the consultation may reproduce sociocultural patterns of power and subordination, leaving no voice for the woman patient (Borges & Waitzkin, 1995; Code, 1995).

I had occasionally had experiences that told me that my tacit clinical knowledge included certain communicative skills, including questions that might give access to further understanding. These skills manifested themselves intuitively and casually, and I was not able to account for what I said or how it worked. Realizing that my ways of asking might lead to major differences as a key unlocking my understanding of the woman's problem, I became inspired to identify and refine specific components of my communicative style. I wanted to find out how my occasionally successful experiences could be generalized, by looking for core elements of communicative action that could lead to shared knowledge in various situations with various patients, knowledge that could preferably be applied not only by me but also by my colleagues.

I decided to systematize this by developing a clinical communicative method intended to empower the voices of female patients who suffered from "unexplained" problems. My hypothesis was that this kind of empowerment would promote the exchange of medically relevant information. Key questions became my tools. My approach was to construct simple communicative clues inviting the patient to share her knowledge. The key questions were designed as speech acts, conversational elements that hold a potential to promote action (Austin, 1982). By reading more about speech acts, I later found that my ideas belonged to a theoretical tradition of pragmatic linguistics; however, I still believe that such theoretical knowledge is not necessary for colleagues who want to apply the clinical method.

My clinical experience advised me to use a stepwise design focusing on four different key questions to invite the woman to share her knowledge about problem definition, causal beliefs, expected actions from the physician, and previous experiences of management. This was not intended as a clinical questionnaire, with all four questions posed in one consultation, but rather as subprojects exploring the potential and limitations separately for each of the four key questions. The idea was to develop various components of the communicative tool, making it later possible to choose the assumedly most purposeful of these in the individual encounter. An action research design based on qualitative evaluation made it possible to describe and analyze the *process* (development and characteristics of the key questions) as well as the *outcome* (the answers from the women when the key question was used).

Design—Action Research—Material

A conceptual challenge related to the notion of "method" appears in research projects on development and use of innovative clinical strategies and methods. The *research method* is the tool to describe and analyze the *clinical method*. A scientific approach requires that these two levels of method not be confused or merged. There is certainly a close relationship between the two levels of method: The research method must be adequate for the task of capturing the matters it is supposed to describe and analyze. In the case of this project, the clinical method is the key questions and the research method is the qualitative approach I used to study the key questions and their outcomes.

The research method of the project I present here belongs to the tradition of *action research*—the study of a social situation, intended to improve the quality of action (Malterud, 1995a; Winter, 1989). The two central concerns, improvement in practice and increased knowledge and understanding, are linked together in an integrated and dynamic cycle of activities, in which each phase learns from the previous one and in turn shapes the next (Winter, 1989). My approach can be labeled as *qualitative formative evaluation,* and it is intended to focus on the characteristics of process and matters rather than on results and traditional outcomes (Patton, 1990). The design for each of the subprojects was identical, with a two-step procedure including an initial period when the key question was developed (*process*) followed by a period when the key question was applied (*outcome*). According to the different objectives of these two steps, different methodology and material were used to evaluate these two steps (see Figure 17.1).

The most challenging part was the first step, the process analysis intended to capture the subtle nuances related to different ways of linguistic behavior. Within this field, I found scarce support in the method literature. Along the way, I developed a pragmatic approach, in which brief field notes were taken during and immediately after consultations where different versions of the key question were elaborated. Field notes and analysis focused on linguistic and contextual elements that seemed to make a difference regarding the intended objective: the development of a key question that most often gave rise to conversations where useful material for further medical understanding was provided. While talking to the patient, I jotted down a couple of lines on paper, capturing my impression of how things worked out. A typical note might go like this: "10/07/90—F 1934—Low back pain—Too embarrassing for her to suggest something, shame on her if she is wrong—safe environment needed to admit specific

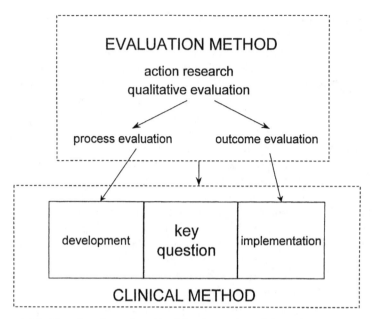

Figure 17.1. Two-Step Procedure Used for the Design of the Subprojects

wishes." Or I might just more literally write down her answer and add my feeling of how or why it worked out, just after she had left my office. No audiotaping or transcribing was done at this step.

I was inspired by speech act theory and used no formal theoretical classification system: The objective of the analysis was to tell myself and my colleagues how a powerful question could be phrased and situated. The findings were presented in three different ways, meant to complement each other:

1. a *narrative* of how different ways of asking led to different types of responses;

2. a *summarized list* of the conversational elements supposed to contribute to this; and

3. the *final version of the question,* intended as an example of how the experiences above could be expressed.

It was an easier task to capture the outcome of the key questions. I audiotaped the answers of the women when the key question had been posed and did a more traditional qualitative analysis to find out which kind of phenomena the women spoke about.

I consider the first step, the process evaluation, as the most original one, the most clinical one, and also the most complicated to share. In this presentation, I shall therefore emphasize the process evaluation. The second part, the outcome evaluation, will serve partly as an illustration of the context where this was going on, partly as an example of the very selective, but nevertheless purposeful, sampling of material in this project and partly (finally) as a presentation of outcome subsequent to application of the key questions.

What I Did: Process Evaluation

Each of the subprojects was devoted to developing one key question in each of the following areas: problem definition, causal beliefs, expected actions from the physician, and previous experiences of management. The key questions were elaborated through a specific procedure illustrated in Figure 17.2, taking successful incidents recognized by introspection as a point of departure (Malterud, 1994). Seeing my own patients in consecutive, everyday consultations, I rephrased each question repeatedly to learn successively more from an increasing variety of woman patients about, for instance, what the patient expects the physician to do. The subproject about actions expected from the physician will be described here to demonstrate how each of the subprojects was accomplished.

From introspection, I recalled the following phrase as a previously successful expression that served as my *point of departure* in this subproject:

"What kind of examination or treatment do you want?"

During the development process, the question was elaborated into this *key question:*

What do you think I should do with x?* I'm sure you have thought of that before you came here.

The question was revisited during 35 consecutive consultations with women 40 to 69 years old. Between these two ways of asking—the point of departure and the key question—I recall from my field notes turns, responses, and changes experienced along the way. From previous subprojects, I had the experience that the key question had to be *open ended.* However, the initial phrasing seemed to be too open, as I understood from responses telling me to clarify what I meant by saying so. Some of the

---

* "X" was the expression used by the patient to describe her symptoms and problems, regardless of my medical interpretation of them.

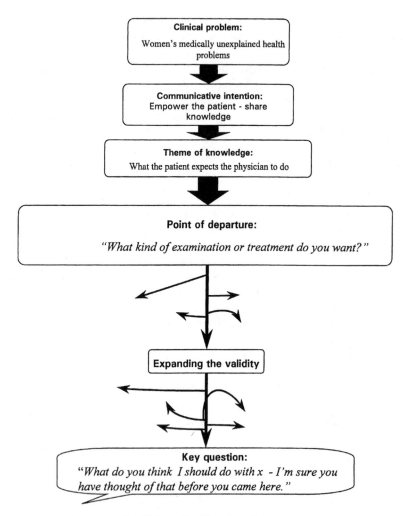

Figure 17.2. Procedure for Elaborating Key Questions

women also seemed more eager to reveal my conception of examination and treatment rather than telling me about their own. This led me to ask more explicitly whether the woman expected me to do something about her complaint or whether it was more important to know what it was. However, this kind of "either/or" choice turned out to be inadequate and more closing than intended, as several women clearly stated that naming the problems might be part of treating them.

Initially, I found it easier to elicit a response when I introduced my question by "Let me hear. . . ." or "I would like to know. . . ," an experience

I interpreted as a need to state explicitly that I was actually interested in listening to the woman's version. Later on, such phrases were not needed to obtain the same atmosphere, probably because my interest by then had been sufficiently implicitly included in the question. I tried to ask what the women wanted but found that this often led to a somehow embarrassed response where my request was returned: "I am not the one to decide, I guess it is up to the physician to decide." Responses became more vivid when I suggested that she certainly had imagined something more specific, a way of asking that invited her to share her fantasies, perhaps, more than her wishes. This might create less of a context of obligation, allowing the patient a role wherein she could not be taken to require this or that. I found it useful to choose words meant to indicate that I did not intend to abdicate my medical responsibility by asking her to share her thoughts (". . . that I might do. . . ."). Using verbs in the past tense (". . . have you thought. . . in advance, before you came here. . . .") gave access to the possibility of a dignified retreat in cases where my plans turned out to be very different from what the woman had expected. In such cases, it seemed important to create an atmosphere without any shameful connotations related to such discrepancies. The hypothetical phrasing in the subjunctive mood (". . . should do. . . .") also seemed to support such matters, and it signaled perhaps also an acknowledgment from me about the woman's previous experiences and mental preparations before she came. Still, my impression was, nevertheless, that several women seemed embarrassed by being expected to tell what they had imagined.

What finally broke the ice was an additional phrase indicating that I knew I was not the only one who had thought about what should be done (". . . because you have certainly thought about this before you came here. . . ."). When this phrase was included in the key question, I repeatedly found that the woman laughed cheerfully and relaxed more. Such a humorous invitation to mutuality seemed to make it possible for the woman to put away her fears of being considered a craving person or a patient with incorrect and ridiculous expectations of the physician. Responses about such expectations seemed unavailable if the key question was posed before a common ground for problem definition and causal beliefs had been established. Still, there had to be time enough left in the consultation to employ the knowledge shared by the woman on these matters. I also discovered how important it was for me to be hesitant and not reveal my initial plans prematurely. In consultations where I as the physician won this race, the run was closed and impossible for the patient.

The field notes and the narrative presented above constituted my material for further analysis, identifying linguistic elements assumed to make a change. No formal coding was done, but my theoretical frame of reference reminded me to look for ways of talking related to the intended consequence of disclosing and sharing relevant knowledge through some kind of empowerment. I deliberately chose to express the patterns of the unlocking talk in commonsensical terms because this was what I wanted my colleagues to attend to without further theoretical training on their part.

I summarize my findings from the process analysis as the following recommendations:

- Use an open-ended question, not separating investigation and treatment.
- Implicitly signal the interest of the doctor regarding the thoughts of the female patient.
- Invite the woman to use her imagination.
- Convey that the doctor intended no withdrawal from medical responsibility.
- Create potentials for the female patient for dignified retreat without shame.
- Acknowledge the mental preparations of the patient as her contributions to the consultation.
- Use humor as an invitation to mutual and harmless exchange of information.

What I Heard: Outcome Evaluation

The question was applied and audiotape-recorded in a total of 27 consecutive consultations with women 40 to 69 years old. I transcribed selected specific parts of the consultation, namely what the women answered when I had asked the key question. These pieces of texts of two to 30 written lines were used in the qualitative analysis, with an approach that probably could be called the immersion/crystallization style of Miller and Crabtree (Chapter 7), although I did not know of this concept at the time. I read the texts, sorting the patterns of different kinds of expectations the women had toward their physician. I must admit that at that time, I was not aware of any theoretical frame of reference that supported my reading. In retrospect, I assume I was guided by pragmatic thinking (Skagestad, 1981), exploring patterns of consequence that would tell me what to do as a doctor (Malterud, 1992). Below, I will present some findings from this analysis, mostly to illustrate the potential outcome of the key question approach and to set the context of the process analysis that I have described above. Each of the categories or themes denotes different patterns of expectations and is displayed with a subtitle, a short summary, and a typical quote—thus answered the woman:

Specific Expectation—But I Leave It to the Doctor to Decide

Some of the women were not able to express their expectations in more detail; however, by answering the key question, they nevertheless made it perfectly clear that they came to the doctor with very particular anticipations that most often would be about "getting to know." To illustrate:

The patient (age 65) had been tired for awhile, and previously her creatinine level had been increased. At the next test, her values were normal. She came back to discuss what to do. Her answer to the key question was:

> I leave it completely to the doctor—I don't even think of it. I just needed to have an answer.

Is It Dangerous to Wait and See?

The patient does not always anticipate further investigation or treatment, even though her symptoms may be bothering her. Sometimes, her most significant request is to have the physician make an assessment that probably concludes by confirming that she will not suffer any loss or have a reason to worry if she just waits and sees. This is a way to escape the responsibility that something specific should have been done. To illustrate:

Four weeks before the visit, this woman, 59 years old, hit her head on the luggage rack of a train. When she returned home, she went to her physician, who told her that she had a minor concussion. She recovered steadily but still felt dizzy and had a headache in stressed situations. This was her answer to the key question:

> I just wanted to know whether you usually feel like this in such situations. Because my friend's daughter experienced something similar, I guess nearly 2 years ago. She just turned 37. And she was told to lie down, but I guess she did not follow the advice as strictly as she should. So she came on disability pension due to this. I was afraid that if I did not take this sufficiently seriously, I might also maintain my symptoms and not be able to do anything at all.

There were no neurological findings, and she was clearly feeling better. Her friends thought she needed an X ray, but she was prepared to wait unless that would be risky for her.

Clinical Examination—Safe and Simple Clarification

A symptom can produce a very specific perception in the patient of what is wrong with her. She may have considered what is needed to confirm or discard this conception, often very simple actions with a potential for providing safety, if only the physician knows about these thoughts. To illustrate:

I had previously seen this patient, age 65, several times for her back-aches. The X rays demonstrated degenerative signs of aging. She visited me because the pain had become worse in the last week. Her answer was this:

> I thought that maybe you would examine my back. If perhaps you found a lump or something. It feels as if I had a knife in my back which was pulled out. Yes—just find out whether there is something abnormal—I can't reach around there, so I won't be able to find out myself.

No lump could be found, but her muscles were very tense and painful at the left upper lumbar area where the "knife" had been felt.

Prepared for a Possible Series of Investigation or Intervention

The patient may have very definite ideas of what could be done to find an explanation of her symptoms. This does not necessarily mean that she prefers further referral to happen, although she may have prepared herself for this possibility:

This 62-year-old woman was healthy until, a few days before her visit, she fell against the frame of a door and hit her back. She showed signs of pain but did not seem to be especially worried. Her answer to the key question was this:

> You know, my only concern is to have a proper examination. It feels like something pressing on. And then—if you find an X ray to be necessary—well—if I should admit that I thought of anything at all, that is what came to my thoughts.

She was relieved when I concluded after the clinical exam that I did not think she would need a referral. A week later she called and said she was fully recovered and doing her usual things.

I Know What Works for Me

Treatment experiences provide significant contributions to the shaping of the woman's expectations of what should be done. If she previously went through actions that gave her small benefit, she would not be happy to repeat the same procedure. Effectual approaches may be more tempting, even when the actual problem is something other than the treatment was intended for:

This woman (66 years old) had for years been suffering from a painful hip and periods of pain from her left shoulder. Her appointment was made to discuss the shoulder, but during the visit, she said that the hip was perhaps even more troublesome. She answered the key question like this:

> As for my hip—I had treatments like heat and massage. That is many years ago, but it kept me well for a long time. That might perhaps help me? You would know—I was here previously with my shoulder. I was told that I should go home, lift my iron and move it all around. But I did that, and still—I am not able to lift the arm as I would like to. And it is painful when I stretch to put on my bra. So I don't know what to do with this arm—I really don't know. No, if I am going to treatment, I will need massage. No electric devices.

It would not have made sense to suggest that this woman should go home and do exercises for her shoulder. It was useful for me to hear about her reluctance regarding ultrasound and electrotherapy, which might have activated her uneasiness toward any kind of physiotherapy. I referred her for heat, massage, and selected exercises.

Someone Who Will Listen to Me

Women often listen to others and share responsibility for other people's problems and worries. At the same time, they hope that someone will listen to their worries when they are in need themselves. If they have the impression that there is no space for them and their problems, it may feel like being abandoned. Perhaps the most important expectation of the woman is the hope that her physician will give her the space she needs:

This woman of 45 years started by briefly describing her considerable family problems and told me that she recently had felt dizzy and tired. She had previously seen another physician for these matters but felt that she had not been helped. Her presentation demonstrated a clear insight into the connections between her symptoms and her life situation. I thought that maybe she still wanted a somatic investigation. However, her answer to the key question was this:

> You know, I was wondering quite a lot—somehow, I don't know what to do, because it makes no sense to speak to the physician I saw before. He sat there, writing at his computer—didn't talk to me at all—writing while I talked, so I kept wondering whether it was about what I said, or about other patients he had just seen an hour ago or something. It was very frustrating.

At my last visit, I felt he urged me out of his office—he put on his shoes and seemed to be on his way home. There were still a lot of people at the waiting room—no system in the line or something, and a woman asked to come before me, because she was supposed to have her appointment an hour earlier. So I felt frustrated and decided that I could not continue seeing that doctor. He gives me no understanding. I just had an instant of needing someone who would listen to me.

We talked for 15 minutes, and I did not say much. She had her husband join her for her visit with the family counselor, and later she returned to me for other problems.

*What Is Really Needed Cannot
Be Provided by a Physician*

Sometimes the patient knows very well that the physician cannot solve her problems. Still, she goes in for a visit. This might mislead the provider to believe that the woman does not trust her own coping abilities. Perhaps her need is to use the physician as one to whom she can declare her own strength:

This 51-year-old woman was on a long-term sick leave after a period of burn-out at work. She loved her demanding job, although it had taken all her energy, beyond the capacity of her body. Her feelings of responsibility toward her work were large, and it was not easy for her to refuse tasks where the resources were too small for appropriate accomplishment. She responded like this:

I guess I am the one who needs to do something to stop this race. Although this is not easy, considering all these people to whom we are accountable.

My role during her sick leave was to support her in developing a strategy where she gradually learned how far she wanted to stretch herself, elaborating methods for putting up limits when needed.

**Theoretical Frames of Reference:
Related Approaches**

I was certainly not the first one to realize that practical knowledge, accomplished and elaborated in clinical situations, can be valuable and available even though we do not know exactly what is going on. Expert knowledge, developed through experience and practice, can take tacit and unarticulated forms and still constitute significant components of expert knowledge (Polanyi, 1983). The practical knowledge is gradually developed to a more advanced capacity as the practitioner moves on from novice to a more experienced level (Dreyfus & Dreyfus, 1986). In clinical work, tacit knowing constitutes an important part of diagnostic reasoning and judgment of medical conditions (Widdershoven-Heerding, 1987). As practitioners, we apply a broad range of experiential knowledge and strategies that are hardly mentioned in the textbooks. The experienced clinician holds a variety of strategies for diagnostic problem solving, several of them beyond the logic of hypothetic-deductive approaches (McGuire, 1985). Belonging to medicine, a discipline that is proud of its scientific foundations, the family physician should thus be eager to explore these fields and look for ways of describing and analyzing what is going on. The randomized, controlled trial and the traditional procedures for evidence-based medicine are not well suited for such purposes (Malterud, 1995a).

In this project, I approached my tacit knowledge of doing something by saying something. I decided to have a closer look at phenomena Austin (1982) would have called *speech acts* and gradually elaborate my ways of asking by moving from Schön's (1991) unconscious level of "reflection-in-action" to the more focused level of "reflection-on-action." This is not to say that we should always know and be able to tell what we are doing; it is to invite you as my colleagues to the abundant field of using curiosity, experience, and research methods to understand more of what is going on in clinical practice.

This is why, in this chapter, I have given priority to presenting the methodology of the process evaluation rather than the outcome evaluation. Although communicative action is an integral component of clinical work, we do not actually know much about our skills and follies as medical professionals. Social scientists, linguists, and anthropologists have provided important contributions to the field of medical communication (Cicourel, 1973; Kleinman, 1980; Mishler, 1984), but insider knowledge focusing on the art of improving your own talk as a physician is still rare. Inherent skills are, however, not at all rare among my colleagues and deserve to be identified and shared.

I believe in the power of introspection and reflection, and I have realized that qualitative research methods can constitute tools for transforming heuristic approaches into systematic knowledge. Heading for new areas of medical knowledge in the core of clinical work, you will probably discover, as I did, that existing coding systems for the study of communication may not catch the phenomena you want to explore. Through the process of this project, within a design representing high feasibility and low costs, I have learned to enjoy the strengths and benefits of pragmatic approaches to qualitative research that gave access to the study of everyday phenomena in my own practice. The key question design has later been repeated in a study where I, together with my Danish colleague Hanne Hollnagel, developed and applied key questions about patients' self-assessed personal health resources (Malterud & Hollnagel, 1997, 1998).

METHODOLOGICAL CHALLENGES

Although this book probably is not the place in which to argue for the adequacy and trustworthiness of qualitative research methods, you deserve to know that it takes a lot of energy and knowledge to legitimize research approaches like the one I have described within the culture of medical research. If you want an easy journey, you should rather choose a more traditional research strategy, even among the qualitative methods. But if you are prepared to enter the jungle and go for exciting treasures, you will need a commitment to critical reflection and systematic procedures. A humble understanding of the limitations of "truth" and "facts" is needed, as well as an ability to share with others the paths you have followed (Malterud, 1993a).

Although the design presented here represents an $N = 1$, the number of patients and visits where the key questions were used allows for considerations about external validity. Instead of claiming that my outcomes are repeatable by any physician, my choice on transferability assessment was to scrutinize potential limitations of the method related to me as the person doing it: how special am I, doing this, and how special is my patient population who gave me these answers? If your conditions for developing a clinical method are very personal, you should not waste your time by pretending an unrealistic level of transferability. However, developing a personal approach may certainly include elements that can be transferred to contexts beyond the one where it was first designed. The potential for this will depend on your ability to assess and validate the role of your personal involvement. For the key question method, my conclusion was that I do not believe my colleagues will receive exactly the same responses as I got when I used the questions, but I consider the principles of the method to be repeatable by others. Still, my conclusion is that this method requires a certain level of clinical experience and is therefore not recommended for young students and inexperienced residents.

Although I prefer to identify myself as a holistic and patient-centered health care provider, I realize that any research method, even the qualitative ones, will only give access to selected parts of reality. I also admit that the deliberate use of specific questions, even open-ended ones, may imply a level of physician control of the communication. Rather than dismissing communicative approaches and qualitative methods for these reasons, I suggest that we use them for what they are worth and admit that they do not tell the whole truth. I realize that there is still a lot left for which we do not have the imagination, ears, words, or creativity to observe and share. We may still ask whether our perspectives are relevant, adequate, and useful, and for which purposes. The key question design is a cross-sectional exploration of a dynamic human interaction, and the purposeful sampling of material will only open a small window to what is going on.

A methodological pitfall within the presented approach is to believe or claim that the questions are causing the answers. This is not a design that allows for causal conclusions because we do not know what would have been said if the question had not been posed. It is a descriptive design, presenting what was said by the patient subsequent to the physician's question, representing an intention of empowerment and shared knowledge within a specified context. The internal validity—what the study is intended to study—relates to this limited objective. I did not even mean to embrace the whole world of emotions and social context embedded in the communication; I accept the role of the family physician as a part-time participant in the life of people. Finding out how to deal with the questions our patients regard as most significant is an art belonging to the heart of family practice and research.

Metapositions

Qualitative research requires that the researcher be capable of grasping her or his own role in the research process and considering the consequences of this for the findings, interpretations, and conclusions. In the design presented here, this is especially important due to the dual role of clinician/researcher. Especially for the process evaluation, your role as an observing participant requires reflective skills and certain techniques. Do not try to deny your own involvement; rather, do your best to consider its impact. You will need to step aside, look at your own case, and appreciate your own involvement. A metaposition is a perspective where the distance needed for this can be obtained (Malterud & Kristiansen, 1995).

Collecting material from your own practice means that you will have to explore and expose the more intimate and sometimes embarrassing parts of your professional work. Even the most humanistic physician sometimes happens to be rude or stupid with her or his patients. You will not be allowed to exclude such elements from your material, and some exercise on sharing audiotapes or transcripts with a colleague might prepare you for that. I found it very important to be able to develop a somewhat humorous approach to my own faults, without defending them.

It may certainly be tempting to choose your favorite patients for key questions or to do your research in consultations where you feel most comfortable. In the design presented above, this will imply bias restricting the applicability of your findings and is, therefore, not advised. My choice was to define, follow, and describe my procedures rather rigorously, to prevent myself from just having fun and to make the procedures transparent for others. I introduced the principle of consecutiveness in sampling, never believing that my sample was a randomized one, but to ensure that my clinical method was exposed to all kinds of clinical situations. During analysis, I directed myself toward an attitude more descriptive than interpretive, realizing that it would be a very hard task to decipher the underlying meanings of my own behavior. Learning from experience, I eventually preferred doing the analysis together with someone when the design was repeated on self-assessed health resources. I do not think consensus warrants truth or validity, but four eyes can read a text more creatively than only your own two eyes and prevent you from neglecting your own blind spots.

Validity

From working myself through this project, I have learned to appreciate the challenges of validity questions, even in a qualitative research project (Kvale, 1996). I realize that my findings represent only a temporary and limited view of the world. Still, certain fundamental questions need to be discussed and partly answered: What is this actually about? Can it be shared? How? Can it be used? For what? By whom? And why? I am convinced that the quality of my clinical work in general has been improved through research experiences that taught me to ask such questions continuously.

Good luck!

PART
VI

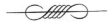

Summary

18

Standards of Qualitative Research

Richard M. Frankel

God is in the details.
R. Preston, 1994, p. 298

The devil is in the details.
Popular adage

I t seems as if the details of qualitative research can lead simultaneously to God or the devil, and if the contexts of study are ambiguous enough to be heaven or hell, how can there be standards of research that are trustworthy and well accepted in the scholarly community? I have four goals in this chapter. The first is to comment briefly on some of the paradigm assumptions about qualitative research using material from the preceding chapters as well as my own experience as a qualitative researcher. Beyond the question of what counts as evidence for a variety of qualitative approaches, I want also to comment on what, in my opinion, differentiates studies using the *same* methods from one another. In this respect I would apply George Orwell's (1946) famous dictum from *Animal Farm* to

AUTHOR'S NOTE: I would like to thank Vicki James, Benjamin Crabtree, and William Miller for their thoughtful reading and commitment to this chapter.

333

qualitative research: "All qualitative studies are equal, but some are more equal than others." What criteria differentiate good (adequate) studies from great studies? Next, I return to the question of generic assessment of qualitative research studies. I end with a summary and thoughts about standards of research in the context of primary care medicine.

PARADIGM ISSUES

That quantitative and nonquantitative approaches to research differ in assumptions, methods, and outlook is not in question. The differences in approach to social science research have been documented by many scholars (Cicourel, 1964; Crabtree & Miller, Introduction to this book; Patton, 1990). In the broader context of the history and philosophy of science, Kuhn (1962) asserts that such paradigmatic differences are a fundamental basis for change and innovation. They are also a source of conflict.

Perhaps working from within such a view, Poses and Isen (1998) recently published a rather stinging critique of qualitative research in clinical medicine. The authors made a number of useful observations, but what caught my attention was their assumption that qualitative research is a single thing governed by uniform canons of evidence. One need only refer to chapters in this volume by Gilchrist and Williams on key informant interviews, Miller and Crabtree on depth interviews, and Brown on focus group interviews to get a sense of the rich variety of approaches and roles for data gathering using interviews. From these chapters on different forms of qualitative interviewing, it is easy to see that there are clearly very different standards on what makes a good focus group and what makes a good depth interview. Chapters by Kuzel on sampling, Muller on narrative approaches, Thesen and Kuzel on participatory research, Aita and McIlvain on case study research, and Elderkin-Thompson and Waitzkin on the use of video recordings provide additional descriptions of the range of traditions and approaches and the criteria of adequacy and appropriateness that are applied to them. Indiscriminately citing and comparing evidence from a variety of studies simply because they are nonstatistically based is like saying one is going to judge the value of Samuel Beckett's *Waiting for Godot* on the basis of Mary Shelley's *Frankenstein*. To claim that there is a single standard for judging an entire paradigm, be it in literature or qualitative research, is, in a word, absurd. What is required is a specification of each of the approaches or traditions that make up a paradigm or approach, a description of the rules or canons of evidence used in each, and an account of its success or failure in persuading the reader or reviewer of its goodness (Altheide & Johnson, 1994; Creswell, 1998; Mays & Pope, 1995b). Beyond these canons of evidence, it is useful to consider what makes for greatness.

GREATNESS IN
QUALITATIVE RESEARCH

I believe there is reasonably good consensus about issues like adequacy, appropriateness, and completeness within each of the qualitative research traditions (e.g., see Creswell, 1998). Different traditions, such as ethnography (Bernard, 1995; Fetterman, 1998; Pelto & Pelto, 1978), case study research (see Chapter 14; Merriam, 1998; Stake, 1995), ethnomethodology (Cicourel, 1964; Garfinkel, 1967), and grounded theory (Strauss & Corbin, 1990), as well as particular methods, such as focus groups (Chapter 6; Morgan, 1988, 1992a), participant observation (Chapter 3; Spradley, 1980), and depth interviews (Chapter 5; McCracken, 1988), each have canons of evidence for both researchers and readers to follow. There have even been numerous discussions in the clinical research literature about these canons of evidence (Elder & Miller, 1995; Inui & Frankel, 1991; Kuzel, Engel, Addison, & Bogdewic, 1994; Kuzel & Like, 1991; Mays & Pope, 1995a), with some common agreement that verification procedures include tactics such as triangulation, prolonged engagement, peer debriefing, thick description, member checking, external audits, and searching for confirming and disconfirming cases (e.g., see Creswell, 1998; Kuzel & Like, 1991). Creswell (1998) suggests that at least two of these should be present in any given study, but the ultimate test is that the report carries "sufficient conviction to enable someone else to have the same experience as the original observer and appreciate the truth of the account" (Mays & Pope, 1995b, p. 111).

There is much less agreement on what makes for greatness. In a way, it's like the books one sees on how to make a million dollars in the stock market. If you follow the author's formula exactly, the chances of making a million dollars in the stock market are exceedingly low (somewhere between zero and none). Likewise, if you use a textbook like this as a recipe and apply it mechanically, the chances that you will produce an awardwinning study are slim to none. It's not that the investment ideas or research methods are bad, it's that a host of intervening and sometimes transforming factors have come into play, not the least of which may be the transforming influence the book or study has had on people's perceptions of the world. Below are some of the qualities that characterize outstanding qualitative studies.

Does the Use of the Approach Represent
a "First" or a Breakthrough?

Consider, as an example, physician-assisted suicide. Although this was an issue that had visibility among some segments of the medical community (ethicists and hospice doctors, primarily), that was transformed overnight by the publication of a single case study by Timothy Quill (1991) in the *New England Journal of Medicine*. In that case study, Quill admitted that he had prescribed enough narcotics for his patient (Diane) to kill herself. Quill went on to state what everyone in the medical community already knew: that this was, if not common, at least a well-recognized practice. Quill was brought before a grand jury that declined to press charges despite a call from the State Attorney General in New York to indict him. A subsequent case brought by Quill and others in New York State was argued all the way to the Supreme Court.

For the current discussion of research standards, there are two important lessons to derive. One is that a single case analysis under the right circumstances can have profound institutional and even societal effects. The second is that once the world has been transformed, the same method may be viewed differently. *The New England Journal* was not interested in publishing the second single case analysis of assisted suicide. One aspect of greatness is competitive—it is being the first to point to or map a new territory.

Is the Approach Used in a Novel or Creative Way?

A second quality that differentiates studies using similar methods is creativity. Miller and Crabtree, in Chapter 7, "The Dance of Interpretation," state that "Interpretation is a complex and dynamic craft, with as much creative artistry as technical exactitude, and it requires an abundance of patient plodding, fortitude, and discipline" (Chapter 7, p. 128). When I review qualitative research studies, creativity is a quality that ranks high on my list.

A wonderful example of the creative use of film and video as a research tool can be found in a study by Erickson and Shultz (1982). The researchers were interested in the effects of ethnicity in counseling. They began by noting that Caucasian counselors often complained about African American counselees who didn't seem to "get" the points they were making, although their Caucasian counterparts had no such difficulty. African American counselees, by contrast, complained that Caucasian counselors treated them as if they were stupid and repeated their points over and over again. Taken at face value, the researcher might have concluded that the Caucasian interviewers were discriminating against African American counselees.

In addition to their real-time observations, the researchers filmed the sessions and invited each dyad to review the films, independently stopping the film "anytime something new or different occurred." As reported anecdotally, the Caucasian-Caucasian pairs had no difficulty. The Caucasian-Black pairs independently stopped the films in exactly the same places, but each came away with dramatically different interpretations of the event. On closer inspection, the investigators discovered a critical nonverbal difference between the Caucasian and Black counselees' responses during the sessions. Whereas Caucasian counselees would shake their heads vigorously up and down to show acknowledgment of the counselor's points, the same signal, although present, was displayed in greatly reduced form among the Black counselees. The result was that the Caucasian counselors were systematically missing signs of acknowledgment from the Black counselees and repeating themselves as a consequence.

The creative use of a standard qualitative tool (film), plus involving the participants in evaluating the data of their own performance, led the researchers to an elegant solution to a pressing practical problem. The result was increased understanding and sensitivity on the counselors' part in working with clients from different ethnic groups. The technique was adapted for use in primary care research by Frankel and Beckman (1982) as a means for exploring the differences in perspective between physician trainees, faculty, and patients. It has also been used to explore communication dynamics among parents and professionals providing care and services to children with autism and other developmental disabilities (Frankel, Leary, & Kilman, 1987) and, most recently, to better understand the perspectives of physicians and patients around issues of HIV risk during the clinical interview (Epstein et al., 1998).

Is the Approach Parsimonious?

Sometimes a qualitative study attains greatness because it represents a more practical or economical approach to a problem. In the early days of survey research, individual interviews and questionnaires were used extensively to sample Americans' attitudes and values on a range of issues from race relations to fluoridation. Although useful, large-scale surveys are expensive to conduct and often take a long time to complete. One consequence is that the issue around which the survey is focused may have shifted or taken on a different relevance by the time the analysis is completed.

The post-World War II period in American saw rapid economic, social, and political change and, with it, increasing demands for accurate and useful information about consumer opinion leaders and their voting preferences. In addition to representative sampling of attitudes and values, social scientists began to focus on how selected groups in a society went about making decisions, again across a range of issues from voting preferences to buying a particular brand of shoe polish. Exploring the interface between survey and market research, Merton, Fiske, and Kendall published an article in 1956 titled *The Focused Interview*. In it, they argued the utility of interviewing small groups of like individuals to explore their response to, acceptance or rejection of, or suggestions for improving an issue, product, or person.

The focused interview of today is called a focus group, and it has gained enormous popularity in business, politics, and social science research, in large measure because it is inexpensive compared with other methodologies, and because it produces useful results. Chapter 6, by Judith Belle Brown, details the use of focus groups in the modern clinical context. In the past decade alone, she has identified well over 100 primary care research studies from around the globe based on focus group methodology. It would not be surprising to see that number triple or quadruple over the next 10 years.

Does the Study Get to the Heart of the Question?

Another quality that I look for in assessing qualitative studies is the extent to which the analysis has core significance and gets to the heart or essence of the research question. From the end of World War II onward, there has been great interest among social scientists in the phenomenon of authority and expectations. Stanley Milgram (1963, 1965), in a series of experiments, showed that obedience to authority frequently overrode the common sense of subjects who were willing to apply a near fatal electric shock at the urging of an experimenter. This particularly troubling result went to the heart not only of a specific experimental question that was posed but to that of a much deeper and more troubling question (about the rise of Nazism and the Holocaust that followed), as well.

In a much less dramatic but equally interesting experiment, Rosenthal and Jacobson (1968) set out to study the effects of expectations on teacher performance. The researchers matched two sets of students for IQ and school performance. To the teacher of one set, they described the students as "well below average," with poor prospects for improved performance during the year. To the teacher of the second set, the students were described as "high achievers," with very bright prospects for achievement throughout the year. Even though both sets of students started out the year equally in objective terms, they ended the year at two extremes in terms of performance. The students who were characterized as poor achievers did poorly; those who were expected to perform well did so. Rosenthal and Jacobson's study stands as a classic example of the role of social context in shaping performance outcomes.

In the clinical arena, the role of context and expectations in interpreting behavior was explored to great effect by Rosenhahn (1973), who, unbeknownst to the staff of a psychiatric facility, arranged to have several of his graduate students admitted for "observation." The students were all quite normal, in fact. In the context of having been admitted to a psychiatric ward, however, many of their behaviors (taking field notes, for instance) were viewed by the staff as psychiatric symptomatology (paranoid behavior). Framing the question in terms of how normal behavior would be "read" in the context of a psychiatric setting allowed Rosenhahn to get to the heart of a critically important question: What effect(s) do institutional contexts exert on the perception and labeling of behavior or, as the title of his paper implies, "On Being Sane in Insane Places?"

Two recent qualitative studies are worth mentioning in terms of getting to a core question or concept in clinical medicine. The first, *The Discourse of Medicine* by Elliot Mishler (1984), explored the language used by physicians and that used by patients to characterize their activities. Drawing on the traditions of sociolinguistic analysis and critical theory, Mishler identified two distinct "voices," the "voice of medicine" and the "voice of the life world." In painstaking detail, Mishler showed that the voice of medicine tends to decontextualize the patient and reduce him or her to signs, symptoms, and disease, the effect of which is to miss the fact that in the life world, persons suffer with illness and disease, get frightened, and often desire empathy and support in addition to technically competent treatment. Again, the effect of Mishler's study was to get to the heart of what prevents many physicians and patients from entering into more meaningful and productive relationships.

The study by Rich and Stone (1996) focused on the narratives of young Black males presenting to the Emergency Department at Boston City Hospital as victims of violence. The medical history has always been valued, in the modern era at least, as crucial to making an accurate diagnosis, but there has been little focus on patient narrative as having predictive value beyond establishing the diagnosis.

Using principles of microinteractional analysis, Rich and Stone began investigating the link between patient narratives and subsequent visits to the Emergency Department for violence-related problems. For example, a patient who describes having been shot because he was walking unprotected in a rival gang's territory and as a result wants to get out of gang life altogether is assigned a low probability score for subsequent violence-related ED visits. By contrast, a patient who describes the same situation and vows to kill the person who shot him is assigned a high probability of return to the ED for violence-related visits. The use of patient narratives to predict subsequent behavior gets to the heart of a critically important question for young Black males—where and how to intervene in a cycle of violence that puts them at greater or lesser risk of additional violence.

GENERIC ELEMENTS OF
QUALITATIVE RESEARCH STUDIES

My goal in the preceding section was to illuminate some of the more subjective dimensions that I, and I believe others, use in evaluating the quality of qualitative research. Differences along four dimensions—innovation, creativity, economy, and core significance—tend to differentiate adequate from outstanding studies. In the next section, I return to the more generic question of evaluating any type of qualitative research study. I first describe three elements of qualitative research: setting the question, selection of methods and samples, and presentation of results. These same criteria were used by William Miller and Benjamin Crabtree, who developed a document for the Information Mastery Working Group to identify articles worth reviewing for the *Journal of Family Practice* and *Evidence-Based Practice*. Articles that meet the criteria in Figure 18.1 are reviewed and considered Patient Oriented Evidence that Matters (POEMs). Next, I discuss the criteria or standards as they apply to each element. Finally, I pose some questions designed to help uncover design flaws or barriers to successful publication of qualitative studies.

Setting the Research Question

Virtually every text one reads on how to conduct qualitative research stresses the importance of this element of the research process. Yet, it is interesting that little concrete attention is paid to this activity and less still to criteria for knowing that one has asked a good, and potentially great, question. In many cases, the clarity and obviousness of the question are a key to its quality. I recall many years ago coming across an article in *Scientific American* titled "Why Doesn't the Stomach Digest Itself?" The question posed by the authors was simple, obvious, and intriguing, so much so that I remember thinking to myself: "That's a great question. Given what the stomach does to food, why *doesn't* it digest itself?" Two decades later, as a graduate student in sociology, my mentor and teacher Harvey Sacks (1974) wrote a paper titled "Everyone Has to Lie," in which he analyzed the ritual response to telephone conversation openings that contained "bad news." Despite the news that was eventually delivered, the overwhelming response to the question "How are you?" was "Fine," which was interactionally appropriate but also a lie. Sacks's paper struck the same chord in me, although the topic and context were entirely different. In general, I try to evaluate the quality and depth of the research question based on its importance, timeliness, and relevance. Similarly, the POEM worksheet (Figure 18.1) asks if the problem is common and if the information will require the reader to change his or her practice.

Another approach to question setting is to determine whether it has appeal to others. This can be done in small group settings or among peers and colleagues. I personally try to discuss research questions that I am interested in pursuing with groups of peers, persons who are senior to me, and also those who are more junior. In that way, I get useful feedback at

1. **Determine relevance:** Is this article worth taking the time to read? If the answer to any of these questions is No, it may be better to read other articles first. Based on the conclusion of the abstract:

   A. **Did the authors study an outcome that patients would care about? (Be careful to avoid results that require extrapolation to an outcome that truly matters to patients.)**

      Yes (go on)   No (stop)

   B. **Is the problem common to your practice, and is the intervention feasible?**

      Yes (go on)   No (stop)

   C. **Will this information, if true, require you to change your current practice?**

      Yes (go on)   No (stop)

2. **Determine validity:** If the answer to all three questions above is Yes, then continued assessment is mandatory. Study design flaws are common; fatal flaws are arresting.

   D. **Was the appropriate method used to answer the**   Yes   No (Stop)
   question?
   Interviews, such as depth, group, or life history should be used to study perceptions. Observation methods are required to evaluate behaviors.

   E. **Was appropriate and adequate sampling used to get**   Yes   No (Stop)
   the best information?
   Participants, events, and so on are selected to maximize appropriate information, the richest information relevant to the research question. Random sampling is rarely used. Assurance that enough people were studied to provide sufficient information should be found in the description. Negative or disconfirming evidence is sought.

   F. **Was an iterative process of collecting and analyzing**   Yes   No (Stop)
   data used and data saturation achieved?
   In qualitative research, the investigative team learns about the topic as the research progresses. The study design should consist of data collection and analysis, followed by more data collection and analysis, in an iterative fashion, until no new information is obtained.

   G. **Was a thorough analysis presented?**   Yes   No (Stop)
   A good qualitative study not only presents the findings but provides a thorough analysis of the data. Beware studies that simply present superficial descriptions without interpretation. Something new is learned.

   H. **Are the background, training, and preconceptions**   Yes   No (Stop)
   of the investigators described?
   Because the investigators are being relied on for analysis of the data, we must know their training and biases. Knowing these characteristics, we can use them to evaluate their conclusions. Their original preconceptions are changed or surprised by the study results as they emerge.

Figure 18.1. A Worksheet for Assessing Qualitative Articles

SOURCE: Worksheet developed by William Miller and Benjamin Crabtree for *The Journal of Family Practice*.

all levels before making any final decisions. Generally speaking, the amount of time spent setting the question is directly proportional to the quality and relevance of the question. Although it is not a criterion for evaluation of qualitative research, I often counsel prospective researchers to choose a question and area that they are fundamentally interested in, as the research process often takes months and sometimes years to complete. Chapter 8 in this volume, by Richard Addison, is a good case in point. Addison spent many months collecting, refining, and corroborating his observations. He then spent an equal if not greater amount of time in iterative reflection, deepening his understanding and appreciation of the data and experiences he was engaged in. In essence, he became "wedded" to his data through an iterative self-reflective process.

Two other considerations inform the selection of a problem: when to review the literature and whether to select a basic or applied problem. In terms of literature review, there is no ideal solution. Setting a problem without a thorough review of the literature may lead to duplication or a limited view of the research domain. On the other hand, premature review of the literature can stifle creativity and bias the researcher to take a very conventional approach to the problem. Sometimes the approach one takes does have a recommended approach. In Chapter 5, "Depth Interviewing," Miller and Crabtree perform an initial review of the literature to "identify existing descriptive theoretical and analytic categories." This is important for depth interviewing because the literature review helps to set the foundation for the interview guide (McCracken, 1988). I do a lot of sequential analysis of taped exchanges during medical encounters and don't do much depth interviewing, so I tend not to do a lot of literature review during the phase of problem identification. Instead, I try to immerse myself in the data or the context I'm interested in and learn as much as I can by listening and looking at tapes or transcripts. I try to let the data "speak for itself." This is merely my personal preference, and it works well for the approach I have chosen. I believe excellent question setting can be done either way with respect to the existing literature.

The final consideration is the type of problem one is undertaking to study. If one is studying doctor-patient communication as an instance of stranger-stranger interaction, one is likely to be asking a theoretically informed, basic social science question that is not driven by a preexisting social problem. On the other hand, if one is studying the effect of ethnicity on rates of adherence in diabetes, one is asking a fundamentally different question based on a different set of key assumptions or presuppositions. The selection of a basic or applied question nearly always determines the audience and, therefore, the journal(s) or publisher(s) and funding agencies who are likely to be interested in the study and its results. Obviously, it pays to think carefully about who the intended audience is: clinicians, other social scientists, policy makers, and so on.

Methods and Sampling

If there is a single consistent message in this book, it is this: The research question should always determine the method and not the other way around (see Figure 18.1). Designing a good fit between methods, sample selection, and the research question is both an art and a practical skill that takes into account budgets, personnel, resource use, and intuition.

Many excellent research questions suffer from poor selection of methods and sampling. For example, in designing a qualitative study of the impact of managed care on the doctor-patient relationship, it would make little sense to use a mailed fixed-choice questionnaire, especially as it relates to the patient's lived experience of care. Fixed-choice questions would be likely to reflect the biases of the researchers who constructed the questionnaire and would automatically limit the range of patient responses. In the absence of exploratory studies, one might, as suggested by Brown in Chapter 6, begin by convening a series of focus groups to explore the impact of managed care on patients' experiences of care. For comparative purposes, the research team might write down its assumptions and predictions about what focus group participants are likely to say and then compare their predictions with what patients actually say.

Similarly, sample selection decisions will largely determine the scope and generalizability of the discussion. Some qualitative researchers, ethnomethodologists in particular, hold that it is inappropriate to generalize beyond the particulars of the particular situation one is studying (Garfinkel, 1967). Others, such as grounded theorists and ethnographers, stress the importance of collecting and synthesizing multiple observations on multiple occasions. Investigators who subscribe to these approaches generally argue the importance of remaining true to the samples under study and not generalizing beyond them.

More recently, large-scale qualitative research projects, such as Levinson, Roter, et al.'s (1997) study of communication aspects of medical malpractice, have been based on sampling strategies more frequently found in quantitative studies. These studies may use techniques such as randomization, blinding, and crossover designs that make the results much more amenable to generalization. Such qualitative designs may be well suited to multimethod research (Crabtree, Miller, et al., 1998; Stange, Zyzanski, Smith, et al., 1998).

Other qualities of methodological rigor in qualitative research include the use of member checks (see Chapters 8 and 16), field notes and journals (see Chapter 3), confirming and disconfirming cases (see Chapter 2), audit trails (see Chapter 16), and skeptical peer review (see Chapter 4). The goal of all of these procedures is to provide checks and balances on the accuracy and trustworthiness of data and analysis (Creswell, 1998). Perhaps most important and telling as a criterion for methodological adequacy is consideration of so-called "deviant cases," analytic categories or occurrences that don't fit the dominant theme or pattern. We recently completed a focus group study of patients' and providers' experiences of receiving and giving bad news in the context of cancer (Frankel, Speice, et al., 1997). Among faculty, there was universal agreement that bad news should never be given over the telephone. Virtually all patients subscribed to the same view; however, we did find two patients who said that they preferred getting the news over the telephone and that it would have made them very uncomfortable to receive it face to face. Our conclusion, after having analyzed these two "deviant cases," was that it was inappropriate to establish a hard and fast rule about where and how to deliver bad news over the phone. Instead, given the fact that there were a few patients who preferred it that way, the more appropriate strategy is to inquire about preferences and negotiate them in advance of a situation in which bad news is to be delivered.

Presentation of Results

One of the biggest obstacles facing qualitative researchers who wish to publish in mainstream medical journals is severe restrictions on space. The often vast amounts of information that are collected, and qualitative research traditions that strongly encourage, if not require, segments of primary data to be displayed as part of the analysis, make presentation in limited space challenging at best. Short of being able to present data in detail, one useful strategy that some researchers are adopting is to offer to make primary data available on line or by request from the principal investigator. *The Journal of Family Practice* now has a web page in which supplementary materials for published articles can be placed, and the journal guarantees they will remain accessible (www.jfp.denver.co.us). This acts as something akin to an external audit. Another option is to divide study results into different domains, such as theory, methods, and practice, and make each into a separate paper with different audiences and publication outlets. Clinicians are likely to be interested in the practical results or applications of a study, methodologists in the detailed steps involved in doing the analysis, and theorists in a discussion of different perspectives on the phenomena of interest. This was the strategy used by the editors of this volume when they published the methods for a study using in-depth interviews (Crabtree & Miller, 1991) prior to the publication of the results of the study (Miller, Yanoshik, et al., 1994).

Another criterion or tenet for presentation of results is the logic and integrity of analytic steps and their relationship to the question under investigation (Questions 2F through 2G in Figure 18.1). Inui and Frankel (1991) identified desirable features of manuscripts describing qualitative research results. Manuscripts should begin with a description of the history of the inquiry, the investigator's role, perception at the beginning of the research process, and all the methods of analysis employed. Inferences and judgments should be presented in sufficient detail and richness to support the overall result(s) and to persuade the average interested but skeptical reader. The results should demonstrate coherence, that is, internal consistency making thorough sense of the phenomenon of interest and relatedness and boundedness, which essentially locate the work in the context of previous investigations of the same or similar topics. Salience and verisimilitude are criteria that relate to the credibility and relevance of the study and its findings. Generativity refers to the extent to which new territories, opportunities for further exploration, are uncovered by the research. Finally, there are qualities of scholarship that apply generically—brevity, clarity, and accessibility. These are especially important in any emerging area of scholarship and have particular relevance to qualitative research, which has developed a technical language of its own that may be difficult for clinicians and lay persons to decipher. A helpful criterion in this regard is to ask, If a Martian were to read this manuscript, would it be able to make sense of the logic and importance of the question, analysis, and conclusions drawn? If not, how could I edit the text to make it utterly simple and available to such a person?

CONCLUSION

As I reflect on nearly 30 years of doing qualitative research, I find myself endlessly fascinated by the various ways of knowing that social scientists, basic scientists, and clinicians have devised for understanding the human condition. Much earlier in my career, I was a "methodological imperialist," asserting that the only "proper" approach to research was based on a single theory and a single method. In late midcareer, I have become much more pragmatic and, in fact, much more interested in what works and generates new knowledge. I no longer subscribe to a single theory or single method of doing research (although I do believe that the approach I was taught is elegant, rigorous, and reproducible). By analogy, I could compare my own growth and development as a social scientist to that of my physician colleagues, who were taught, and now reject, a unicausal model of disease.

Perhaps, like Ludwig Wittgenstein, the philosopher of language, we are destined to slowly and inexorably change our position 180 degrees over the course of an academic career. Regardless, in the time that I've been doing research, I've had the opportunity to work with a dazzling array of qualitative and, more recently, quantitative researchers who approach their task with awe, humility, and good humor.

The primary lessons that I have taken away from these encounters are these:

1. It is a goal of qualitative research to use yourself as a research instrument. It pays to work in teams and to develop a system of checks and balances on your work, but ultimately it is important to learn to trust your own judgment, intuition, and inner voice when it comes to making important decisions about setting the research question and deciding on methods.

2. The best way to judge the quality of qualitative research is to let go of specious distinctions between research traditions that encourage conflict and disagreement and to look instead at how any method relates to the problem at hand.

3. Science and satisfaction are not mutually exclusive. It is possible to be creative and critical and, at the same time, thoroughly enjoy the process. The only limitations that exist to doing creative integrative research that explores new territories and horizons are those that are self-imposed.

As the editors and other authors before me have, we invite you to discover the diversity and dynamism of qualitative research and its growing influence and popularity in the medical community. Clinicians will especially appreciate the bridge that qualitative research methods offer between the experience of providing care to individual patients and doing so using the language of probabilistic thinking and population data. Under the best of circumstances, the two blend together seamlessly and patients feel cared for. More characteristically these days, there is tension between these two ways of knowing, and the relationship between physician and patient suffers. Creative, relevant research (both qualitative and multimethod) in this area is desperately needed to restore vitality, caring, and mutual respect to the relationship.

19

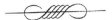

Qualitative Research

Perspectives on the Future

Lucy M. Candib
Kurt C. Stange
Wendy Levinson

W hat does it all mean? We have built our craft and reached the water's edge and are now ready to enter the sea of primary care research. But how will our craft and crew handle the inevitable squalls, calms, and sandbars? How does qualitative research fit into the present and future realities of primary care? How does it affect our lives? What changes need to occur? Where do we need to go from here?

In this chapter, as in all the preceding ones, we start with the questions that arise from personal experience and follow them wherever they lead. We join with all those we find along the way, changing them, ourselves, and the water around us, the world in which we live, love, and work. This chapter begins with the experiential questions that coaxed Wendy Levinson, a practicing primary care internist, to use qualitative methods. She shares her journey and looks at the promise that qualitative methods have for addressing the complex problems that primary care physicians face each day. Kurt Stange, a family physician researcher, then explores the cultural and institutional changes that are necessary for achieving a new integrative, multimethod, transdisciplinary research culture that can address these living questions. Finally, family practice clinician Lucy Candib reminds us that, even as qualitative methods achieve greater acceptance and the research culture begins to change, we cannot afford complacency. If research is for all of us, then all of us need to be empowered participants in the research process. She points the way toward real emancipatory research.

The circle of inquiry never ceases turning. The direction in which it moves is up to us. If we step off the ladder of universal truth, turn our global eyes toward home, recognize how like our patients we are, and join in the dance of living more meaningful, empowered lives together, then we will have offered real hope to life on our beautiful blue planet. Begin your voyage. Many of us will be there with you.

A PRACTICING PHYSICIAN'S REFLECTIONS ON QUALITATIVE RESEARCH (WENDY LEVINSON)

As a practicing physician, I have often marveled at the complexity of the task of seeing patients and delivering high-quality medical care. Sometimes I sit back and think about the multiple facets of this work, including the incredible amount of new medical knowledge, the translation of this sophisticated knowledge into caring for the patients in routine primary care practice, the relationships with patients, and the interaction with my colleagues in the medical practice setting. In my career, I have been particularly fascinated with the nature of the relationship between my patients and me. What really allows patients to trust me? What are the emotional and psychological issues leading patients to present with symptoms, and how can I discover them? What are my own feelings in caring for patients—why do I feel very connected to some and dislike a few? I have tried to reflect on my own work in an effort to understand what makes me effective as a doctor and what the barriers are to my delivering the best care. My scientific teaching and the medical culture led me to believe that the way to understand things is with the scientific method, using the tools of research—randomized control trials, case control studies, and, more recently (because fashions change all the time), meta-analysis and N of 1 trials. I value these methods to answer some important questions about treatment, causation, or prognosis, but I have found that they have not helped me explore many of the questions that arise in the examination room with patients. I had no training in how to study these aspects of needed care.

In the absence of tools, I sometimes turned to thinking about individual patients' stories to better understand what happened between me and a particular patient and to draw from that experience lessons I could use with other patients. For example, I learned about "mining for gold" from a patient I disliked (Levinson, 1993). I sought help from a colleague to reflect about a "drug-seeking, chronic pain patient who was calling me all the time and driving me nuts." My colleague told me to look for something I liked about her—mine for gold. When I discovered that she was a loving mother invested in her child's track and field activities, I found that my feelings for her changed considerably, and my visits with her changed dramatically. I respected her parenting and started to ask and learn more about her children, in addition to discussing her pain. In another case, when I just could not figure out why the patient wasn't following any of my suggestions, I learned about the "invisible third person in the room." This is the person who has much more influence on the patient than me; it's the person who coaches the patient and shapes his or her beliefs about the cause of illness and the appropriate treatment. Discovering the beliefs of the invisible health care advisor allowed me to understand my patient in a different way that was more effective in explaining suggested treatments.

In trying to understand my relationship with patients like these, I guess I have been doing qualitative research. I've tried to extract the nuggets from caring for individual patients and then test their use with a broader group of patients and situations.

Qualitative methods like those described in this book have offered different approaches to scientific inquiry and new methods that may help illuminate some of these questions. As a nonexpert, I have dabbled in some of these methods. For example, I have used in-depth interviews to better understand physicians' experiences of making mistakes. We don't talk about this topic with our colleagues, so it's hard to learn from each other. More recently, I have worked with a colleague, Richard Frankel, to study aspects of physician-patient communication as it relates to medical malpractice. We have tried to understand what patterns of communication are used by primary care physicians and surgeons who have had medical malpractice claims in the past, compared to doctors who have never had claims against them. These efforts have introduced me to more formal qualitative research methods.

I share all this because my reflections may be useful in thinking about what qualitative methods offer at present and what they may offer researchers and practicing doctors in the future.

What have I learned? Most certainly, I understand now that the researcher is part of the process of research. This is a foreign concept to physician scientists trained in the present medical culture. I realize that the process of studying my patients depends on my personal experience in the relationship with the patient, reflecting about it, asking what worked and what did not, and then trying something new. This requires me to bring my own emotions and reactions to the conscious level and incorporate them into the medical care process. This is just not the process of new inquiry I learned about in medical school, my residency, and my fellowship, and beyond. It was and is a shift in thinking that is not easy to make. It needs to be experienced, not just explained to doctors/researchers.

I have also been impressed with the jargon developing in the field of qualitative research, and I wonder if it helps or whether, perhaps, it makes the methods less available to a novice like me. At a recent scientific meeting, I saw a young researcher who is studying the effect of financial conflict of interest on the doctor-patient relationship talking to a very established qualitative researcher about "trustworthiness," "snowball sampling techniques," and "immersion/crystallization." The experienced senior researcher looked puzzled but eager to learn, and I wasn't sure if the junior person was using jargon to "show his stuff" or because he was truly educating the colleague. Perhaps a new field needs to establish its own language to communicate concepts effectively, but sometimes I am not sure if it is helpful.

Multimethod research using both quantitative and qualitative methods offers exciting possibilities, but I rarely see a mixture of these methods in research projects. In my experience, often the quantitative researchers in health services research at a particular institution don't even know the researchers using qualitative methods to examine similar problems. They are sometimes in different departments, often in different campus locations. In this recent project on physician-patient communication and medical malpractice, I asked both a quantitative researcher and a qualitative researcher who were both very involved in this field of study to participate in the research team. I naively didn't appreciate that they had never worked together before and weren't quite sure whether to trust each other. In fact, the project ultimately benefited enormously from the interweaving of methods, but I think it came as a bit of a surprise to the members of the team. I think we are only at the beginning of learning how to mix methods to deepen our work and that we need to experiment with different approaches.

Over time, I anticipate that some qualitative methods will prove to be extremely useful in understanding common medical problems. These methods will become better known, well accepted, and ultimately integrated into the standard package of tools used by doctor-scientists. Other methods are likely to be abandoned as not particularly useful. Overall, I am encouraged by the prospect that newer qualitative methods will allow us to understand the rich and complex nature of medical care, which I experienced early in my office. More and more I see traditional physician-researchers, like myself, intrigued by the possibility that these methods may illuminate the answers to important questions.

QUALITATIVE RESEARCH:
A CHANGE IN CULTURE
(KURT C. STANGE)

This book calls for a change in the predominant research cultures, in which questions (and their answers) are frequently constrained by the disciplinary and methodological paradigms of the researchers. The text shows *why* it is necessary to change the current research approaches. More important, the individual chapters provide a blueprint on *how* to actualize a new research paradigm that is driven by the pursuit of knowledge and understanding and is served by, rather than driven or limited by, the chosen methods. The editors and authors explode the false dichotomy between quantitative and qualitative research approaches by making the qualitative research process transparent and explicit. In so doing, they point the way toward integrating a wide range of research traditions into true multimethod, transdisciplinary research (Crabtree, Addison, Gilchrist, & Kuzel, 1994). This book challenges researchers to make explicit the goals of lines of inquiry that are likely to involve both discovery and hypothesis testing, both induction and deduction. This second edition is even more grounded than the first in the actual experience of conducting primary care research, which is the generation of new knowledge in the primary care setting, from a primary care perspective (Stange, 1996). Although grounded in their own experience in primary care settings, the authors' approach has the potential to transform and integrate the entire biomedicosocial research endeavor.

How might a new integrative, multimethod, transdisciplinary research culture be actualized? What are its implications for the future? This new research culture involves beginning a line of inquiry and following that line in the direction dictated by new discoveries and the context in which they will be used. Researchers in this new culture start with an initial question but are not limited by the initial question or its implied methods. This means that multiple methods will almost certainly be needed during the inquiry, often being used simultaneously and nearly always sequentially over time (Stange, Miller, et al., 1994). Although the emerging multimethod research tradition will breed a new generation of researchers who are comfortable with a wide range of research approaches, no one researcher is likely to be skilled in all the methods required by a line of inquiry. In addition, even the highly skilled multimethodologist will require different perspectives afforded by diverse content experts and study participants. Thus, multimethod research nearly always requires *trans*disciplinary collaboration. This is distinguished from *multi*disciplinary research, in which participants bring diverse expertise but retain their disciplinary perspectives (Crabtree, Addison, et al., 1994). Rather, in true transdisciplinary research, diverse expertise is brought to bear on a research trajectory in an integrated way in which each participant becomes part of a larger whole that transcends the perspective that each participant initially brought to the enterprise. This requires a tolerance for ambiguity and frustration and a high degree of learning on the part of all participants. However, a transdisciplinary approach gives back to each participant and to the larger process by creating a transforming experience. My own experience with transdisciplinary research, involving the coeditors and others, confirms the exciting, transforming, creative and productive nature of transdisciplinary teams. They are entities to be fostered and treasured.

Appropriately configured transdisciplinary teams develop research questions that are grounded in the experience of the research "subjects." The direct involvement of participants as true collaborators in the question generation, discovery, interpretation, and dissemination processes is a logical consequence of a transdisciplinary approach and is a major advantage (see Chapter 15 of this book; Macaulay et al., 1998). The potential approached by participatory research to dissolve the boundaries between discovery, education, dissemination, and transformation is profound.

An amalgamation of alternative research paradigms, aims, and styles, embodied by the sequential or simultaneous use of multiple methods (Stange, Miller, et al., 1994), has the potential to increase the innovation, relevance, and efficiency of the research enterprise. For example, researchers who are coming toward this integrated, transdisciplinary research paradigm from a traditionally quantitative, materialistic, biomedical research tradition often bring the strengths of the experimental and survey research styles. The traditional aims of their inquiries are explanation, testing, prescription, and control (see Chapter 1). However, the simultaneous or sequential incorporation of field and philosophic research styles of inquiry would foster a more grounded explanation of the phenomenon under study, as well as greater understanding of context and meaning of the treatment and control lines of inquiry. Combining materialist inquiry into natural laws with constructivist and ecological paradigms would put the discovery of these laws into the context of their interactions with the complexities of culture, context, and environment embodied in the constructivist and critical/ecological paradigms of inquiry. Likewise, researchers who approach this new integrated research model from a traditionally qualitative constructivist paradigm often bring the strengths of field or documentary-historical research styles. The typical aims of their inquiry are identification, qualitative description, or explanation-testing/prediction. Sequentially or simultaneously invoking survey or experimental styles would open the inquiry to identification of natural laws and allow greater generalization of findings to other contexts.

What will it take to make such multimethod, transdisciplinary, participatory teams a common feature of the modern research landscape? Changes are needed in attitudes, relationships among researchers and other research participants, the structure of the institutions that support research, the methods used to generate new knowledge, and the options available to transmit this new knowledge.

Attitudes must change to decrease the arrogant judgmentalism that sometimes stems from parochial, unidisciplinary worldviews. Judgmentalism must be replaced by a critical openness to tailoring the research methods to the question. Researchers must sustain a greater willingness to allow the questions to emerge as part of the research trajectory. Researchers must be willing to join with study participants to understand the phenomena under study from alternate perspectives. When researchers are working to isolate some of the phenomena from their context, they must simultaneously work to understand the importance of that context. Relationships between researchers and the communities and individuals who participate in the research must be built over time so that the dichotomy between the generation and dissemination of knowledge can be diminished.

For multimethod research to thrive, the institutions that support research must change. Bridges must be built across the disciplinary boundaries that are so useful in generating specialized expertise but that reinforce intellectual parochialism. The multidisciplinary National Institutes of Health (NIH) centers programs, which support centers for research on cancer, arthritis, AIDS, and other diseases, are excellent models. Imagine the progress in generating a science base for caring for the problems that affect most of the people most of the time (Nutting & Green, 1994) that could be achieved by the creation of a centers program for primary care and community health research! Likewise, the categorical structure of the NIH and most other funding agencies, although useful for the generation of specialized knowledge, stifles researchers with research questions that transcend a narrow disease or specific population focus. True peer review for research designed to answer questions with a broad primary care or community focus must be developed if this new research paradigm is to emerge.

In addition, the scope of institutions involved in the systematic generation of new knowledge must be expanded. The generation of practice-based research networks of primary care clinicians (Green, Hames, & Nutting, 1994; Hickner, 1993; Nutting & Green, 1994; Stange, 1993) is an important development that must be expanded and provided with support for infrastructure as well as specific projects. Practitioners and trainees must be seen not only as passive receptacles for new knowledge but as participants in its generation. Community-oriented primary care (Mettee, Martin, & Williams, 1998; Nutting, 1987) and participatory research approaches are needed to diminish the we/they dichotomy of researchers and subjects. These approaches, which integrate community grounding with expertise in health service and research methods, have an established theoretical basis but limited implementation. Limitations in funding, failures in transdisciplinary relationships, and fear of innovative thinking must be overcome.

Multimethod trandisciplinary research implementation has been constrained by the lack of methods development. This book fills an important void by describing qualitative methods in an accessible fashion that is ripe for integration with quantitative research traditions. Training programs that include this integrated approach as an acceptable paradigm, and increasingly model its use, are needed to develop a new generation of multimethod researchers. Within the existing community of researchers, opportunities for cross-fertilization of ideas, methods, and emergent research findings must be developed. Current professional meetings and scholarly journals often foster isolation rather than integration of perspectives. The three Agency for Health Care Policy and Research (AHCPR) primary care research conferences (Hibbard, Nutting, & Grady, 1991; Mayfield & Grady, 1990) and the AHCPR-sponsored conference on multimethod research (Crabtree, Addison, et al., 1994) were excellent prototypes. A regular and sustained transdisciplinary multimethod research forum would be worthy of support from philanthropic and governmental institutions interested in increasing the community and population relevance, applicability, and innovation of biomedicosocial research.

Multimethod researchers must have the courage to challenge the research dissemination vehicles by presenting and writing their research in a fashion that integrates quantitative and qualitative findings. As this becomes commonplace, future editions of this book will be able to draw on examples of scholarly work in which the (multi-)methods are well specified and described and the findings include both numbers and narratives. The next generation of scholarly writing will tie in the perspectives of the relevant literature, the researchers, and the study participants. The increasing openness of traditional medical journals to qualitative research and the innovative integration of print and permanent website media pioneered by *The Journal of Family Practice* show that the time is ripe for scholars to creatively develop unified communication vehicles that integrate multiple methods, diverse perspectives, and findings that both summarize and deeply describe. In addition, researchers should increase their creativity in interactively disseminating findings and seeking interpretation and direction from the populations and individuals who are affected by the research but who do not attend to traditional scholarly dissemination vehicles.

What are the implications of a new integrative, multimethod, transdisciplinary research culture? Disciplinary bounds and methods-based constraints will be broken. New lines of inquiry will be opened. The perspectives of traditional research subjects will be incorporated into the asking and answering of questions. The false dichotomy between discovery and dissemination will be blurred as researchers are transformed by their research subjects and colleagues and vice versa. Research findings will deal less with finding fault and more with finding and evaluating solutions that are acceptable to those involved. Definitions of quality of care will be broadened as evidence-based research guidelines increasingly recognize the importance of context. The importance of research in primary care settings from a primary care perspective will become increasingly apparent. The study of traditionally underserved and disenfranchised populations will increase. Type 3 and 4 errors will become less common in the published research literature. The environment for creation of a generalist research funding institute as a common good to balance the overemphasis on reductionistic, materialistic research approaches fostered by categorical funding will become increasingly favorable. The ability to generalize the findings from randomized clinical trials to other populations and to understand limitations in the applicability of research findings will increase. Increased attention to sampling issues will improve understanding of the transportability of studies of culture and meaning. The efficiency of circles of discovery and validation and application will increase. Research will become increasingly approachable for clinicians and the population.

This book gives us the tools to develop a new, integrative, multimethod, transdisciplinary research culture. However, tools are only as useful as the vision and skill of the craftspersons who use them. It is time for researchers to expand their vision to create a new multimethod research culture. Using the tools in this book, together we can create transdisciplinary teams that will integrate diverse methods and perspectives to create new knowledge that is focused on the most important problems faced by people in need. We can train the next generation of researchers in a new integrated paradigm. We can involve those traditionally thought of as research subjects or consumers as active participants in the process of generating new knowledge. This process will require courage. Progress will be made incrementally, through small successes and learning from failures. The time to begin is with the next research question. The time is now.

TOWARD EMANCIPATORY RESEARCH
(LUCY M. CANDIB)

Prediction is a fool's game. To attempt to predict the future of qualitative research is a gamble—it could be right or wrong. Instead, what seems imperative is to point in the direction that qualitative research must go, given the social, political, and economic realities that dominate the world today. Why do we do research? We do it because it is interesting to us; it grabs us. We feel energized in the process of posing problems, devising methods to address them, doing the project, and getting some answers. Of course, we also do it because it is our work; some of us are paid to do it, at least some of the time. For some, the recognition is important; for others, being successful at bringing grant money to our institution is a reward in itself that guarantees future promotion and success. Research also has historically justified itself by claiming to discover the truth and to be able to make life better for people. Qualitative research in particular has claimed the goal of meaning making; this interpretive function—of revealing that the world makes sense—seems enough to justify the work.

This claim must be held up against the realization that most research, including qualitative work, has reproduced the power relations in society: wealthy over poor, educated over less educated, healthy over sick, entitled over disempowered. Research constructed by researchers to study others inevitably objectifies those studied; they are "othered" by the very process intended, in qualitative work, to reveal their reality. Often those studied— the poor, sick, disabled, troubled—appear to be "the problem" rather than the social and political context in which their difficulties emerge. In many cases, the research process, although it will have jumped the hurdle of the institutional review board or internal ethics committee, is not necessarily understandable, much less empowering, to most participants (LoVerde, Prochazka, & Byyny, 1989). Often in the course of conducting research we find ourselves trying to obfuscate what we are really doing so that our "subjects" or "informants" will act normally, thus generating the material we need to do our research (see Chapter 3). We may find that doing the research means acting as if we are friends with those we study, leading them to believe, by virtue of our interest in them, that we are real friends. The old order of power relations between researcher and researched remains unchanged.

And the benefits of research for those studied has been ambiguous. Many disadvantaged groups—communities of color, disabled people, psychiatric patients—feel that not only have they been exploited in the research process (witness the Tuskegee Experiment) but that the outcome of the research has been used against their interests. Despite our best intentions, more often it is the researcher who reaps the benefits, not necessarily the family or community where the work is done. Though the researcher may be fully engaged during the course of the investigation, she or he can and usually does pull out of the participants' world afterwards and is not confined to the situation or conditions of the research context in the same way that the participants are—for example, studying working class communities (Cornwell, 1984; Fine & Weis, 1996) or women having their first babies (Oakley, 1981). The researcher may make tight and meaningful connections with key informants, but those connections always bear the dual and sometimes conflictual role of serving the research, as well as the friendship. As Judith Stacey (1988) put it, after the death of a key informant, even the funeral was "grist for the ethnographic mill. . . . Conflicts of interest and emotion between the ethnographer as authentic, related person (i.e., participant), and as exploiting researcher (i.e., observer) are also an inescapable feature of ethnographic method" (p. 23). Thus even qualitative research can be manipulative and controlling toward research subjects because of the "inherently unequal reciprocity" (p. 26), despite the ultimate goal of better exploring and revealing subjects' reality.

Consider the following scenario: a Native American group seeks some assistance in investigating their health status from some physicians affiliated with the local medical school. Some of the physicians assume that the findings should be published. The Native American group refuses. How could that be? Wouldn't it be good for people to know the needs of the Native American population? reasoned the doctors. The reasoning of the Native American group is presumably quite different; if it turns out that the health indicators are bad (e.g., high infant mortality, low frequency of Pap smears, low frequency of mammography), then Native Americans would once again look like an uneducated and disadvantaged people. If, on the other hand, the indicators are good, that could be used to imply that Native Americans don't need any help getting their health needs met. The Native American community, having lived as a racially discriminated group, presumably considers that no matter how any research turned out, it could be used against the interests of their people. They choose not to make their findings public. The physicians are confused because they do not share the same vulnerability to and therefore suspicion of publication of research findings. Research in this context is highly problematic.

Clearly a kind of research that chooses to confront and change oppressive power relations would be preferable. A variety of researchers from different disciplines are now calling for such a change in direction—toward emancipatory research (Heron & Reason, 1997; Lather, 1988; Stone & Priestley, 1996). In a discussion of research on disability, Stone and Priestley (1996) set forth six principles of emancipatory research. First, the research must locate what is studied within the social context, not as an individual's pathology, a medical problem, or a personal tragedy. The experience of oppression is created by the social and cultural setting that itself must be critically examined. Second, the research must be committed to the development of a movement to empower those studied, not to a notion of detached objectivity. Third, the research must result in improvement in the condition of those studied, as determined by those affected. Such work is tied to political action rather than to observation or monitoring. Fourth, the process of the research must reverse the social relations of usual research production by putting the research skills at the disposal of those studied to undo the passivity, marginalization, and exclusion resulting from business as usual. Fifth, the subjective realities of individuals studied must be highlighted as well as the collective experience; emancipation must attend to both the personal and the political. Sixth, a plurality of approaches, qualitative and quantitative, micro- and macro-level, are necessary to do emancipatory research. Choice of the most appropriate research methods will depend on the work to be done. Emancipatory research focuses on the lives and experience of disempowered people, with the goal of using the power of the truth on behalf of those studied. Rejecting the positivist assumptions of a value-free social science, emancipatory research goes "beyond criticizing what is to change what is, to side unapologetically with the less powerful and voiceless" (Maguire, 1996, p. 113). The research is for the participants. Emancipatory research has the potential to have a transforming effect on the world—in the interests of those studied, others like them, and, indeed, even the researchers themselves.

One form of research that is often constructed to be explicitly empowering is participatory action research (see Chapter 15). Here the research is of and by the participants. Research may be initiated *by* outside professionals *or* jointly, by professionals and the community. Nurses have taken the lead in participatory action research within the health fields, perhaps because of their sensitivity to the power issues in medicine and because of their sense of advocacy for patients, families, and communities (Clarke & Mass, 1998; McKibbin & Castle, 1996; Rains & Ray, 1995). Such projects join with the community or group affected by the problem to define exactly what the problem is, enlist the community or group in the solution, and swing the resources of the research establishment under the control of the community so that the outcome serves them and not the principal investigator. Participatory inquiry moves beyond the old subject-object dichotomy to the cocreation of knowledge, where both join together in an unruly process that necessarily challenges preconceived ideas and ways of relating. Participatory action research projects with native peoples, for instance, have led to transformations in how native health workers were empowered (Hecker, 1997) and how clinical illness could best be understood and addressed (Herbert, 1996). Such research has the potential to fulfill the criteria of all six principles described above.

Participatory action research places the highest priority on process. Consistently and persistently confronting the standard power relationships between the researcher and those studied, putting into practice the fourth principle above, is a major challenge in this work. Nevertheless, participatory action research itself has been subject to criticism for not acknowledging the way that gender shapes how men and women can enter into the process of research in the community context (Maguire, 1996). In the course of the work, the entitlements of class, race, education, and gender must be examined as well as the more subtle divisions between the sick and the well, the temporarily able-bodied and those physically or mentally challenged. As Thesen and Kuzel (Chapter 15) point out, power issues weave their way throughout participatory action research, and the investigators must be constantly aware of the tendency for professionals to dominate, often without an awareness of it happening. Participatory action studies of the meaning of diabetes to native peoples (Boston et al., 1997; Herbert, 1996), of the problems of disabled adults (Stone & Priestley, 1996), of people with learning disabilities (Richardson, 1997), and of the needs of parents with learning-disabled children (Malekoff, Johnson, & Klappersack, 1991) reveal the struggle of preventing the usual power relations from further disempowering those studied. Only when these power relationships are revealed and considered critically by researchers and participants alike does action research reach its potential to be emancipatory. As almost anyone who has engaged in it has discovered, such work has a transforming effect on the researcher.

Emancipatory research must be committed to empowerment of both those for whom it is done and those who participate in it (second and third principles). All clinical research may claim the general goal benefiting those who suffer from a disease or those for whom a disease might be prevented or delayed in onset; nevertheless, the benefits are remote from those who participate in the research. If work in qualitative research is really to be meaning making, then it needs to be made available to those who need to understand that meaning. Results need to be formulated in such a way that they are available to participants or others like them (i.e., they must be suitably readable and not technical). Publishing in professional journals does not necessarily achieve this end, although on some occasions it might. For research to be empowering to a group or community, it needs to be under the control of the people to whom it belongs. Maria Mies (1983) made this clear in her very preliminary writings about how to do research on battered women. Some feminist researchers have accomplished this goal by publishing lay books as well as academic books about their research, thereby transmitting the benefit from those they studied to other lay people, not just to other sociologists (see Lather & Smithies, 1997; Oakley, 1980). In some instances of participatory action research, participants review and rewrite drafts and conduct presentations of the materials to assure that the content reflects what all the participants intended (Traylen, 1994; Whitmore, 1994).

Participatory action research is a typical kind of emancipatory research, but other kinds of qualitative (Shields & Dervin, 1993) and even quantitative research can be emancipatory (the sixth principle). For instance, an aboriginal community may choose to do a quantitative study of health indicators for their own reasons. In this book (Chapter 17), a one-to-one research project within the doctor-patient relationship demonstrates the characteristics of emancipatory research at the micro-level. Kirsti Malterud, a Norwegian general practitioner, deliberately chose to investigate what questions would empower her women patients to speak, and she chose a method that involved testing these questions in such a way that the patients' own responses shaped what questions evolved. Both her motivational goal and her process meet the criteria of empowerment. When framing her key questions to her women patients, she was able to focus on which questions worked to get patients to talk about what was happening in their lives, what understandings they had about their illnesses, what hypotheses they had formed, what expectations they held of the physician, and what they had already done to manage their illnesses. In other words, what she was looking for and what she focused on in the very construction of her project was empowering to patients. The process of answering the questions was empowering for the patients who participated, and the responses they gave enabled Malterud to elaborate the questions further, such that future patients were empowered. Malterud worked hard to make sure that patients would not interpret anything she said as possibly critical and allowed them room for dignified retreat and humorous escape. How often do we build these strategies into our research methods? Not often enough, I would venture. Malterud's project demonstrates that empowerment research can be conducted at the level of attention to individual dialog as well as the level of community engagement.

When we turn to the hierarchical and oppressive world of health care, the need for an emancipatory research practice is evident. Lather (1988) holds that the goal of feminist research in the human sciences is "to correct both the *invisibility* and *distortion* of female experience in ways relevant to ending women's unequal social position" (p. 571, italics in original). Emancipatory research in medicine, in parallel, would work to correct both the invisibility and the distortion of patients' experience in ways relevant to ending their unequal social position. Much of qualitative research in medicine has helped us to see the world from patients' points of view, but this is not enough. It does not seem to change us or the medical system enough to make it lastingly different for other patients. And the experience of those health care workers at the bottom of the hierarchy who have the most intimate acquaintance with patient care remains invisible. To change the world, we all need to be transformed by an understanding of those most oppressed in it. Doctors need an intimate awareness of suffering, trainers must apprehend the grueling and dehumanizing aspects of the training they conduct, administrators need to know what it is like to be a nursing assistant, and sick people need to be able to share their reality with others with similar conditions. To be changed, we need to know the details: mothers of malnourished children spend hours daily in the work of feeding their families, do not receive enough money to buy nourishing food, and cannot travel to where the prices are better (Travers, 1996, 1997). Professionals and educators may aim our "help" at individuals, yet it is a whole system that requires change. To open up the possibility of meaningful change, emancipatory research must consider how the specifics of gender, class, race, and education circumscribe people's potential (first principle).

Participatory action research as an example of emancipatory work contains within it the vision of a better future: the possibility of human flourishing (Heron & Reason, 1997). It is not enough to identify and criticize the power inequalities of our current social and economic systems; it is necessary to build into our work the understanding that we contain the potential for a better future. In the individual arena, Malterud and Hollnagel (1997, 1998) have turned their attention to the development of questions that, rather than fixating on patients' health risks, instead examine the personal resources that patients bring to their health. Within North American society, whereas work with disempowered individuals may reveal the desperation and hopelessness of individual conditions, work with groups in community reveals strengths and successes:

> If individual interviews produce the most despairing stories, evince the most minimal sense of possibility, present identities of victimization, and voice stances of hopelessness, in focus groups with the same people the despair begins to evaporate, a sense of possibility sneaks through. . . . In these like-minded communities that come together to trade despair and build hope, we see and hear a cacophony of voices filled with spirit, possibility, and a sense of vitality absent in the individual data. (Fine & Weis, 1996, pp. 267-268)

For qualitative research to move on to become emancipatory research, we need to draw on "the critical and empowering roots of a research paradigm openly committed to critiquing the status quo and building a more just society" (Lather, 1988, note 6, p. 578). We now understand that we bring ourselves into the research that we do, carrying with us the power inequities of the society whenever we engage in studying others. From here we need to continue to question ourselves and our work: Can qualitative research be transformative? Can it give patients more control over their lives and their illnesses? Can it show us how to join with patients in pursuit of healthier lives rather than how to manage them? Can it show us what it means to be sick and change us so that we honor that meaning every time we talk to someone with an illness? Can it help us cross the great divide that separates doctors from patients? Will it help us accompany people to their death with less fear? If we join with people in communities to do research together, will we let ourselves relinquish control and allow ourselves to let the community control the project? Doing research changes us. Can it change us to be better people? Can it change the world to be a better place? Emancipatory research offers us the possibility of answering these questions in the affirmative.

References

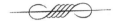

Abram, J. (1996). *The spell of the sensuous.* New York: Random House.

Addison, R. B. (1984). *Surviving the residency: A grounded interpretive investigation of physician socialization.* Berkeley: University of California, Berkeley.

Addison, R. B. (1989a). Covering-over and over-reflecting during residency training: Using personal and professional development groups to integrate dysfunctional modes of being. In M. J. Little & J. E. Midtling (Eds.), *Becoming a family physician.* New York: Springer-Verlag.

Addison, R. B. (1989b). Grounded interpretive research: An investigation of physician socialization. In M. J. Packer & R. B. Addison (Eds.), *Entering the circle: Hermeneutic investigation in psychology* (pp. 39-57). Albany: State University of New York Press.

Addison, R. B. (1992). Grounded hermeneutic research. In B. F. Crabtree & W. L. Miller (Eds.), *Doing qualitative research* (pp. 110-124). Newbury Park, CA: Sage.

Adler, L. M., Ware, J. E., & Enelow, A. J. (1970). Changes in medicine interviewing style after instruction with two closed-circuit television techniques. *Journal of Medical Education, 45,* 21-28.

Agar, M. H. (1980). *The professional stranger: An informal introduction to ethnography.* New York: Academic.

Agar, M. H. (1986). *Speaking of ethnography* (Vol. 2). Beverly Hills, CA: Sage.

Alexander, D. A., Knox, J.D.E., & Morrison, A. T. (1977). Medical students talking to patients. *Medical Education, 11,* 390-393.

Allen, M. N., & Jenson, L. (1990). Hermeneutical inquiry: Meaning and scope. *Western Journal of Nursing Research, 12*(2), 241-253.

Altheide, D. L. (1987). Ethnographic content analysis. *Qualitative Sociology, 10,* 65-77.

Altheide, D. L., & Johnson, J. M. (1994). Criteria for assessing interpretive validity in qualitative research. In N. K. Denzin & Y. S. Lincoln (Eds.), *Handbook of qualitative research* (pp. 485-499). Newbury Park, CA: Sage.

American Academy of Family Physicians. (1991). *Directory of Family Practice Residency Programs.* Kansas City, MO: Author.

American Medical Association Task Force of the Council on Ethical and Judicial Affairs. (1991). Gender disparities in clinical decision making. *Journal of the American Medical Association, 266,* 559-562.

American Psychiatric Association. (1994). *Diagnostic and statistical manual of mental disorders* (4th ed.). Washington, DC: Author.

Annells, M. (1997a). Grounded theory method, Part I: Within the five moments of qualitative research. *Nursing Inquiry, 4,* 120-129.

Annells, M. (1997b). Grounded theory method, Part II: Options for users of the method. *Nursing Inquiry, 4,* 176-180.

Anthony, W. A. (1993). Recovery from mental illness: The guiding vision of the mental health service system in the 1990s. *Psychosocial Rehabilitation Journal, 16,* 11-23.

Arborelius, E., & Timpka, T. (1990). In what way may videotapes be used to get significant information about the patient-physician relationship? *Medical Teacher, 12,* 197-208.

Arborelius, E., & Timpka, T. (1991). Comparison of patients' and doctors' comments on video-recorded consultations. *Scandinavian Journal of Primary Health Care, 9,* 71-77.

Argyris, C., & Schön, D. (1974). *Theory in practice: Increasing professional effectiveness.* San Francisco: Jossey-Bass.

Armitage, K. J., Schneiderman, L. J., & Bass, R. A. (1979). Response of physicians to medical complaints in men and women. *Journal of the American Medical Association, 241,* 2186-2187.

Ashworth, P. D. (1997a). The variety of qualitative research. Part one: Introduction to the problem. *Nurse Education Today, 17,* 215-218.

Ashworth, P. D. (1997b). The variety of qualitative research. Part two: Non-positivist approaches. *Nurse Education Today, 17,* 219-224.

Austin, J. L. (1982). *How to do things with words* (2nd ed.). Oxford: Oxford University Press.

Babbie, E. R. (1979). *The practice of social research* (2nd ed.). Belmont, CA: Wadsworth.

Badger, L., deGruy, F., Harman, J., Plant, M., Leeper, J., Anderson, R., Ficken, R., Gaskins, S., Maxwell, H., & Rand, E. (1994). Patient presentation, interview content, and the detection of depression by primary care physicians. *Psychosomatic Medicine, 56,* 128-135.

Bain, J., & Mackay, N.S.D. (1993). Videotaping general practice consultations [Letter to the editor]. *British Medical Journal, 307,* 504-505.

Baird, A. G., & Gillies, J. C. (1993). Assessing GP's performance: Videotape assessment is threatening [Letter to the editor]. *British Medical Journal, 307,* 60.

Baldwin, C. D., Levine, H. G., & McCormick, D. P. (1995). Meeting the faculty development needs of generalist physicians in academia. *Academic Medicine, 70*(1, Suppl.), s97-s103.

Balint, M. (1957). *The doctor, his patient and the illness.* London: Pitman.

Bandura, A. (1977). *Social learning theory.* Englewood Cliffs, NJ: Prentice Hall.

Barbour, R. S. (1995). Using focus groups in general practice research. *Family Practice, 12*(3), 328-334.

Bargagliotti, L. A. (1983). The scientific method and phenomonology: Toward their peaceful coesixtence in nursing. *Journal of Nursing Research, 5,* 409-411.

Barker, G. K., & Rich, S. (1992). Influences on adolescent sexuality in Nigeria and Kenya: Findings from recent focus-group discussions. *Studies in Family Planning, 23*(3), 199-210.

Barker, L. R., Burton, J. R., & Zieve, P. D. (1991). *Principles of ambulatory medicine* (3rd ed.). Baltimore: Williams & Wilkins.

Barker, R. G. (1968). *Ecological psychology: Concepts and methods for studying the environment of human behavior.* Stanford, CA: Stanford University Press.

Barnhouse, A. H., Kilodychuk, G. R., Pankratz, C., & Olinger, D. A. (1988). Evaluation of acute pain: A comparison of patient and nurse perspectives. *Journal of Nursing Quality Assurance, 2,* 54-63.

Bassett, R., Cox, S., & Rauch, U. (1995, May). The emperor's new clothes: Is there more to NUD*IST than meets the eye? A response to Wall's concerns about software for qualitative data analysis. *Society, 19*(2).

Basso, K. (1984). "Stalking with stories": Names, places, and moral narratives among the western Apache. In E. Bruner (Ed.), *Text, play, and story: The construction and reconstruction of self and society* (pp. 19-55). Washington, DC: American Ethnological Society.

Bateson, G. (1979). *Mind and nature: A necessary unity.* Toronto, Canada: Bantam.

Becker, G. (1997). *Disrupted lives.* Berkeley: University of California Press.

Becker, H. S., Geer, B., Hughes, E., & Strauss, A. (1961). *Boys in white: Student culture in medical school.* Chicago: Chicago University Press.

Bee, R., & Crabtree, B. (1992). Using ETHNOGRAPH in field note management. In M. Boone & J. Wood (Eds.), *Computer applications for anthropologists.* Belmont, CA: Wadsworth.

Beeson, D. (1997). Nuance, complexity, and context: Qualitative methods in genetic counseling research. *Journal of Genetic Counseling, 6*(1), 21-43.

Behar, R. (1996). *The vulnerable observer: Anthrolopogy that breaks your heart.* Boston, MA: Beacon.

Bennett, J. W. (1996). Applied and action anthropology: Ideological and conceptual aspects. *Current Anthropology, 37*(Suppl.), S23-S39.

Bensing, J. M., & Dronkers, J. (1992). Instrumental and affective aspects of physician behavior. *Medical Care, 30*(4), 283-298.

Berelson, B. (1971). *Content analysis in communication research.* New York: Hafner.

Berger, P. L., & Luckman, T. (1967). *The social construction of reality: A treatise in the sociology of knowledge.* Garden City, NJ: Doubleday.

Bernard, H. R. (1988). *Research methods in cultural anthropology.* Newbury Park, CA: Sage.

Bernard, H. R. (1994). *Research methods in anthropology.* Newbury Park, CA: Sage.

Bernard, H. R. (1995). *Research methods in anthropology: Qualitative and quantitative approaches* (2nd ed.). Walnut Creek, CA: Alta Mira.

Bernstein, B. (1981). Physicians' attitudes toward female patients. *Medical Care, 19,* 600-607.

Bernstein, R. J. (1983). *Beyond objectivism and relativism: Science, hermeneutics, and praxis.* Philadelphia: University of Pennsylvania Press.

Berry, D. S., & Pennebaker, J. W. (1993). Nonverbal and verbal emotional expression and health. *Psychotherapy and Psychosomatics, 59,* 1-19.

Birdwell, B. G., Herbers, J. E., & Kroenke, K. (1993). Evaluating chest pain: The patient's presentation style alters the physician's diagnostic approach. *Archives of Internal Medicine, 153,* 1991-1995.

Birdwhistell, R. L. (1970). *Kinesics and context.* Philadelphia: University of Pennsylvania Press.

Blake, R. L., & Bertuso, D. D. (1988). The life space drawing as a measure of social relationships. *Family Medicine, 20*(4), 295-297.

Blanch, A., Fisher, D., Tucker, W., Walsh, D., & Chassman, J. (1993). Consumer-practitioners and psychiatrists share insights about recovery and coping. *Disabilities Studies Quarterly, 13*(2), 17-20.

Bleicher, J. (1980). *Contemporary hermeneutics: Hermeneutics as method, philosophy and critique.* London: Routledge & Kegan Paul.

Bleicher, J. (1982). *The hermeneutic imagination: Outline of a positive critique of scientism and sociology.* London: Routledge & Kegan Paul.

Block, P. (1993). *Stewardship: Choosing service over self-interest.* San Francisco: Berrett-Koehler.

Bloom, S. W. (1963). The process of becoming a physician. *Annals of the American Academy of Political and Social Science, 346,* 77-87.

Blumer, H. (1954). What's wrong with social theory? *American Sociological Review, 19,* 3-10.

Blumer, H. (1969). *Symbolic interactionism.* Englewood Cliffs, NJ: Prentice Hall.

Bogdan, R. C. (1972). *Participant observation in organizational settings.* Syracuse, NY: Syracuse University Press.

Bogdan, R. C., & Biklen, S. K. (1982). *Qualitative research for education: An introduction to theory and methods.* Boston: Allyn & Bacon.

Bogdewic, S. P. (1987). *On becoming a family physician: The stages and characteristics of identity formation in family medicine residency training.* Unpublished doctoral dissertation, University of North Carolina, Chapel Hill.

Bogdewic, S. P. (1992). Participant observation. In B. F. Crabtree & W. L. Miller (Eds.), *Doing qualitative research.* Newbury Park, CA: Sage.

Borges, S., & Waitzkin, H. (1995). Women's narratives in primary care medical encounters. *Women & Health, 23*(1), 29-56.

Borkan, J., Quirk, M., & Sullivan, M. (1991). Finding meaning after the fall: Injury narratives from elderly hip fracture patients. *Social Science and Medicine, 33,* 947-957.

Borkan, J., Reis, S., Hermoni, D., & Biderman, A. (1995). Talking about the pain: A patient-centered study of low back pain in primary care. *Social Science and Medicine, 40*(7), 977-988.

Borkan, J. M., Miller, W. L., Neher, J. O., Cushman, R., & Crabtree, B. F. (1997). Evaluating family practice residencies: A new method for qualitative assessment. *Family Medicine, 29*(9), 640-647.

Bosk, C. L. (1979). *Forgive and remember: Managing medical failure.* Chicago, IL: University of Chicago Press.

Boston, P., Jordan, S., MacNamara, E., Kozolanka, K., Bobbish-Rondeau, E., Iserhoff, H., Mianscum, S., Mianscum-Trapper, R., Mistacheesick, I., Petawabano, B., Sheshamush-Masty, M., Wapachee, R., & Weapenicappo, J. (1997). Using participatory action research to understand the meanings aboriginal Canadians attribute to the rising incidence of diabetes. *Chronic Diseases in Canada, 18*(1), 5-12.

Bowers, C. A. (1997). *The culture of denial.* Albany: State University of New York Press.

Branch, W.T.J. (1990). Teaching models in an ambulatory training program. *Journal of General Internal Medicine, 4,* 515-526.

Bråten, S. (1988). Between dialogic mind and monologic reason. In C. Miriam (Ed.), *Between rationality and cognition.* Turin, Italy: Albert Meynier.

Brewer, J., & Hunter, A. (1989). *Multimethod research: A synthesis of styles.* Newbury Park, CA: Sage.

Briggs, C. (1986). *Learning to ask.* Cambridge, UK: Cambridge University Press.

Brigley, S., Young, Y., Littlejohns, P., & McEwen, J. (1997). Continuing education for medical professionals: A reflective model. *Postgraduate Medical Journal, 73*(855), 23-26.

Brock, S. C. (1995). Narrative and medical genetics: On ethics and therapeutics. *Qualitative Health Research, 5*(2), 150-168.

Brody, H. (1987). *Stories of sickness.* New Haven, CT: Yale University Press.

Brown, J. B., Dickie, I., Brown, L., & Biehn, J. (1997). Long-term attendance at a family practice teaching unit: Qualitative study of patients' views. *Canadian Family Physician, 43,* 901-906.

Brown, J. B., Harris, S., & Sangster, L. M. (1997, November 12-15). *Clinical practice guidelines: Family physicians' experience in patients with atrial fibrillation.* Paper presented at the North American Primary Care Research Group, Orlando, FL.

Brown, J. B., McWilliam, C. L., & Mai, V. (1997). Barriers and facilitators to seniors' independence: Perceptions of seniors, caregivers, and health care providers. *Canadian Family Physician, 43,* 469-475.

Brown, J. B., Sangster, M., & Swift, J. (1998). Factors influencing palliative care: Qualitative study of family physicians' practices. *Canadian Family Physician, 44,* 1028-1034.

Brown, J. B., Sas, G., & Lent, B. (1993). Identifying and treating wife abuse. *Journal of Family Practice, 36*(2), 185-191.

Bruner, J. (1986). *Actual minds, possible worlds.* Cambridge, MA: Harvard University Press.

Bruner, J. (1990). *Acts of meaning.* Cambridge, MA: Harvard University Press.

Burack, J. H., Irby, D. M., Carline, J. D., Ambrozy, D. M., Ellsbury, K. E., & Stritter, F. T. (1997). A study of medical students' specialty-choice pathways: Trying on possible selves. *Academic Medicine, 72*(6), 534-541.

Burkett, G. L. (1990). Classifying basic research designs. *Family Medicine, 22*(2), 143-148.

Burkett, G. L. (1991). Culture, illness, and the biopsychosocial model. *Family Medicine, 23,* 287-291.

Butler, D. J., Seidl, J. J., Holloway, R. L., & Robertson, R. G. (1995). Family practice residents' learning needs and beliefs about office-based psychological counseling. *Family Medicine, 27*(6), 371-375.

Butler, O. J. (1996). Informed consent for videotaping. *Academic Medicine, 71,* 1276-1277.

Calderhead, J. (1981). Stimulated recall: A method for research on teaching. *British Journal of Educational Psychology, 51,* 211-217.

Calhoun, E. F. (1993, October). Action research: Three approaches. *Educational Leadership, 51,* 62-65.

Callahan, E. J., & Bertakis, K. D. (1991). Development and validation of the Davis Observation Code. *Family Medicine, 23*(1), 19-24.

Candib, L. M. (1995). *Medicine and the family: A feminist perspective.* New York: Basic Books.

Caputo, J. D. (1987). *Radical hermeneutics: Repetition, deconstruction, and the hermeneutic project.* Bloomington: University of Indiana Press.

Cassata, D. M., Conroy, R. M., & Clements, P. W. (1977). A program for enhancing medical interviewing using video-tape feedback in the family practice residency. *Journal of Family Practice, 4,* 763-677.

Cassell, E. J. (1985). *Talking with patients.* Cambridge, MA: MIT Press.

Cave, A., Maharaj, U., Gibson, N., & Jackson, E. (1995). Physicians and immigrant patients: Cross-cultural communication. *Canadian Family Physician, 41,* 1685-1690.

Charon, R. (1994). Narrative contributions to medical ethics. In E. DuBose, R. Hamel, & L. O'Connell (Eds.), *A matter of principles? Ferment in U.S. bioethics* (pp. 260-283). Valley Forge, PA: Trinity.

Charon, R., Banks, J. T., Connelly, J. E., Hawkins, A. H., Hunter, K. M., Jones, A. H., Montello, M., & Poirer, S. (1995). Literature and medicine: Contributions to clinical practice. *Annals of Internal Medicine, 122,* 599-606.

Chelimsky, E., & Shadish, W. R. (Eds.). (1997). *Evaluation for the 21st century: A handbook.* Thousand Oaks, CA: Sage.

Chen, A. M., Wismer, B. A., Lew, R., Kang, S. H., Min, K., Moskowitz, J. M., & Tager, I. B. (1997). Health is strength: A research collaboration involving Korean Americans in Alameda County. *American Journal of Preventive Medicine, 13*(6, Suppl.), 93-100.

Chenitz, W. C., & Swanson, J. M. (Eds.). (1986). *From practice to grounded theory: Qualitative research in nursing.* Menlo Park, CA: Addison-Wesley.

Churchill, L., & Churchill, S. (1982). Storytelling in medical arenas: The art of self-determination. *Literature and Medicine, 1,* 73-79.

Cicourel, A. (1964). *Method and measurement in sociology.* New York: Free Press.

Cicourel, A. V. (1973). *Cognitive sociology: Language and meaning in social interactions.* Harmondsworth/Middlesex: Penguin Education.

Clandinin, D. J., & Connelly, F. M. (1995, April). *Storying and restoring ourselves: Narrative and reflection.* Paper presented at the Annual Meeting of the American Educational Research Association, San Francisco.

Clarke, H. F., & Mass, H. (1998). Comox Valley Nursing Centre: From collaboration to empowerment. *Public Health Nursing, 15*(3), 216-224.

Clemens, E., Wetle, T., Feltes, M., Crabtree, B., & Dubitzky, D. (1994). Contradictions in case management: Client-centered theory and directive practice. *Journal of Aging and Health, 6*(1), 70-88.

Code, L. (1995). *Rhetorical spaces: Essays on gendered locations.* New York: Routledge.

Cogswell, B., & Eggert, M. S. (1993). People want doctors to give more preventive care: A qualitative study of health care consumers. *Archives of Family Medicine, 2*(6), 611-619.

Cohen, M., Woodward, C. A., Ferrier, B., & Williams, A. P. (1995). Sanctions against sexual abuse of patients by doctors: Sex differences in attitudes among young family physicians. *Canadian Medical Association Journal, 153*(2), 169-176.

Colaizzi, P. (1978). Psychological research as the phenomonologist views it. In R. Vale & M. King (Eds.), *Existential-phenomonological alternatives for psychology* (pp. 48-71). New York: Oxford University Press.

Cornwell, J. (1984). *Hard-earned lives: Accounts of health and illness from East London.* New York: Tavistock.

Couser, G. T. (1997). *Recovering bodies: Illness, disability and life writing.* Madison: University of Wisconsin Press.

Coward, D. D. (1990). Critical multiplism: A research strategy for nursing science. *Image, 22,* 163-167.

Crabtree, B. F., Addison, M. W., Gilchrist, V. J., & Kuzel, A. (1994). *Exploring collaborative research in primary care.* Newbury Park, CA: Sage.

Crabtree, B. F., & Miller, W. L. (1991). A qualitative approach to primary care research: The long interview. *Family Medicine, 23*(2), 145-151.

Crabtree, B. F., Miller, W. L., Aita, V. A., Flocke, S. A., & Stange, K. C. (1998). Primary care practice organization and preventive services delivery: A qualitative analysis. *Journal of Family Practice, 46*(5), 403-409.

Craft, N. (1997). Women's health is a global issue. *British Medical Journal, 315,* 1154-1157.

Creswell, J. W. (1998). *Qualitative inquiry and research design: Choosing among five traditions.* Thousand Oaks, CA: Sage.

Curry, R. H., & Makoul, G. (1996). An active-learning approach to basic clinical skills. *Academic Medicine, 71,* 41-44.

Cushing, A. M., & Jones, A. (1995). Evaluation of a breaking bad news course for medical students. *Medical Education, 29,* 430-435.

Czarniawska, B. (1998). *A narrative approach to organizational studies* (Vol. 43). Thousand Oaks, CA: Sage.

Davis, K. (1988). *Power under the microscope.* Providence, RI: Foris.

Deegan, P. (1996). Recovery as a journey of the heart. *Psychiatric Rehabilitation Journal, 19*(3), 91-97.

Deegan, P. (1997). Recovery and empowerment for people with psychiatric disabilities. *Social Work Health Care, 25*(3), 11-24.

Del Mar, C., & Isaacs, G. (1992). Teaching consultation skills by videotaping interviews: A study of student opinion. *Medical Teaching, 14,* 53-58.

Deming, W. E. (1986). *Out of the crisis.* Boston, MA: MIT Center for Advanced Engineering.

Denzin, N. K. (1989a). *Interpretive biography.* Newbury Park, CA: Sage.

Denzin, N. K. (1989b). *Interpretive interactionism.* Newbury Park, CA: Sage.

Denzin, N. K. (1997). *Interpretive ethnography: Ethnographic practices for the 21st century.* Thousand Oaks, CA: Sage.

Denzin, N. K., & Lincoln, Y. S. (Eds.). (1994). *Handbook of qualitative research.* Newbury Park, CA: Sage.

Dewey, J. (1929). *The quest for certainty.* New York: Minton, Balch.

Dey, I. (1993). *Qualitative data analysis: A user-friendly guide for social scientists* (Vol. 1). London: Routledge.

Diamond, E. L., & Grauer, K. (1986). The physician's reaction to patients with chronic pain. *American Family Physician, 34,* 117-122.

Diers, D. (1979). *Research in nursing practice.* Philadelphia: J. B. Lippincott.

DiGiacomo, J. C., Hoff, W. S., Rotondo, M. F., Martin, K., Kauder, D. R., Anderson, H. L. III, Phillips, G. R. III, & Schwab, C. W. (1997). Barrier precautions in trauma resuscitation: Real-time analysis utilizing videotape review. *American Journal of Emergency Medicine, 15,* 34-39.

DiMatteo, M. R., Prince, L. M., & Hays, R. (1986a). Nonverbal communication in the medical context: The physician-patient relationship. In P. D. Blanck, R. Buck, & R. Rosenthal (Eds.), *Nonverbal communication in the clinical context* (pp. 74-98). University Park: Pennsylvania State University Press.

DiMatteo, M. R., Prince, L. M., & Hays, R. (1986b). Relationship of physicians' nonverbal communication skill to patient satisfaction, appointment noncompliance, and physician workload. *Health Psychology, 5,* 581-594.

DiMatteo, M. R., Taranta, A., Friedman, H., & Prince, L. M. (1980). Predicting patient satisfaction from physicians' nonverbal communication skills. *Medical Care, 18,* 376-387.

Dobbert, M. L. (1982). *Ethnographic research: Theory and application for modern schools and societies.* New York: Praeger.

Doblin, B. H., & Klamen, D. L. (1997). The ability of first-year medical students to correctly identify and directly respond to patients' observed behaviors. *Academic Medicine, 72,* 631-634.

Douglas, J. D. (1985). *Creative interviewing.* Beverly Hills, CA: Sage.

Douglas, M. (1982). *Natural symbols: Explorations in cosmology.* New York: Pantheon.

Dozor, R. B., & Addison, R. B. (1992). Toward a good death: An interpretive investigation of family practice residents' practices with dying patients. *Family Medicine, 24*(7), 538-543.

Dreyfus, H. L. (1986). Why studies of human capacities modeled on ideal natural science can never achieve their goal. In J. Margolis, M. Krausz, & R. M. Burian (Eds.), *Rationality, relativism and the human sciences* (pp. 3-22). Dordrecht, Holland: Martinus Nijhoff.

Dreyfus, H. L. (1991). *Being-in-the-world: A commentary on Heidegger's* Being and Time, *Division I.* Cambridge, MA: MIT Press.

Dreyfus, H. L., & Dreyfus, S. E. (1986). Putting computers in their place. *Social Research, 53,* 57-76.

Edwards, A., Tzelepis, A., Klingbeil, C., Melgar, T., Speece, M., Schubiner, H., & Burack, R. (1996). Fifteen years of a videotape review program for internal medicine and medicine-pediatrics residents [Letter to the editor]. *Academic Medicine, 71,* 744-748.

Edwards, D. (1997). *Discourse and cognition.* Thousand Oaks, CA: Sage.

Eibl-Eibesfeldt, I. (1989). *Human ethology.* New York: Aldine de Gruyter.

Elder, N. C., & Miller, W. L. (1995). Reading and evaluating qualitative research studies. *Journal of Family Practice, 41*(3), 279-285.

Elderkin-Thompson, V. (1996). Narrative and nonverbal communication of somatizing and nonsomatizing patients in a primary care setting. *Dissertation Abstracts International, 57,* 6568B.

Elderkin-Thompson, V., Silver, R. C., & Waitzkin, H. (1998a). Narratives of somatizing and non-somatizing patients in a primary care setting. *Journal of Health Psychology, 3,* 407-428.

Elderkin-Thompson, V., Silver, R. C., & Waitzkin, H. (1998b). *Nonverbal behavior of English and Spanish-speaking somatizing patients in a primary care setting.* Unpublished manuscript, University of California, Irvine.

Elderkin-Thompson, V., Silver, R. C., & Waitzkin, H. (1998c). *When nurses double as interpreters.* Unpublished manuscript, University of California, Irvine.

Elderkin-Thompson, V., & Waitzkin, H. (1991). Differences in clinical communication by gender: Are there diagnostic and treatment implications? *Journal of General Internal Medicine, 14,* 112-121.

Ellen, R. F. (1984). *Ethnographic research: A guide to general conduct.* New York: Academic Press.

Elliott, J. (1991). *Action research for educational change.* Milton Keynes, PA: Open University Press.

Ely, M., Anzul, M., Friedman, T., Garner, D., & Steinmetz, A. M. (1991). *Doing qualitative research: Circles within circles.* London: Palmer.

Emmel, N. D., & O'Keefe, P. (1996). Participatory analysis for redefining health delivery in a Bombay slum. *Journal of Public Health Medicine, 18*(3), 301-307.

Enelow, A. J., Adler, L. M., & Wexler, M. (1970). Programmed instruction in interviewing: An experiment in medical education. *Journal of the American Medical Association, 212,* 1843-1846.

Engelhardt, H. T., & Spicker, S. F. (Eds.). (1975). *Evaluation and explanation in the biomedical sciences: Proceedings of the First Trans-Disciplinary Symposium on Philosophy and Medicine held at Galveston May 9-11, 1974.* Boston: Reidel.

Epstein, R. M., Morse, D. S., Frankel, R. M., Frarey, L., Anderson, K., & Beckman, H. B. (1998). Awkward moments in patient-physician communication about HIV risk. *Annals of Internal Medicine, 128,* 435-442.

Erickson, F., & Shultz, J. (1982). *The counselor as gatekeeper.* New York: Academic.

Escobar, J., Rubio-Stipec, M., Canino, G., & Karno, M. (1989). Somatic symptom index (SSI): A new and abridged somatization construct: Prevalence and epidemiological correlates in two large community samples. *Journal of Nervous and Mental Diseases, 177,* 140-146.

Fagerhaugh, S. Y., & Strauss, A. (1977). *Politics of pain management: Staff-patient interaction.* Menlo Park, CA: Addison-Wesley.

Fahy, K. (1997). Postmodern feminist emancipatory research: Is it an oxymoron? *Nursing Inquiry, 4,* 27-33.

Fals-Borda, O., & Rahman, M. A. (Eds.). (1991). *Action and knowledge: Breaking the monopoly with participatory action research.* New York: Intermediate Technology/Apex.

Fardy, H. J., & Jeffs, D. (1994). Focus groups: A method for developing consensus guidelines in general practice. *Family Practice, 11*(3), 325-329.

Faulkner, A., Argent, J., Jones, A., & O'Keeffe, C. (1995). Improving the skills of doctors in giving distressing information. *Medical Education, 29,* 303-307.

Faust, J., & Melamed, B. G. (1984). Influence of arousal, previous experience, and age on surgery preparation of same day surgery and in-hospital pediatric patients. *Journal of Consulting and Clinical Psychology, 52,* 359-365.

Fay, B. (1987). *Critical social science*. Ithaca, NY: Cornell University Press.

Feltes, M., Clemens, E., Wetle, T., & Crabtree, B. (1994). Communication between physicians and case managers. *Journal of the American Geriatric Society, 42*, 5-10.

Fetterman, D. M. (1989). *Ethnography: Step-by-step*. Newbury Park, CA: Sage.

Fetterman, D. M. (1994). Steps of empowerment evaluation: From California to Cape Town. *Evaluation and Program Planning, 17*(3), 305-313.

Fetterman, D. M. (1998). *Ethnography* (2nd ed.). Thousand Oaks, CA: Sage.

Fetterman, D. M., Kaftarian, S. J., & Wandersman, A. (Eds.). (1996). *Empowerment evaluation*. Newbury Park, CA: Sage.

Fielding, N. G., & Lee, R. M. (Eds.). (1991). *Using computers in qualitative research*. Newbury Park, CA: Sage.

Fields, H. L. (1987). *Pain*. New York: McGraw-Hill.

Fine, M. (1992). *Disruptive voices: The possibilities of feminist research*. Ann Arbor: University of Michigan Press.

Fine, M., & Weis, L. (1996). Writing the "wrongs" of fieldwork: Confronting our own research/writing dilemmas in urban ethnographies. *Qualitative Inquiry, 2*, 251-274.

Fisher, S. (1984). Doctor-patient communication: A social and micro-political performance. *Sociology of Health and Illness, 6*, 1-29.

Fontana, A., & Frey, J. (1994). Interviewing: The art of science. In N. Denzin & Y. Lincoln (Eds.), *Handbook of qualitative research*. Newbury Park, CA: Sage.

Fossen, Ø. (1994). *Action research as reflective practice*. Doctoral thesis, University of Trondheim, Norwegian Institute of Technology.

Foster, P. (1989). Improving the doctor/patient relationship: A feminist perspective. *Journal of Social Policy, 18*, 337-361.

Foucault, M. (1984). Introduction. In P. Rabinow (Ed.), *The Foucault reader: An introduction to Foucault's thought*. New York: Pantheon.

Frank, A. (1995). *The wounded storyteller*. Chicago: University of Chicago Press.

Frank, A. (1998). Just listening: Narrative and deep illness. *Family, Systems & Health, 16*(3), 197-212.

Frank, A.J.M., Moll, J.M.H., & Hurt, J. F. (1982). A comparison of three ways of measuring pain. *Rheumatology and Rehabilitation, 21*, 211-217.

Frankel, R. (1984). From sentence to sequence: Understanding the medical encounter through micro-interactional analysis. *Discourse Processes, 7*, 135-170.

Frankel, R. M., & Beckman, H. B. (1982). IMPACT: An interaction based method for preserving and analyzing clinical transactions. In L. S. Pettegrew (Ed.), *Straight talk: Explorations in provider and patient interaction* (pp. 71-85). Nashville, TN: Humana.

Frankel, R. M., Leary, M., & Kilman, B. (1987). Building social skills through pragmatic analysis: Assess and treatment implications for children with autism. In D. Cohen & A. Donnellan (Eds.), *Handbook of autism and AT development*. New York: Wiley.

Frankel, R. M., Speice, J., Branca, L., Roter, D., Kornblith, A. B., Holland, J. C., Ahles, T., Winer, E., Fleishman, S., Luber, P., Zevon, M., McQuellon, R., Treif, P., Finkel, J., & Spira, J. (1997, April). Oncology providers' and patients' experiences with communication problems. Poster presented at the meeting of the American Society of Clinical Oncology, Denver, CO.

Frasier, P. Y., Slatt, L., Kowlowitz, V., Kollisch, D. O., & Mintzer, M. (1997). Focus groups: A useful tool for curriculum evaluation. *Family Medicine, 29*(7), 500-507.

Freemon, B., Negrete, V. F., Davis, M., & Korsch, B. M. (1971). Gaps in doctor-patient communications: Doctor-patient interaction analysis. *Pediatric Research, 5*, 298-311.

Freire, P. (1993). *Pedagogy of the oppressed*. London: Penguin.

Friedrichs, J., & Ludtke, H. (1974). *Participant observation: Theory and practice*. Westmead, UK: Saxon House.

Fuller, F. F., & Manning, B. A. (1973). Self-confrontation reviewed: A conceptualization for video playback in teacher education. *Review of Educational Research, 43,* 469-528.

Gadamer, H. G. (1976). *Philosophical hermeneutics.* Berkeley: University of California Press.

Garcia, B. (1997). Concepts and methods in teaching oppression courses. *Journal of Progressive Human Services, 8*(1), 23-40.

Garfinkel, H. (1967). *Studies in ethnomethodology.* Englewood Cliffs, NJ: Prentice Hall.

Garro, L. (1994). Narrative representations of chronic illness experience: Cultural models of illness, mind, and body in stories concerning the temporomandibular joint (TMJ). *Social Science and Medicine, 38*(6), 775-788.

Gee, J. (1985). The narrativization of experience in the oral style. *Journal of Education, 167,* 9-35.

Geer, B., Haas, J., ViVona, C., Miller, S., Woods, C., & Becker, H. (1968). Learning the ropes: Situational learning in four occupational training programs. In I. Deutscher & E. Thompson (Eds.), *Among the people: Encounters with the poor* (pp. 209-233). New York: Basic Books.

Geertz, C. (1973). *Interpretation of cultures.* New York: Basic Books.

Geertz, C. (1983). *Local knowledge: Further essays in interpretive anthropology.* New York: Basic Books.

Geertz, C. (1988). *Works and lives: The anthropologist as author.* Stanford, CA: Stanford University Press.

Gergen, K. J. (1986). Correspondence versus autonomy in the language of understanding human action. In D. W. Fiske & R. A. Shweder (Eds.), *Metatheory in social science.* Chicago: University of Chicago Press.

Gilchrist, V. J. (1992). Key informant interviews. In B. F. Crabtree & W. L. Miller (Eds.), *Doing qualitative research* (pp. 70-89). Newbury Park, CA: Sage.

Giorgi, A. (1970). *Psychology as a human science: A phenomonologically based approach.* New York: Harper & Row.

Girón, M., Manjón-Arce, P., Puerto-Barber, J., Sánches-García, E., & Gómez-Beneyto, M. (1998). Clinical interview skills and identification of emotional disorders in primary care. *American Journal of Psychiatry, 155,* 530-535.

Gladwin, C. H. (1989). *Ethnographic decision tree modeling.* Newbury Park, CA: Sage.

Glaser, B. (1978). *Theoretical sensitivity.* Mill Valley, CA: Sociology Press.

Glaser, B. (1992). *Basics of grounded theory analysis.* Mill Valley, CA: Sociology Press.

Glaser, B., & Strauss, A. L. (1967). *The discovery of grounded theory.* New York: Aldine.

Glasgow, R. E., La Chance, P. A., Toobert, D. J., Brown, J., Hampson, S. E., & Riddle, M. C. (1997). Long-term effects and cost of brief behavioural dietary intervention for patients with diabetes delivered from the medical office. *Patient Education and Counseling, 32,* 175-184.

Glasgow, R. E., Toobert, D. J., & Hampson, S. E. (1996). Effects of a brief office-based intervention to facilitate diabetes dietary self-management. *Diabetes Care, 19,* 835-842.

Gluckman, M. (Ed.). (1963). *Essays on the ritual of social relations.* Manchester, UK: Manchester University Press.

Goetz, J. P., & LeCompte, M. D. (1984). *Ethnography and qualitative design in educational research.* Orlando, FL: Academic Press.

Good, B. (1994). *Medicine, rationality and experience.* New York: Cambridge University Press.

Good, M. J. (1995). *American medicine: The quest for competence.* Berkeley: University of California Press.

Good, M. J. D. V., Munakata, T., Kobayashi, Y., Mattingly, C., & Good, B. (1994). Oncology and narrative time. *Social Science and Medicine, 38*(6), 775-788.

Goodman, N. (1984). *Of mind and other matters.* Cambridge, MA: Harvard University Press.

Goodwin, C. (1981). *Conversational organization: Interaction between speakers and hearers.* New York: Academic Press.

Gordon, D. R. (1988). Tenacious assumptions in Western medicine. In M. Lock & D. Gordon (Eds.), *Biomedicine examined* (pp. 19-56). Boston: Reidel.

Gordon, D. R., & Paci, E. (1995). Narrative and quality of life. In B. Spilker (Ed.), *Quality of life and pharmoeconomics in clinical trials* (2nd ed., pp. 387-395). New York: Raven.

Gordon, J. J., Saunders, N. A., Hennrikus, D., & Sanson-Fisher, R. W. (1992). Interns' performances with simulated patients at the beginning and the end of the intern year. *Journal of General Internal Medicine, 7,* 57-62.

Gordon, R. L. (1975). *Interviewing: Strategy, techniques and tactics.* Homewood, IL: Dorsey.

Gottlieb, M. (1986). *Interview.* New York: Longman.

Green, L., Hames, C. G., & Nutting, P. A. (1994). Potential of practice-based research networks: Experiences from ASPN. *Journal of Family Practice, 38,* 400-406.

Greenfield, S., Kaplan, S. H., Ware, J. E., Yano, E. M., & Frank, H.J.L. (1988). Patients' participation in medical care: Effects on blood sugar control and quality of life in diabetes. *Journal of General Internal Medicine, 3,* 448-457.

Gregor, S., & Galazka, S. S. (1990). The use of key informant networks in the assessment of community health. *Family Medicine, 22*(2), 118-121.

Guba, E. G. (1990). *The paradigm dialog.* Newbury Park, CA: Sage.

Guba, E. G., & Lincoln, Y. S. (1989). *Fourth generation evaluation.* Newbury Park, CA: Sage.

Gumperz, J. J., & Hymes, D. (Eds.). (1972). *Directions in sociolinguistics: The ethnography of communication.* New York: Holt, Rinehart & Winston.

Habermas, J. (1968). *Knowledge and human interests.* Boston: Beacon.

Habermas, J. (1977). A review of Gadamer's *Truth and Method.* In F. R. Dallmayr & T. A. McCarthy (Eds.), *Understanding and social inquiry.* Notre Dame, IN: University of Notre Dame Press.

Hall, E. T. (1974). *Handbook for proxemic research.* Washington, DC: Society for the Anthropology of Visual Communication.

Hall, J. A., Irish, J. T., Roter, D. L., Ehrlich, C. M., & Miller, L. H. (1994). Gender in medical encounters: An analysis of physician and patient communication in a primary care setting. *Health Psychology, 13,* 384-392.

Hall, J. A., Roter, D. L., Milburn, M. A., & Daltroy, L. H. (1996). Patients' health as a predictor of physician and patient behavior in medical visits: A synthesis of four studies. *Medical Care, 34,* 1205-1218.

Hamel, J., Dufour, S., & Fortin, D. (1993). *Case study method* (Vol. 32). Newbury Park, CA: Sage.

Hammersley, M. (1992). *What's wrong with ethnography? Methodological explorations.* London: Routledge.

Hammersley, M., & Atkinson, P. (1983). *Ethnography: Principles in practice.* New York: Tavistock.

Hardin, G. (1985). *Filters against folly.* New York: Penguin.

Harding, C. M., & Zahniser, J. H. (1994). Empirical correction of seven myths about schizophrenia with implications for treatment. *Acta Psychiatrica Scandinavica, 90*(Suppl. 384), 140-146.

Harrigan, J. A., & Rosenthal, R. (1986). Nonverbal aspects of empathy and rapport in physician-patient interaction. In R. D. Blanck, R. Buck, & R. Rosenthal (Eds.), *Nonverbal communication in the clinical context* (pp. 36-71). University Park: Pennsylvania State University Press.

Harris, M. (1966). The cultural ecology of India's sacred cattle. *Current Anthropology, 7,* 51-66.

Hawkins, A. H. (1993). *Reconstructing illness: Studies in pathography.* West Lafayette, IN: Purdue University Press.

Hecker, R. (1997). Participatory action research as a strategy for empowering aboriginal health workers. *Australian and New Zealand Journal of Public Health, 21*(7), 784-788.

Heidegger, M. (1962). *Being and time.* New York: Harper & Row. (Original work published 1927)

Helman, C. G. (1991). Research in primary care: The qualitative approach. In P. Norton, M. Stewart, F. Tudiver, M. Bass, & E. Dunn (Ed.), *Primary care research: Traditional and innovative approaches* (pp. 105-124). Newbury Park, CA: Sage.

Helseth, L., Susman, J., Crabtree, B., & O'Connor, P. (1999). Primary care physicians' perceptions of diabetes management: A balancing act. *Journal of Family Practice, 48*(1), 37-42.

Henderson, D. J. (1995). Consciousness raising in participatory research: Method and methodology for emancipatory nursing inquiry. *Advances in Nursing Science, 17*(3), 58-69.

Henley, N. (1977). *Body politics: Power, sex, and nonverbal communication.* Englewood Cliffs, NJ: Prentice Hall.

Herbert, C. P. (1996). Community-based research as a tool for empowerment: The Haida Gwaii diabetes project example. *Canadian Journal of Public Health, Revue Canadienne de Sante Publique, 87*(2), 109-112.

Heron, J. (1996). *Co-operative inquiry: Research into the human condition.* Newbury Park, CA: Sage.

Heron, J., & Reason, P. (1997). A participatory inquiry paradigm. *Qualitative Inquiry, 3,* 274-294.

Hibbard, H., Nutting, P. A., & Grady, M. (1991). *Primary care research: Theory and methods.* Washington, DC: U.S. Department of Health and Human Services, Public Health Service, Agency for Health Care Policy and Research.

Hickner, J. (1993). Practice-based network research. In M. Bass, E. Dunn, P. Norton, M. Stewart, & F. Tudiver (Eds.), *Conducting research in the practice setting* (Vol. 5, pp. 126-139). Newbury Park, CA: Sage.

Hilbert, R. A. (1984). The acultural dimensions of chronic pain: Flawed reality construction and the problem of meaning. *Social Problems, 31,* 365-378.

Hildebrandt, E. (1994). A model for community involvement in health (CIH) program development. *Social Science and Medicine, 39*(2), 247-254.

Holstein, J., & Gubrium, J. (1995). *The active interview.* Newbury Park, CA: Sage.

Houts, A., Cook, T., & Shadish, W. (1986). The person-situation debate: A critical multiplist perspective. *Journal of Personality, 54,* 53-107.

Huberman, A. M., & Miles, M. (1998). Data management and analysis methods. In N. Denzin & Y. Lincoln (Eds.), *Collecting and interpreting qualitative materials.* Thousand Oaks, CA: Sage.

Huberman, A. M., & Miles, M. B. (1994). Data management and analysis methods. In N. K. Denzin & Y. S. Lincoln (Eds.), *Handbook of qualitative research* (pp. 428-444). Newbury Park, CA: Sage.

Hunt, L. (1994). Practicing oncology in provincial Mexico: A narrative analysis. *Social Science and Medicine, 38*(6), 843-853.

Hunter, K. M. (1991). *Doctors' stories.* Princeton, NJ: Princeton University Press.

Hursh, D. (1997). Critical, collaborative action research in politically contested times. In S. Hollingsworth (Ed.), *International action research: A casebook for educational reform* (pp. 124-134). London: Falmer.

Husserl, E. (1931). *Ideas: A general introduction to pure phenomenology.* New York: Humanities.

Inui, T. S., & Frankel, R. M. (1991). Evaluating the quality of qualitative research. *Journal of General Internal Medicine, 6*(5), 485-486.

Irish, J., & Hall, J. (1995). Interruptive patterns in medical visits: The effects of role, status and gender. *Social Science and Medicine, 41,* 873-881.

Ivey, A. E. (1971). *Microcounseling: Innovations in interviewing training.* Springfield, IL: Charles C Thomas.

Jackson, L., & Yuan, L. (1997). Family physicians managing tuberculosis: Qualitative study of overcoming barriers. *Canadian Family Physician, 43,* 649-655.

Jaeger, R. M. (1988). *Complementary methods for research in education.* Washington, DC: American Educational Research Association.

Johnson, J. D. (1990). *Selecting ethnographic informants.* Newbury Park, CA: Sage.

Jones, A. H. (1997). Literature and medicine: Narrative ethics. *Lancet, 349,* 1243-1246.

Jorgensen, D. L. (1989). *Participant observation: A methodology for human studies.* Newbury Park, CA: Sage.

Junek, W., Burra, P., & Leichner, P. (1979). Teaching interviewing skills by encountering patients. *Journal of Medical Education, 54,* 402-407.

Junker, B. H. (1960). *Field work: An introduction to the social sciences.* Chicago: University of Chicago Press.

Kahn, G., Cohen, B., & Jason, H. (1979). The teaching of interpersonal skills in the US medical schools. *Journal of Medical Education, 54,* 29-35.

Kaufman, S. (1993). *The healer's tale.* Madison: University of Wisconsin Press.

Kaufman, S. (1997). Construction and practice of medical responsibility: Dilemmas and narratives from geriatrics. *Culture, Medicine, and Psychiatry, 21,* 1-26.

Kelley, H. H. (1967). Attribution theory in social psychology. In D. Levine (Ed.), *Nebraska symposium on motivation.* Lincoln: University of Nebraska Press.

Kemmis, S., & McTaggart, R. (Eds.). (1988). *The action research planner.* Geelong, Australia: Deakin University Press.

Kendall, S., & Tannen, D. (1997). Gender and language in the workplace. In R. Wodak (Ed.), *Gender and discourse* (pp. 81-106). Thousand Oaks, CA: Sage.

Kiecolt-Glaser, J. K., & Glaser, R. (1985). Behavioral influences on immune function: Evidence for the interplay between stress and health. In T. Field, P. McCabe, & N. Schneiderman (Eds.), *Stress and coping across development* (Vol. 2, pp. 189-205). Hillsdale, NJ: Lawrence Erlbaum.

Klafta, J. M., & Roizen, M. F. (1996). Current understanding of patients' attitudes toward and preparation for anesthesia: A review. *Anesthesia and Analgesia, 83,* 1314-1321.

Kleinman, A. (1980). *Patients and healers in the context of culture: An exploration of the borderland between anthropology, medicine and psychiatry.* Berkeley: University of California Press.

Kleinman, A. (1983). The cultural meanings of social uses of illness. *Journal of Family Practice, 16,* 539-545.

Kleinman, A. (1988). *The illness narratives.* New York: Basic Books.

Kleinman, A., & Good, B. (Eds.). (1985). *Culture and depression: Studies in the anthropology and cross-cultural psychiatry of affect and disorder.* Berkeley: University of California Press.

Koch, T. (1995). Interpretive approaches in nursing research: The influence of Husserl and Heidegger. *Journal of Advanced Nursing, 21,* 827-836.

Konner, M. (1987). *Becoming a doctor: A journey of initiation in medical school.* New York: Viking Penguin.

Korsch, B. M., Freemon, B., & Negrete, V. F. (1971). Practical implications of doctor-patient interaction: Analysis for pediatric practice. *American Journal of Diseases of Children, 121,* 110-114.

Korsch, B. M., Gozzi, E. K., & Francis, V. (1968). Gaps in doctor-patient communication: Doctor-patient interaction and patient satisfaction. *Pediatrics, 42,* 885-871.

Korsnes, O., Andersen, A., & Brate, T. (1997). *Sosiologisk leksikon* (Sociological lexicon). Oslo: Universitetsforlaget.

Koss, T., & Rosenthal, R. (1997). Interactional synchrony, positivity, and patient satisfaction in the physician-patient relationship. *Medical Care, 35,* 1158-1163.

Kotarba, J., & Seidel, J. (1984). Managing the problem pain patient: Compliance or social control. *Social Science and Medicine, 19,* 1393-1400.

Kotarba, J. A. (1983). *Chronic pain: Its social dimensions.* Newbury Park, CA: Sage.

Krueger, R. (1998). *Focus group kit: Moderating focus groups* (Vol. 3). Thousand Oaks, CA: Sage.

Kuhn, T. S. (1962). *The structure of scientific revolutions.* Chicago: University of Chicago Press.

Kuzel, A. J. (1986). Naturalistic inquiry: An appropriate model for family medicine. *Family Medicine, 18*(6), 369-374.

Kuzel, A. J. (1990). Qualitative and quantitative research: The discussion continues. *Family Medicine, 22*(4), 254-256.

Kuzel, A. J. (1992). Sampling in qualitative inquiry. In B. F. Crabtree & W. L. Miller (Eds.), *Doing qualitative research* (pp. 31-44). Newbury Park, CA: Sage.

Kuzel, A. J., Engel, J. D., Addison, R. B., & Bogdewic, S. (1994). Desirable features of qualitative research. *Family Practice Research Journal, 14*(4), 369-378.

Kuzel, A. J., & Like, R. C. (1991). Standards of trustworthiness for qualitative studies in primary care. In P. Norton, M. Stewart, F. Tudiver, M. Bass, & E. Dunn (Eds.), *Primary care research: Traditional and innovative approaches* (pp. 138-158). Newbury Park, CA: Sage.

Kvale, S. (1996). *InterViews: An introduction to qualitative research interviewing.* Newbury Park, CA: Sage.

Labov, W., & Waletsky, J. (1967). Narrative analysis: Oral versions of personal experience. In J. Helm (Ed.), *Essays on the verbal and visual arts: Proceedings of the 1966 annual spring meeting of the American Ethnological Society* (pp. 12-44). Seattle: University of Washington Press.

Last, J. M. (1983). *A dictionary of epidemiology.* New York: Oxford University Press.

Lather, P. (1986). Research as praxis. *Harvard Educational Review, 56*(3), 257-277.

Lather, P. (1988). Feminist perspectives on empowering research methodologies. *Women's Studies International Forum, 11,* 569-581.

Lather, P. (1991). *Getting smart: Feminist research and pedagogy with/in the postmodern.* New York: Routledge.

Lather, P., & Smithies, C. (1997). *Troubling angels: Women living with HIV/AIDS.* Boulder, CO: Westview.

Lavelle-Jones, C., Byrne, D. J., Rice, P., & Cushieri, H. (1993). Factors affecting quality of informed consent. *British Medical Journal, 306,* 885-890.

Levinson, W. (1993). Reflections: Mining for gold. *Journal of General Internal Medicine, 8,* 172.

Levinson, W., Dull, V. T., Roter, D. L., Chaumeton, N., & Frankel, R. M. (1998). Recruiting physicians for office-based research. *Medical Care, 36,* 934-937.

Levinson, W., Roter, D. L., Mullooly, J. P., Dull, V. T., & Frankel, R. M. (1997). Physician-patient communication: The relationship with malpractice claims among primary care physicians and surgeons. *Journal of the American Medical Association, 277,* 553-559.

Levi-Strauss, C. (1963). *Structural anthropology.* New York: Basic Books.

Levy, R. I., & Hollan, D. W. (1998). Person-centered interviewing and observation. In N. R. Bernard (Ed.), *Handbook of methods in cultural anthropology.* Walnut Creek, CA: Alta Mira.

Lewin, K. (1948). *Resolving social conflicts.* New York: Harper.

Li, L. B., Williams, S. D., & Scammon, D. L. (1995). Practicing with the urban underserved. A qualitative analysis of motivations, incentives, and disincentives. *Archives of Family Medicine, 4*(2), 124-133.

Liaw, S. T., Litt, J., & Radford, A. (1992). Patient perceptions of continuity of care: Is there a socioeconomic factor? *Family Practice, 9*(1), 9-14.

Lieberman, L., Meana, M., & Stewart, D. (1998). Cardiac rehabilitation: Gender differences in factors influencing participation. *Journal of Women's Health, 7*(6), 717-723.

Light, R., & Pillemer, D. (1982). Numbers and narrative: Combining their strengths in research reviews. *Harvard Educational Review, 52,* 1-23.

Lin, N. (1976). *Foundations of social research.* New York: McGraw-Hill.

Lincoln, Y. S., & Guba, E. G. (1985). *Naturalistic inquiry.* Newbury Park, CA: Sage.

Lindemann, E. C. (1924). *Social discovery.* New York: Republic.

Lindqvist, K., Timpka, T., & Schelp, L. (1996). Ten years of experiences from a participatory community-based injury prevention program in Motala, Sweden. *Public Health, 110*(6), 339-346.

Lofland, J., & Lofland, L. H. (1995). *Analysing social settings: A guide to qualitative observation and analysis* (3rd ed.). Belmont, CA: Wadsworth.

Lofland, J. G., & Lofland, L. H. (1984). *Analyzing social settings.* Belmont, CA: Wadsworth.

Lorenz, K. (1966). *On aggression.* London: Methuen.

LoVerde, M. E., Prochazka, A. V., & Byyny, R. L. (1989). Research consent forms: Continued unreadability and increasing length. *Journal of General Internal Medicine, 4,* 410-412.

Macaulay, A., Gibson, N., Commanda, L., McCabe, M., Robbins, C., & Twohig, P. (1998). Responsible research with communities: Participatory research in primary care. In press, *British Medical Journal.* Sponsored by North American Primary Care Research Group. Retrieved April 22, 1999 from the World Wide Web: http://views.vcu.edu/views/fap/napcrg98/exec.html

Mackenzie, C. F., Jefferies, N. J., Hunter, W. A., Bernhard, W. M., & Xiao, Y. (1996). Comparison of self-reporting of deficiencies in airway management with video analyses of actual performance. *Human Factors, 38,* 623-635.

Maguire, P. (1996). Considering more feminist participatory research: What's congruency got to do with it? *Qualitative Inquiry, 2,* 106-118.

Malatesta, C. Z., & Culver, C. (1992). Gendered health: Differences between men and women in the relation between physical symptoms and emotion expression behavior. In H. C. Traue & J. W. Pennebaker (Eds.), *Emotion, inhibition and health* (pp. 116-144). Seattle, WA: Hogrefe & Huber.

Malekoff, A., Johnson, H., & Klappersack, B. (1991). Parent-professional collaboration on behalf of children with learning disabilities. *Families in Society, 72*(7), 416-424.

Malinowski, B. (1961). *Argonauts of the western Pacific.* New York: Dutton.

Malterud, K. (1987). Illness and disease in female patients. I. Pitfalls and inadequacies of primary health care classification systems—A theoretical review. *Scandinavian Journal of Primary Health Care, 5,* 205-209.

Malterud, K. (1992). Women's "undefined" disorders: A challenge for clinical communication. *Family Practice, 9,* 299-303.

Malterud, K. (1993a). Shared understanding of the qualitative research process: Guidelines for the medical researcher. *Family Practice, 10,* 201-206.

Malterud, K. (1993b). Strategies for empowering women's voices in the medical culture. *Health Care for Women International, 14,* 365-373.

Malterud, K. (1994). Key questions—A strategy for modifying clinical communication: Transforming tacit skills into a clinical method. *Scandinavian Journal of Primary Health Care, 12,* 121-127.

Malterud, K. (1995a). Action research: A strategy for evaluation of medical interventions. *Family Practice, 12,* 476-481.

Malterud, K. (1995b). The legitimacy of clinical knowledge: Towards a medical epistemology embracing the art of medicine. *Theoretical Medicine, 16,* 183-198.

Malterud, K. (1996). *Kvalitative metoder I medisinsk forskning: en innføring* (Qualitative methods in medical research: An introduction). Oslo: TANO.

Malterud, K., Baerheim, A., Hunskaar, S., & Meland, E. (1997). Focus groups as a path to clinical knowledge about the acutely and severely ill child. *Scandinavian Journal of Primary Health Care, 15*(1), 26-29.

Malterud, K., & Hollnagel, H. (1997). Women's self-assessed personal health resources. *Scandinavian Journal of Primary Health Care, 15,* 163-168.

Malterud, K., & Hollnagel, H. (1998). Talking with women about personal health resources in general practice: Key questions and salutogenesis. *Scandinavian Journal of Primary Health Care, 16,* 66-71.

Malterud, K., & Kristiansen, U. (1995). The reflective metapositions of evaluation: A strategy for development of collaborative competence and clinical knowledge. *Family Systems Medicine, 13,* 79-89.

Malterud, K., & Thesen, J. (1994). Evalueringsverksted: Virkemiddelfor kunnskapsproduksjon I et aksjonsforskningsprosjekt (Evaluation workshop: Tool for knowledge production in an action research project). In A. Gulbrandsen (Ed.). *Universitetspedagogisk utviklingsarbeid i Bergen* (Developing university pedagogical work in Bergen) (pp. 85-105). Bergen: University of Bergen.

Manning, P., & Cullum-Swan, B. (1994). Narrative, content and semiotic analysis. In N. Denzin & Y. Lincoln (Eds.), *Handbook of qualitative research* (pp. 463-477). Newbury Park, CA: Sage.

Manning, P. K. (1987). *Semiotics and fieldwork.* Newbury Park, CA: Sage.

Marchand, L., & Morrow, M. H. (1994). Infant feeding practices: Understanding the decision-making process. *Family Medicine, 26*(5), 319-324.

Marmoreo, J., Brown, J. B., Batty, H. R., Cummings, S., & Powell, M. (1998). Hormone replacement therapy: Determinants of women's decisions. *Patient Education and Counseling, 33,* 289-298.

Marshall, C., & Rossman, G. (1995). *Designing qualitative research* (2nd ed.). Newbury Park, CA: Sage.

Marshall, C., & Rossman, G. (1998). *Designing qualitative research* (3rd ed.). Thousand Oaks, CA: Sage.

Marshall, C., & Rossman, G. B. (1989). *Designing qualitative research.* Newbury Park, CA: Sage.

Marshall, M. N. (1996). Sampling for qualitative research. *Family Practice, 13*(6), 522-525.

Marshall, W. R., Rothenberger, L. A., & Bunnell, S. (1984). The efficacy of personalized audiovisual patient-education materials. *Journal of Family Practice, 19,* 659-663.

Marvel, M. K., Staehling, S., & Hendricks, B. (1991). A taxonomy of clinical research methods: Comparisons of family practice and general medical journals. *Family Medicine, 23*(3), 202-207.

Maslow, A. (1968). *Toward a psychology of being.* New York: Van Nostrand.

Mason, J. (1996). *Qualitative researching.* Newbury Park, CA: Sage.

Mathews, H. F., Lannin, D. R., & Mitchell, J. P. (1994). Coming to terms with advanced breast cancer: Black women's narratives from eastern North Carolina. *Social Science and Medicine, 38*(6), 789-800.

Mattingly, C. (1994). The concept of therapeutic emplotment. *Social Science and Medicine, 38*(6), 811-822.

Mattingly, C. (1998). In search of the good: Narrative reasoning in clinical practice. *Medical Anthropology Quarterly, 12*(3), 273-297.

Mausner, J. S., & Kramer, S. (1985). *Epidemiology: An introductory book* (2nd ed.). Philadelphia: W. B. Saunders.

Maxwell, J. (1996). *Qualitative research design.* Newbury Park, CA: Sage.

Mayfield, J., & Grady, M. (1990). *Primary care research: An agenda for the 90's.* Washington, DC: U.S. Department of Health and Human Services, Public Health Service, Agency for Health Care Policy and Research.

Mays, N., & Pope, C. (1995a). Observational methods in health care settings. *British Medical Journal, 311,* 182-184.

Mays, N., & Pope, C. (1995b). Rigour and qualitative research. *British Medical Journal, 311,* 109-112.

McCarthy, T. (1978). *The critical theory of Jurgen Habermas.* Cambridge, MA: MIT Press.

McCracken, G. (1988). *The long interview.* Newbury Park, CA: Sage.

McCue, K. (1980). Preparing children for medical procedures. In J. Kellerman (Ed.), *Psychological aspects of childhood cancer* (pp. 238-260). Springfield, IL: Charles C Thomas.

McGoldrick, M., & Gerson, R. (1985). *Genogram in family assessment.* New York: W. W. Norton.

McGuire, C. H. (1985). Medical problem-solving: A critique of the literature. *Journal of Medical Education, 60,* 587-595.

McIlvain, H., Crabtree, B., Medder, J., Stange, K. C., & Miller, W. L. (1998). Using practice genograms to understand and describe practice configurations. *Family Medicine, 30*(7), 490-496.

McIlvain, H. E., Crabtree, B. F., Gilbert, C., Havranek, R., & Backer, E. L. (1997). Current trends in tobacco prevention and cessation in Nebraska physicians' offices. *Journal of Family Practice, 44*(2), 193-202.

McKibbin, E. C., & Castle, P. J. (1996). Nurses in action: An introduction to action research in nursing. *Curationis, 19*(4), 35-39.

McLaughlin, M. L. (1984). *Conversation: How talk is organized.* Beverly Hills, CA: Sage.

McTaggart, R. (1997). Guiding principles for participatory action research. In R. McTaggart (Ed.), *Participatory action research: International contexts and consequences* (pp. 25-43). Albany: State University of New York Press.

McVea, K., Crabtree, B. F., Medder, J. D., Susman, J. L., Lukas, L., McIlvain, H. E., Davis, C. M., Gilbert, C. S., & Hawver, M. (1996). An ounce of prevention? Evaluation of the 'put prevention into practice' program. *Journal of Family Practice, 43*(4), 361-369.

McWhinney, I. (1989). An acquaintance with particulars. *Family Medicine, 21*(4), 296-298.

McWhinney, I. R. (1991). Primary care research in the next twenty years. In P. Norton, M. Stewart, F. Tudiver, M. Bass, & E. Dunn (Eds.), *Primary care research: Traditional and innovative approaches.* Newbury Park, CA: Sage.

Mead, G. H. (1934). *Mind, self and society: From the standpoint of a social behaviorist.* Chicago: University of Chicago Press.

Mead, G. H. (1934). *Mind, self and society: From the standpoint of a social behaviorist.* Chicago: University of Chicago Press.

Mehan, H., & Wood, H. (1975). *The reality of ethnomethodology.* New York: Wiley.

Melamed, B., & Seigel, L. (1975). Reduction of anxiety in children facing hospitalization and surgery by use of filmed modeling. *Journal of Consulting and Clinical Psychology, 43,* 511-521.

Melamed, B. G., Yurcheson, R., Fleece, E. L., Hutcherson, S., & Hawes, R. (1978). Effects of film modeling on the reduction of anxiety-related behaviors in individuals varying in level of previous experience in the stress situation. *Journal of Consulting and Clinical Psychology, 46,* 1357-1367.

Mellor, J., & Chambers, N. (1995). Addressing the patient's agenda in the reorganization of antenatal and infant health care: Experience in one general practice. *British Journal of General Practice, 45*(397), 423-425.

Melzack, R. (1975). The McGill pain questionnaire: Major properties and scoring methods. *Pain, 1*(3), 277-299.

Merriam, S. B. (1988). *Case study research in education.* San Francisco: Jossey-Bass.

Merriam, S. B. (1998). *Qualitative research and case study applications in education: Revised and expanded from case study research in education.* San Francisco: Jossey-Bass.

Merton, R. K., Fiske, M., & Kendall, P. L. (1956). *The focused interview: A manual of problems and procedures.* Glencoe, IL: Free Press.

Merton, R. K., & Kendall, P. (1946). The focused interview. *American Journal of Sociology, 51,* 541-557.

Mettee, T. M., Martin, K. B., & Williams, R. L. (1998). Tools for community-oriented primary care: A process for linking practice and community data. *Journal of American Board of Family Practice, 11,* 28-33.

Mies, M. (1983). Towards a methodology for feminist research. In G. Bowles & R. D. Klein (Eds.), *Theories of women's studies* (pp. 117-139). Boston: Routledge & Kegan Paul.

Miles, M. B., & Huberman, A. M. (1984). *Qualitative data analysis: A sourcebook of new methods.* Beverly Hills, CA: Sage.

Miles, M. B., & Huberman, A. M. (1994). *Qualitative data analysis: An expanded sourcebook* (2nd ed.). Newbury Park, CA: Sage.

Milgram, S. (1963). Behavioral study of obedience. *Journal of Abnormal Social Psychology, 67,* 371-378.

Milgram, S. (1965). Some conditions of obedience and disobedience to authority. *Human Relations, 18*(1), 57-76.

Miller, W. L. (1992). Routine, ceremony, or drama: An exploratory field study of the primary care clinical encounter. *Journal of Family Practice, 34*(3), 289-296.

Miller, W. L., & Crabtree, B. F. (1990). Start with the stories. *Family Medicine Research Updates, 9,* 2-3.

Miller, W. L., & Crabtree, B. F. (1992). Primary care research: A multimethod typology and qualitative roadmap. In B. F. Crabtree & W. L. Miller (Eds.), *Doing qualitative research* (1st ed., pp. 3-28). Newbury Park, CA: Sage.

Miller, W. L., & Crabtree, B. F. (1994a). Clinical research. In N. Denzin & Y. Lincoln (Eds.), *Handbook of qualitative research* (pp. 340-352). Newbury Park, CA: Sage.

Miller, W. L., & Crabtree, B. F. (1994b). Qualitative analysis: How to begin making sense. *Family Practice Research Journal, 14*(3), 289-297.

Miller, W. L., Crabtree, B. F., McDaniel, R., & Stange, K. C. (1998). Understanding change in primary care practice using complexity theory. *Journal of Family Practice, 46*(5), 369-376.

Miller, W. L., Yanoshik, M. K., Crabtree, B. F., & Reymond, W. K. (1994). Patients, family physicians, and pain: Visions from interview narratives. *Family Medicine, 26*(3), 179-184.

Mishler, E. G. (1984). *The discourse of medicine: Dialectics of medical interviews.* Norwood, NJ: Ablex.

Mishler, E. G. (1986). *Research interviewing.* Cambridge, MA: Harvard University Press.

Mishler, E. G. (1990). Validation in inquiry-guided research: The role of exemplars in narrative studies. *Harvard Education Review, 60,* 415-442.

Mishler, E. G., Clark, J. A., Ingelfinger, J., & Simon, M. P. (1989). The language of attentive patient care: A comparison of two medical interviews. *Journal of General Internal Medicine, 4*(4), 325-335.

Moerman, M. (1988). *Talking culture: Ethnography and conversation analysis.* Philadelphia: University of Pennsylvania Press.

Moldofsky, H., Broder, I., Davies, G., & Leznoff, A. (1979). Videotape educational program for people with asthma. *Canadian Medical Association Journal, 120,* 669-672.

Monnickendam, S. M., Borkan, J. M., Matalon, A., & Zalewski, S. (1996). Trials and tribulations of country doctors: A qualitative study of doctor-patient relationships in rural Israel. *Israel Journal of Medical Science, 32*(3-4), 239-245.

Morgan, D. (1988). *Focus groups as qualitative research.* Newbury Park, CA: Sage.

Morgan, D. L. (1992a). Designing focus groups research. In M. Stewart, F. Tudiver, M. J. Bass, E. V. Dunn, & P. G. Norton (Eds.), *Tools for primary care research* (pp. 205-230). Newbury Park, CA: Sage.

Morgan, D. L. (1992b). Doctor-caregiver relationships: An exploration using focus groups. In B. F. Crabtree & W. L. Miller (Eds.), *Doing qualitative research* (pp. 205-230). Newbury Park, CA: Sage.

Morgan, D. L. (1993). Qualitative content analysis: A guide to paths not taken. *Qualitative Health Research, 3*(1), 112-121.

Morgan, D. L. (1998a). *Focus group kit: The focus group guidebook* (Vol. 1). Thousand Oaks, CA: Sage.

Morgan, D. L. (1998b). *Focus group kit: Planning focus groups* (Vol. 2). Thousand Oaks, CA: Sage.

Morgan, D. L., & Krueger, R. A. (1998). *The focus group kit.* Thousand Oaks, CA: Sage.

Morse, J. M. (1995). The significance of saturation. *Qualitative Health Research, 5*(2), 147-149.

Mostyn, B. (1985). The content analysis of qualitative research data: A dynamic approach. In M. Brenner, J. Brown, & D. Canter (Eds.), *The research interview: Uses and approaches* (pp. 115-145). New York: Academic.

Moustakas, C. (1990). *Heuristic research: Design, methodology and applications.* Newbury Park, CA: Sage.

Mumford, E. (1970). *Interns: From students to physicians.* Cambridge, MA: Harvard University Press.

Murdock, G. P., Ford, C. S., & Hudson, A. E., et al. (1950). *Outline of cultural materials.* (3rd ed.). New Haven, CT: Human Relations Area Files.

Naber, S. J., Halstead, L. K., Broome, M. E., & Rehwaldt, M. (1995). Communication and control: Parent, child, and health care professional interactions during painful procedures. *Issues in Comprehensive Pediatric Nursing, 18,* 79-90.

Nathanson, C. (1975). Illness and the feminine role: A theoretical review. *Social Science and Medicine, 9,* 57-62.

National Advisory Mental Health Council. (1985). Emotion and motivation. Basic behavioral science research for mental health: A national investment. *American Psychologist, 50,* 838-845.

Nutting, P. A. (1987). *Community-oriented primary care: From principals to practice.* Washington, DC: U.S. Government Printing Office.

Nutting, P. A., & Green, L. A. (1994). Practice-based research networks: Reuniting practice and research around the problems most of the people have most of the time. *Journal of Family Practice, 38,* 335-336.

Oakley, A. (1980). *Becoming a mother.* New York: Schocken.

Oakley, A. (1981). Interviewing women: A contradiction in terms. In H. Roberts (Ed.), *Doing feminist research* (pp. 30-61). Boston, MA: Routledge & Kegan Paul.

O'Connor, P. J. (1990). Normative data: Their definition, interpretation, and importance for primary care physicians. *Family Medicine, 22,* 307-311.

O'Connor, P. J., Crabtree, B. F., & Yanoshik, M. K. (1997). Differences between diabetic patients who do and do not respond to a diabetes care intervention: A qualitative analysis. *Family Medicine, 29*(6), 424-428.

Oiler, C. (1982). The phenomenological approach in nursing research. *Nursing Research, 31*(3), 178-181.

Ornstein, S. M., Musham, C., Reid, A. O., Garr, D. R., Jenkins, R. G., & Zemp, L. D. (1994). Improving a preventive services reminder system using feedback from focus groups. *Archives of Family Medicine, 3*(9), 801-806.

Orwell, G. (1946). *Animal farm.* New York: Harcourt Brace.

Pace, P. W., Henske, J. C., Whitfill, B. J., Andrews, S. M., Russell, M. L., Probstfield, J. L., & Insull, W. Jr. (1983). Videocassette use in diet instructions. *Journal of the American Dietetic Association, 83,* 166-169.

Packer, M. J., & Addison, R. B. (1989). *Entering the circle: Hermeneutic investigation in psychology.* Albany: State University of New York Press.

Padilla, G. V., Grant, M. M., Rains, B. L., Hansen, B. C., Bergstrom, N., Wong, H. L., Hanson, R., & Kubo, W. (1981). Distress reduction and the effects of preparatory teaching films and patient control. *Research in Nursing and Health, 4,* 375-387.

Palmer, R. E. (1969). *Hermeneutics: Interpretation theory in Schleiermacher, Dilthey, Heidegger, and Gadamer.* Evanston, IL: Northwestern University Press.

Pangaro, L. M., Worth-Dickstein, H., Macmillan, M. K., Klass, D. J., & Shatzer, J. H. (1997). Performance of "standardized examinees" in a standardized-patient examination of clinical skills. *Academic Medicine, 72,* 1008-1011.

Parker, E. A., Schultz, A. J., Israel, B. A., & Hollis, R. (1998). Detroit's east side village health worker partnership: Community based lay health advisor intervention in an urban area. *Health Education and Behavior, 25*(1), 24-45.

Parrish, J. M., & Babbitt, R. L. (1991). Video-mediated instruction in medical settings. In P. W. Dowrick (Ed.), *Practical guide to using video in the behavioral sciences* (pp. 166-185). New York: Wiley.

Patterson, J. L. (1983). *Nonverbal behavior: A functional perspective.* New York: Springer-Verlag.

Patton, M. Q. (1980). *Qualitative evaluation methods.* Beverly Hills, CA: Sage.

Patton, M. Q. (1987). *How to use qualitative methods in evaluation.* Beverly Hills, CA: Sage.

Patton, M. Q. (1990). *Qualitative evaluation and research methods* (2nd ed.). Newbury Park, CA: Sage.

Peacock, J. L. (1986). *The anthropological lens: Harsh light, soft focus.* Cambridge, UK: Cambridge University Press.

Pelto, P. J., & Pelto, G. H. (1978). *Anthropological research: The structure of inquiry* (2nd ed.). New York: Cambridge University Press.

Penayo, U., Jacobson, L., Caldera, T., & Burmann, G. (1988). Community attitudes and awareness of mental health disorders: A key informant study in two Nicaraguan towns. *ACTA Psychiatrica Scandinavica, 78,* 561-566.

Pennebaker, J. W., & Traue, H. C. (1992). Inhibition and psychosomatic processes. In H. C. Traue & J. W. Pennebaker (Eds.), *Emotion, inhibition and health* (pp. 145-163). Seattle, WA: Hogrefe & Huber.

Perry, S. W. (1985). Irrational attitudes towards addicts and narcotics. *Bulletin of the New York Academy of Medicine, 61,* 706-723.

Peterson, L., Schultheis, K., Ridley-Johnson, R., Miller, D. J., & Tracy, K. (1984). Comparison of three modeling procedures on the presurgical and postsurgical reactions of children. *Behavior Therapy, 15,* 197-203.

Plavin, M. H. (1988). Effects of presurgical preparation on anxiety of children and their mothers: Support versus information. *Dissertation Abstracts International, 49,* 223A-224A.

Polanyi, M. (1983). *The tacit dimension.* Gloucester, MA: Peter Smith.

Pommerenke, F. A., & Dietrich, A. J. (1992a). Improving and maintaining preventive services. Part 1: Applying the patient model. *Journal of Family Practice, 34*(1), 86-91.

Pommerenke, F. A., & Dietrich, A. J. (1992b). Improving and maintaining preventive services. Part 2: Practical principles for primary care. *Journal of Family Practice, 34*(1), 92-97.

Poses, R. M., & Isen, A. M. (1998). Qualitative research in medicine and health care: Questions and controversy. *Journal of General Internal Medicine, 13,* 32-38.

Potter, J. (1996). *Representing reality: Discourse, rhetoric and social construction.* Newbury Park, CA: Sage.

Preston, R. (1994). *The hot zone.* New York: Random House.

Pringle, M., & Stewart-Evans, C. (1990). Does awareness of being video recorded affect doctors' consultation behavior? *British Journal of General Practice, 40,* 455-458.

Punch, M. (1994). Politics and ethics in qualitative research. In N. Denzin & Y. Lincoln (Eds.), *Handbook of qualitative research.* Newbury Park, CA: Sage.

Quill, T. E. (1991). Death and dignity: A case study of individualized decision making. *New England Journal of Medicine, 324*(10), 691-694.

Quirk, M., & Babineau, R. (1982). Teaching interviewing skills to students in clinical years: A comparative analysis of three strategies. *Journal of Medical Education, 57,* 939-941.

Rabinow, P., & Sullivan, W. M. (Eds.). (1979). *Interpretive social science: A reader.* Berkeley: University of California Press.

Rains, J. W., & Ray, D. W. (1995). Participatory action research for community health promotion. *Public Health Nursing, 12*(4), 256-261.

Reason, P. (1994). Three approaches to participative inquiry. In N. K. Denzin & Y. S. Lincoln (Eds.), *Handbook of qualitative research.* Newbury Park, CA: Sage.

Redman, S., Dickinson, J. A., Cockburn, J., Hennrikus, D., & Sanson-Fisher, R. W. (1989). The assessment of reactivity in direct observations of doctor-patient interactions. *Psychology and Health, 3,* 17-25.

Redman, S., Webb, G., Hennrikus, D., Gordon, J., & Sanson-Fisher, R. (1991). The effects of gender on diagnosis of psychological disturbance. *Journal of Behavioral Medicine, 14,* 527-539.

Reilly, D. (1995). Research homeopathy, and therapeutic consultation. *Alternative Therapies in Health and Medicine, 1*(4), 64-73.

Remen, R. N. (1996). *Kitchen table wisdom.* New York: Riverhead.

Rich, J. A., & Stone, D. A. (1996). The experience of violent injury for young African-American men: The meaning of being a "sucker." *Journal of General Internal Medicine, 11*(2), 77-82.

Richards, L., & Richards, T. (1994a). From filing cabinet to computer. In R. W. Burgess & A. Bryman (Eds.), *Analyzing qualitative data*. London: Routledge.

Richards, L., & Richards, T. (1994b). Using computers in qualitative analysis. In N. K. Denizen & Y. S. Lincoln (Eds.), *Handbook of qualitative research* (pp. 445-462). Newbury Park, CA: Sage.

Richardson, M. (1990). *Writing strategies: Reaching diverse audiences*. Newbury Park, CA: Sage.

Richardson, M. (1997). Participatory research methods: People with learning difficulties. *British Journal of Nursing, 6*(19), 1114-1121.

Ricoeur, P. (1979). The model of the text: Meaningful action considered as a text. In P. Rabinow & W. M. Sullivan (Eds.), *Interpretive social science: A reader* (pp. 73-101). Berkeley: University of California Press.

Ricoeur, P. (1981). *Hermeneutics and the human sciences*. Cambridge, UK: Cambridge University Press.

Ricoeur, P. (1984). *Time and narrative* (Vol. 1). Chicago: University of Chicago Press.

Ricoeur, P. (1991). The human experience of time and narrative. In M. Valdes (Ed.), *A Ricoeur reader: Reflections and imagination* (pp. 98-116). Toronto: University of Toronto Press.

Riessman, C. T. (1993). *Narrative analysis*. Newbury Park, CA: Sage.

Rigg, J. (1979). Five things not to do when making patient videotapes. *Health Care Education, 8*, 22-24.

Robling, M., Kinnersley, P., Houston, H., Hourihan, M., Cohen, D. & Hale, J. (1998). An exploration of GP's use of MRI: A critical incident study. *Family Practice, 15*, 236-243.

Roche, A. M., Guray, C., & Saunders, J. B. (1991). General practitioners' experiences of patients with drug and alcohol problems. *British Journal of Addiction, 86*(3), 263-267.

Rodriguez, M. A., Quiroga, S. S., & Bauer, H. M. (1996). Breaking the silence: Battered women's perspectives on medical care. *Archives of Family Medicine, 5*(3), 153-158.

Rogers, C. (1961). *On becoming a person*. London: Constable.

Rosaldo, R. (1989). *Culture and truth*. Boston: Beacon.

Rosenhahn, D. L. (1973). On being sane in insane places. *Science, 179*, 250-258.

Rosenthal, R., & Jacobson, E. (1968). *Pygmalion in the classroom: Teacher expectation and intellectual development*. New York: Holt, Reinhart and Winston.

Roter, D., Lipkin, M., & Korsgaard, A. (1991). Sex differences in patients' and physicians' communication during primary care medical visits. *Medical Care, 29*, 1083-1093.

Roter, D. L. (1977). Patient participation in the patient-provider interaction: The effects of patient question asking on the quality of interaction, satisfaction and compliance. *Health Education Monographs, 5*, 281-315.

Roter, D. L., Cole, D. A., Kern, D. E., Barker, L. R., & Grayson, M. (1990). An evaluation of residency training in interviewing skills and the psychosocial domain of medical practice. *Journal of General Internal Medicine, 5*, 347-354.

Roter, D. L., Hall, J. A., & Katz, N. R. (1987). Relations between physicians' behaviors and analogue patients' satisfaction, recall, and impressions. *Medical Care, 25*, 437-451.

Roter, D. L., Hall, J. A., Kern, D. E., Barker, L. R., Cole, D. A., & Roca, R. P. (1995). Improving physicians' interviewing skills and reducing patients' emotional distress. *Archives of Internal Medicine, 155*, 1877-1884.

Roter, D. L., Stewart, M., Pubnam, S. M., Lipkin, M. Jr., Stiles, W., & Inui, T. S. (1997). Communication patterns of primary care physicians. *Journal of the American Medical Association, 277*, 350-356.

Rubenstein, R. (1995). Narratives of elder parental death: A structural and cultural analysis. *Medical Anthropology Quarterly, 9*(2), 257-276.

Rubin, H. J., & Rubin, I. S. (1995). *Qualitative interviewing: The art of hearing data.* Newbury Park, CA: Sage.

Ryan, G., Martinez, H., & Pelto, G. (1996). Methodological issues for eliciting local signs/symptoms/illness terms associated with acute respiratory illnesses. *Archives of Medical Research, 27,* 359-365.

Ryan, S. (1995). Learning communities: An alternative to the "expert" model. In S. Chawla & J. Renesch (Eds.), *Learning organizations.* Portland, OR: Productivity.

Sacks, H., Schegloff, E. A., & Jefferson, G. (1974). A systematics for organization of turntaking for conversation. *Language, 50,* 696-735.

Sanjek, R. (Ed.). (1990). *Fieldnotes: The makings of anthropology.* Ithaca, NY: Cornell University Press.

Schattner, P., Shmerling, A., & Murphy, B. (1993). Focus groups: A useful research method in general practice. *Medical Journal of Australia, 158*(9), 622-625.

Schatzman, L., & Strauss, A. L. (1973). *Field research: Strategies for a natural sociology.* Englewood Cliffs, NJ: Prentice Hall.

Schön, D. (1991). *The reflective practitioner: How professionals think in action.* London: Avebury.

Schurman, S. J. (1996). Making the "new American workplace" safe and healthy: A joint labor-management-researcher approach. *American Journal of Industrial Medicine, 29,* 373-377.

Schutz, A. (1967). *Collected papers* (Vol. 1). The Hague: Martinus Nijhoff.

Schwandt, T. (1994). Constructivist, interpretivist approaches to human inquiry. In N. Denzin & Y. Lincoln (Eds.), *Handbook of qualitative research.* Newbury Park, CA: Sage.

Schwartz, W. B. (1998). *Life without disease: The pursuit of medical utopia.* Riverside, CA: University of California Press.

Searle, J. R. (1995). *The construction of social reality.* New York: Free Press.

Seidel, J. V., Kjolseth, R., & Seymour, E. (1988). *THE ETHNOGRAPH: A user's guide* (Version 3.0). Littleton, CO: Qualis Research Associates.

Senge, P. M. (1990). *The fifth discipline.* New York: Currency Doubleday.

Sessions, G. (Ed.). (1995). *Deep ecology for the 21st century.* Boston: Shambhala.

Shafer, A., & Fish, M. P. (1994). A call for narrative: The patient's story and anesthesia training. *Literature and Medicine, 13*(1), 124-142.

Shaffir, W. B., Stebbins, R. A., & Turowetz, A. (1980). *Fieldwork experience.* New York: St. Martin's.

Shapiro, J. (1993). The use of narrative in the doctor-patient encounter. *Family Systems Medicine, 11*(1), 47-53.

Shields, V. R., & Dervin, B. (1993). Sense-making in feminist social science research: A call to enlarge the methodological options of feminist studies. *Women's Studies in International Forum, 16,* 65-81.

Silverman, D. (1993). *Interpreting qualitative data. Methods for analyzing talk, text and interaction.* Newbury Park, CA: Sage.

Singer, M. (1989). The coming of age of critical medical anthropology. *Social Science and Medicine, 28,* 1193-1203.

Singer, M. (1990). Reinventing medical anthropology: Toward a critical realignment. *Social Science and Medicine, 30*(2), 179-187.

Singer, M. (1994). AIDS and the health crisis of the U.S. urban poor: The perspective of critical medical anthropology. *Social Science and Medicine, 39*(7), 931-948.

Skagestad, P. (1981). *The road of inquiry: Charles Peirce's pragmatic realism.* New York: Columbia University Press.

Sleath, B., Svarstad, B., & Roter, D. (1997). Physician vs patient initiation of psychotropic prescribing in primary care settings: A content analysis of audiotapes. *Social Science and Medicine, 44,* 541-548.

SME. (1990, September). *Tilgjengelighet til tjenester for personer med store psykiske lidelser: Bakgrunnsdokument for forsoksordninger i 6 kommuner/fylker* [Accessibility to services for persons with serious mental illness: Background document for demonstration projects in 6 municipalities/counties] (SME nr 1/59). Sosialdepartementet, SME.

Smith, A., & Kleinman, S. (1989). Managing emotions in medical school: Student's contacts with the living and the dead. *Social Psychology Quarterly, 52,* 56-69.

Smith, J. L., Crabtree, B. F., Davis, C. D., Hawver, M., Falk, R., & Paulman, A. (1996). Nebraska family physician approaches to mammograms. *Nebraska Medical Journal, 81*(3), 58-62.

Sommers, P. S., Muller, J. H., Saba, J. W., Draisin, J. A., & Shore, W. B. (1994). Reflections-on-action: Medical students' accounts of their implicit beliefs and strategies in the context of one-to-one clinical teaching. *Academic Medicine, 10*(Suppl. 69), S84-S86.

Spaniol, L., Gagne, C., & Koehler, M. (Eds.). (1997). *Psychological and social aspects of psychiatric disability.* Boston, MA: Center for Psychiatric Rehabilitation.

Spitzer, R. L., Williams, J.B.W., Kroenke, K., Linzer, M., deGruy, F. V. III, Hahn, S. R., Brody, D., & Johnson, J. G. (1994). Utility of a new procedure of diagnosing mental disorders in primary care: The PRIME-MD study. *Journal of the American Medical Association, 272,* 1749-1756.

Spradley, J. P. (1979). *The ethnographic interview.* New York: Holt, Reinhart and Winston.

Spradley, J. P. (1980). *Participant observation.* New York: Holt, Reinhart, & Winston.

Stacey, J. (1988). Can there be a feminist ethnography? *Women's Studies International Forum, 11,* 21-27.

Stake, R. E. (1995). *The art of case study research* (1st ed., Vol. 1). Newbury Park, CA: Sage.

Stange, K. C. (1993). Practice-based research networks: Their current level of validity, generalizability, and potential for wider application. *Archives of Family Medicine, 2,* 921-923.

Stange, K. C. (1996). Primary care research: Barriers and opportunities. *Journal of Family Practice, 42,* 192-198.

Stange, K. C., Miller, W., Crabtree, B. F., O'Connor, P. J., & Zyzanski, S. J. (1994). Multimethod research: Approaches for integrating qualitative and quantitative methods. *Journal of General Internal Medicine, 9*(5), 278-282.

Stange, K. C., Zyzanski, S. J., Jaen, C. R., Callahan, E. J., Kelly, R. B., Gillanders, W. R., Shank, C., Chao, J., Medalie, J. H., Miller, W. L., Crabtree, B. F., Flocke, S. A., Gilchrist, V. J., Langa, D. M., & Goodwin, M. A. (1998). Illuminating the 'black box': A description of 4454 patient visits to 138 family physicians. *Journal of Family Practice, 46*(5), 377-389.

Stange, K. C., Zyzanski, S. J., Smith, T. F., Kelly, R., Langa, D. M., Flocke, S. A., & Jaen, C. R. (1998). How valid are medical records and patient questionnaires for physician profiling and health services research? A comparison with direct observation of patients' visits. *Medical Care, 36*(6), 851-867.

Stein, H. F. (1990). Bridging the gap via context: An ethnographic clinical-training model. In H. F. Stein & M. Apprey (Eds.), *Clinical stories and their translations* (pp. 149-175). Charlottesville: Altheide.

Stein, H. F. (1994). *Listening deeply.* Westview.

Stevens, P. E., & Tighe Doerr, B. (1997). Trauma of discovery: Women's narratives of being informed they are HIV-infected. *AIDS Care, 9*(5), 523-538.

Stewart, D., & Shamdasani, P. (1990). *Focus groups: Theory and practice*. Newbury Park, CA: Sage.

Stewart, M., Brown, J. B., Weston, W. W., McWhinney, I., McWilliam, C., & Freeman, T. (1995). *Patient-centered medicine: Transforming the clinical method*. Newbury Park, CA: Sage.

Stone, E., & Priestley, M. (1996). Parasites, pawns and partners: Disability research and the role of non-disabled researchers. *British Journal of Sociology, 47*(4), 699-716.

Strauss, A., & Corbin, J. (1990). *Basics of qualitative research: Grounded theory procedures and techniques*. Newbury Park, CA: Sage.

Strauss, A. L. (1987). *Qualitative analysis for social scientists*. Cambridge, MA: Cambridge University Press.

Street, A. (1995). *Nursing replay: Researching nursing culture together*. Melbourne, Australia: Churchill Livingstone.

Street, R. L., Jr. (1990). The communicative functions of parlanguage and prosody. In H. Giles & W. Robinson (Eds.), *Handbook of language and social psychology* (pp. 121-140). New York: Wiley.

Street, R. L., Jr., & Buller, D. B. (1987). Nonverbal response patterns in physician-patient interactions: A functional analysis. *Journal of Nonverbal Behavior, 11*, 234-253.

Street, R. L., Jr., Mulack, A., & Weimann, J. M. (1988). Speech evaluation differences as a function of perspective (participant versus observer) and presentational medium. *Human Communication Research, 14*, 333-363.

Stringer, E. T. (1996). *Action research: A handbook for practitioners*. Newbury Park, CA: Sage.

Stubbs, M. (1983). *Discourse analysis: The sociolinguistic analysis of natural language*. Chicago: University of Chicago Press.

Susman, J. L., Crabtree, B. F., & Essink, G. (1995). Depression in rural family practice: Easy to recognize, difficult to diagnose. *Archives of Family Medicine, 4*(5), 427-431.

Taba, H., Brady, E., & Robinson, J. (1952). *Intergroup education in public schools*. Washington, DC: American Council on Education.

Tang, K. C., Davis, A., Sullivan, S., & Fisher, J. (1995). A review of 5 existing guidelines for planning focus groups in GP research. *Australian Family Physician, 24*(2), 184-186.

Tannen, D. (1990). Gender differences in conversational coherence: Physical alignment and topical cohesion. In B. Dorval (Ed.), *Conversational organization and its development: Advances in discourse processes* (pp. 167-206). Norwood, NJ: Ablex.

Temple-Smith, M., Hammond, J., Pyett, P., & Presswell, N. (1996). Barriers to sexual history taking in general practice. *Australian Family Physician, 25*(9, Suppl. 2), S71-S74.

Tesch, R. (1989). Computer software and qualitative analysis: A reassessment. In G. Blank, McCartney, J. L., & Brent, E. (Eds.), *New technology in sociology: Practical applications in research and work* (pp. 141-154). New Brunswick, NJ: Transaction.

Tesch, R. (1990). *Qualitative research: Analysis types and software tools*. New York: Falmer.

Thesen, J. (1994). *Samhandlingsprosjektet: Sluttrapport 1991-1994* (Final report 1991-1994: The collaboration project). Bergen: University of Bergen. Retrieved April 23, 1999 from the World Wide Web: http://www.uib.no/isf/people/samhandl/httoc.htm

Thom, D. H., & Campbell, B. (1997). Patient-physician trust: An exploratory study. *Journal of Family Practice, 44*(2), 169-176.

Thomas, J. (1983). The Chicago school. *Urban Life, 11*(special issue), 908-944.

Thorne, S. E. (1997). Phenomenological positivism and other problematic trends in health science research. *Qualitative Health Research, 7*, 287-293.

Thornton, C. (1996). A focus group inquiry into the perceptions of primary health care teams and the provision of health care for adults with a learning disability living in the community. *Journal of Advanced Nursing, 23*(6), 1168-1176.

Thrower, S. M., Bruce, W. E., & Walton, R. F. (1982). The family circle method for integrating family systems concepts in family medicine. *Journal of Family Practice, 15,* 451-457.

Tickle-Degnen, L., & Rosenthal, R. (1990). The nature of rapport and its nonverbal correlates. *Psychological Inquiry, 1,* 285-290.

Tierney, W. G., & Lincoln, Y. S. (Eds.). (1997). *Representation and the text: Re-framing the narrative voice.* Albany: State University of New York Press.

Tinbergen, N. (1951). *The study of instinct.* London: Oxford University Press.

Torbert, W. R. (1991). *The power of balance: Transforming self, society, and scientific inquiry.* Newbury Park, CA: Sage.

Trautmann, J. (Ed.). (1982). *The healing arts: Literature and medicine.* Carbondale: Southern Illinois University Press.

Travers, K. D. (1996). The social organization of nutritional inequities. *Social Science and Medicine, 43*(4), 543-553.

Travers, K. D. (1997). Reducing inequities through participatory research and community empowerment. *Health Education and Behavior, 24*(3), 344-356.

Traylen, H. (1994). Confronting hidden agendas: Co-operative inquiry with health visitors. In P. Reason (Ed.), *Participation in human inquiry.* Newbury Park, CA: Sage.

Traynor, M. (1997). Postmodern research: No grounding or privilege, just free-floating trouble making. *Nursing Inquiry, 4,* 99-107.

Tudiver, F., Cushman, R. A., & Crabtree, B. F. (1991). Combining quantitative and qualitative methodologies in primary care: Some examples. In P. Norton, M. Stewart, F. Tudiver, M. Bass, & E. Dunn (Eds.), *Primary care research: Traditional and innovative approaches.* Newbury Park, CA: Sage.

Turner, V. W. (1969). *The ritual process: Structure and anti-structure.* Chicago: Aldine.

Twardosz, S., Weddle, K., Borden, L., & Stevens, E. (1986). A comparison of three methods of preparing children for surgery. *Behavior Therapy, 16,* 14-25.

van den Hoonaard, W. (1996). *Working with sensitizing concepts.* Newbury Park, CA: Sage.

Van Dijk, T. A. (Ed.). (1985). *Handtools of discourse analysis* (Vol. 4). London: Academic Press.

Van Kaam, A. L. (1969). *Existential foundations of psychology.* New York: Doubleday.

Van Mannen, J. (Ed.). (1979). *Qualitative methodology.* Beverly Hills, CA: Sage.

van Wijk, C.M.T.G., Kolk, A. M., van den Bosch, W.J.H.M., & van den Hoogen, H.J.M. (1992). Male and female morbidity in general practice: The nature of sex differences. *Social Science and Medicine, 35,* 665-678.

Ventres, W. B. (1994). Hearing the patient's story: Exploring physician-patient communication using narrative case reports. *Family Practice Research Journal, 14*(2), 139-147.

Vernon, D. T. (1974). Modeling and birth order in response to painful stimuli. *Journal of Personality and Social Psychology, 29,* 794-799.

Vernon, D. T., & Bailey, W. C. (1974). The use of motion pictures in the psychological preparation of children for induction of anesthesia. *Anesthesiology, 40,* 68-72.

Vidich, A., & Lyman, S. (1994). Qualitative methods: Their history in sociology and anthropology. In N. K. Denzin & Y. S. Lincoln (Eds.) *Handbook of qualitative research* (pp. 23-59). Thousand Oaks, CA: Sage.

Wagstaff, L., Schreier, A., Shuenyane, F., & Ahmed, N. (1990). Televised paediatric consultations: A student evaluation of a multipurpose learning strategy. *Medical Education, 24,* 244-251.

Waitzkin, H. (1979). Medicine, superstructure and micropolitics. *Social Science and Medicine, 13A*, 601-609.

Waitzkin, H. (1990). On studying the discourse of medical encounters: A critique of quantitative and qualitative methods and a proposal for reasonable compromise. *Medical Care, 28*, 473-488.

Waitzkin, H. (1991). *The politics of medical encounters: How patients and doctors deal with social problems.* New Haven, CT: Yale University Press.

Waitzkin, H., & Silver, R. C. (1992). *Somatization in refugees and others seeking primary care* (NIMH Grant #1 RO1 47536). Washington, DC: Agency for Health Care Policy and Research, National Institute of Mental Health.

Wallen, J., Waitzkin, H., & Stoeckle, J. D. (1979). Physician stereotypes about female health and illness: A study of patients' sex and the informative process during medical interviews. *Women & Health, 4*, 135-146.

Ward, J. D., Garlant, J. F., Paterson, G., Bone, V., & Hicks, B. H. (1984). Video cassette programmes in diabetes education. *Diabetes Educator, 10*, 48-50.

Watson, L. C., & Watson-Franke, M. B. (1985). *Interpreting life histories: An anthropological inquiry.* New Brunswick, NJ: Rutgers University Press.

Weber, M. (1968). *Economy and society.* New York: Bedminster.

Weber, R. P. (1985). *Basic content analysis.* Beverly Hills, CA: Sage.

Weick, K. (1993). The collapse of sensemaking in organizations: The Mann Gulch disaster. *Administrative Science Quarterly, 38*(4), 628-652.

Weitzman, E. A., & Miles, M. B. (1995). *Computer programs for qualitative data analysis.* Newbury Park, CA: Sage.

Weller, S. C., & Romney, K. A. (1988). *Systematic data collection.* Newbury Park, CA: Sage.

Werner, O., & Schoepfle, G. M. (1987a). *Systematic fieldwork: Ethnographic analysis and data management.* Newbury Park, CA: Sage.

Werner, O., & Schoepfle, G. M. (1987b). *Systematic fieldwork: Foundations of ethnography and interviewing.* Newbury Park, CA: Sage.

West, C. (1984). *Routine complications: Troubles with talk between doctors and patients.* Bloomington: Indiana University Press.

White, H. (1987). *The content of the form: Narrative discourse and historical representation.* Baltimore, MD: Johns Hopkins University Press.

White, L. (1959). *The evolution of culture.* New York: McGraw-Hill.

Whitmore, E. (1994). To tell the truth: Working with oppressed groups in participatory approaches to inquiry. In P. Reason (Ed.), *Participation in human inquiry* (pp. 82-98). Newbury Park, CA: Sage.

Whyte, W. F. (1984). *Learning from the field: A guide from experience.* Beverly Hills, CA: Sage.

Widdershoven-Heerding, I. (1987). Medicine as a form of practical understanding. *Theoretical Medicine, 8*, 179-185.

Widdicombe, S. (1995). Identity, politics and talk: A case for the mundane and everyday. In S. Wilkinson & C. Kitzinger (Eds.), *Feminism and discourse.* Newbury Park, CA: Sage.

Willems, E. P., & Rausch, H. L. (1969). *Naturalistic viewpoints in psychological research.* New York: Holt, Rinehart & Winston.

Williams, G. H., & Wood, P.H.N. (1986). Common-sense beliefs about illness: A mediating role for the doctor. *Lancet, 2*(8521-8522), 1435-1437.

Williams, R. L., Snider, R., Ryan, M. J., & the Cleveland COPC Group. (1994). A key informant "tree" as a tool for community-oriented primary care. *Family Practice Research Journal, 14*(3), 273-280.

Willms, D. G., Best, J. A., Taylor, D. W., Gilbert, J. R., Wilson, D. M. C., & Singer, J. (1990). A systematic approach for using qualitative methods in primary prevention research. *Medical Anthropology Quarterly, 4*(4), 391-409.

Willms, D. G., & Stebbins, K. R. (1991). Anthropology of smoking. *Social Science and Medicine, 33*(12), 1315-1316.

Wilson, A. (1991). Consultation length in general practice: A review. *British Journal of General Practice, 4,* 119-122.

Wilson, D. G., Allan, B. J., Wilon, D.M.C., Gilbert, J. R., Taylor, D. W., Lindsay, E., Singer, J., & Johnson, N. A. (1991). Patients' perspectives of a physician-delivered smoking cessation intervention. *American Journal of Preventive Medicine, 7*(2), 95-100.

Wilson, D. M., Taylor, D. W., Gilbert, J. R., Best, J. A., Lindsay, E. A., Willms, D. G., & Singer, J. (1988). A randomized trial of a family physician intervention for smoking cessation. *Journal of the American Medical Association, 260*(11), 1570-1574.

Winter, R. (1989). *Learning from experience: Principles and practice in action-research.* London: Falmer.

Wissow, L. S., Roter, D. L., & Wilson, M. E. (1994). Pediatrician interview style and mothers' disclosure of psychosocial issues. *Pediatrics, 93,* 289-295.

Wolcott, H. F. (1990). *Writing up qualitative research.* Newbury Park, CA: Sage.

Wolcott, H. F. (1995). *The art of fieldwork.* Walnut Creek, CA: Alta Mira.

Wood, M. L. (1993). Communication between cancer specialists and family doctors. *Canadian Family Physician, 39,* 49-57.

Yin, R. K. (1989). *Case study research: Design and methods* (2nd ed., Vol. 5). Newbury Park: Sage.

Yin, R. K. (1993). *Applications of case study research* (Vol. 34). Newbury Park, CA: Sage.

Yin, R. K. (1994). *Case study research: Design and methods* (2nd ed.). Newbury Park, CA: Sage.

Index

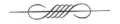

391

About the Editors

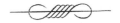

BENJAMIN F. CRABTREE, PhD, is Professor and Director of Research, Department of Family Medicine, University of Nebraska Medical Center, where he is also a medical anthropologist. He has written and contributed to numerous articles and chapters on both qualitative and quantitative methods, covering topics ranging from time series analysis and log-linear models to in-depth interviews, case study research, and qualitative analysis strategies. He is Coeditor of *Exploring Collaborative Research in Primary Care.*

WILLIAM L. MILLER, MD, MA, is Chair and Program Director, Department of Family Medicine, Lehigh Valley Hospital, Allentown, Pennsylvania; he is also a family physician anthropologist. He is active in an effort to make qualitative research more accessible to health care researchers. He has written and contributed to book chapters and articles detailing step-by-step applications of qualitative methods, including the chapter on clinical research in *The Handbook of Qualitative Research,* which he wrote. His research interests center on the role of the patient-physician relationship in health care, on physician and patient understanding of pain and pain management, and on hypertension. In his current work, he is using case study designs to model primary care practices as nonlinear complex adaptive systems.

About the Contributors

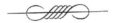

RICHARD B. ADDISON, PhD, is Associate Clinical Professor in the Department of Family and Community Medicine, University of California, San Francisco, School of Medicine, and a faculty member of the Family Practice Residency Program, Sutter Medical Center, Santa Rosa, California. He maintains an independent clinical practice as a licensed psychologist specializing in seeing physicians and their spouses. He is also a consultant for health care professionals, medical groups, and community health centers on local, national and international levels. He has coedited two books: *Entering the Circle: Hermeneutic Investigation in Psychology,* an anthology of exemplary hermeneutic research, and *Exploring Collaborative Research in Primary Care,* a book describing conjoint qualitative and quantitative approaches in primary care research. His other published research includes his work on meaning in medicine, personal and professional development groups for physicians, the professional socialization of family physicians, physician stress and impairment, physician vulnerability, marital stress among physicians and their spouses, support services for resident physicians, how physicians deal with dying patients, and qualitative research strategies.

VIRGINIA A. AITA, RN, PhD, is Assistant Professor, Department of Family Medicine, University of Nebraska Medical Center. In the past, she has worked as a public health nurse and in nursing education. Her more recent work has been in the areas of medical ethics and history. Her current research focuses on the qualitative aspects of preventive health services delivery in primary care. Her interest in quality of care also extends into the realm of clinical ethics consultation and teaching medical students and residents.

STEPHEN P. BOGDEWIC, PhD, is Associate Professor and Vice-Chair, Department of Family Medicine, Indiana University. His research interests include the culture of organizations, professional socialization, and faculty development. His publications have appeared in such journals as *Academic Medicine, Family Medicine,* and *Health Care Management Review.*

JEFFREY BORKAN, MD, PhD, is Director of Research in the Department of Family Medicine at Ben-Gurion University of the Negev and a medical anthropologist and family physician. He divides his professional time between clinical family practice in a remote desert area of southern Israel, research, writing, and teaching. For many years, he coordinated the RAMBAM Israeli Family Practice Research Network, which he helped to found. He has conducted numerous qualitative and mixed qualitative-quantitative studies on a variety of topics in primary care, from low back pain, hip fracture, and alternative medicine to rural physician "burn-out." He lives on a kibbutz with his wife, Suzanne, a clinical social worker and dairy woman, and his three children, Ariela, Noa, and Aidan.

JUDITH BELLE BROWN, PhD, is Associate Professor, Centre for Studies in Family Medicine, Department of Family Medicine, University of Western Ontario and School of Social Work, King's College, London, Ontario, Canada. She conducts research in the areas of patient-doctor communication, physician well-being, physician practice behavior (obstetrics, palliative care, clinical practice guidelines, cancer care), empowerment of the chronically ill elderly, the influence of culture on health, and women abuse. She uses both quantitative and qualitative methods in her research, and the focus group technique has been a key component in over 10 of her many research projects. She has presented papers and conducted workshops both nationally and internationally (Canada, United States, United Kingdom, Holland, Spain, Hong King, Sweden, New Zealand) on many of her research interests but most specifically on the patient-centered clinical method. She coauthored the book *Patient-Centered Medicine: Transforming the Clinical Method.* She was made an Honorary Member of the College of Family Physicians of Canada in 1996.

LUCY M. CANDIB, MD, is Professor of Family Medicine and Community Health at the University of Massachusetts Medical School. She is a family physician who has taught and practiced family medicine, including obstetrics, in an urban neighborhood health center in Worcester, Massachusetts, for over 20 years. She has focused attention on the concerns of women trainees and practitioners in her work with family practice residents and has lectured widely on the topics of sexual abuse and violence against women. She has introduced a feminist critique of medical theory in numerous articles and in her book *Medicine and the Family: A Feminist Perspective* (1995).

DIANE M. DODENDORF, PhD, is Project Coordinator, Research Division, Department of Family Medicine, University of Nebraska Medical Center. She was the central researcher on an intervention study (prevention) with several practices and is Principal Investigator on another intervention study that focuses on women's health and prevention. She has worked in family medicine education and research for 15 years; her interests are organizational and computer tools, women's health, and qualitative research design and data.

VIRGINIA ELDERKIN-THOMPSON, PhD, is a postdoctoral scholar at the University of California, Irvine, investigating the effects of stress and adaptation on individuals' cognitive and behavioral resources. She recently completed a study of the behavior and narratives of somatizing, depressed, and traumatized patients who presented at a primary care clinic for the purpose of analyzing the verbal and nonverbal communicative deficits associated with the emotional disorders. This effort resulted in several manuscripts that are in various stages of publication. Following the study, she analyzed the stress perceived by patients living in a community that had been exposed to several hazardous waste products to understand the community's distrust of an environmental health clinic and its physician staff, who were evaluating the health effects on the community. Currently, she is developing research projects within the Institute on Brain Aging and Dementia to study the cognitive and behavioral effects that accompany the onset of different forms of dementia and the preventive or compensatory measures used by patients to minimize their cognitive and social losses.

RICHARD M. FRANKEL, PhD, is Professor of Medicine, University of Rochester School of Medicine and Dentistry, and Director, Primary Care Institute, University of Rochester. In addition, he is Co-Director, University of Rochester Program for Biopsychosocial Studies. He has been a postdoctoral fellow in qualitative approaches to mental health research at Boston University, and in 1986, he was a Fulbright Senior Research Fellow in social medicine and communication studies at the University of Uppsala, Sweden. He has also held visiting professorships in Holland, Great Britain, Finland, Norway, Canada, and the United States. He has lectured and published extensively on face-to-face communication in a number of contexts and recently participated in a multiyear research project funded by the Agency for Health Care Policy Research exploring communication aspects of medical malpractice. He is the recipient of the American Academy on Physician and Patients' 1999-2000 Prize for contributions to research on physician/patient communication.

VALERIE J. GILCHRIST, MD, is Professor and Chair, Department of Family Medicine, Northeastern Ohio Universities of Medicine. She completed a teaching fellowship at the University of North Carolina, Chapel Hill from 1982 to 1983. She is also active in practice and is Associate Program Director, Aultman Hospital Family Practice Residency Program. Her areas of publication and research interest include qualitative methodology, practice-based research networks, prevention, and women's health care.

ANTON J. KUZEL, MD, is Vice Chairman and Coordinator of Graduate Programs, Department of Family Practice, Medical College of Virginia campus, Virginia Commonwealth University, Richmond. His interest in qualitative research began during graduate studies with John Engel at the Center for Educational Development of the University of Illinois, and he has grown through continuing collaboration with many of the authors of this volume, particularly William Miller and Benjamin Crabtree.

WENDY LEVINSON, MD, is Professor of Medicine and Chief of General Internal Medicine, University of Chicago. Prior to joining the University of Chicago, she was Assistant Chief of Medicine, Good Samaritan Hospital, and Professor of Medicine, Oregon Health Sciences University, Portland. She was a Robert Wood Johnson Clinical Scholar at McGill University, Montreal and is now Director, Robert Wood Johnson Clinical Scholars Program, University of Chicago. She specializes in primary care and does research in physician-patient communication. She is Principal Investigator of a study for the Agency for Health Care Policy and Research (AHCPR) that is investigating the relationship between physician communication behaviors and malpractice history. She is a nationally acclaimed trainer and expert in physician-patient communication and has also conducted programs on this topic in Canada, Japan, and Great Britain. She has published widely in the professional, peer-reviewed literature on communication as well as on training programs in medical education, women in medicine, and other health issues.

KIRSTI MALTERUD, MD, PhD, is Professor of Family Medicine, Department of Public Health and Primary Health Care, University of Bergen, Norway. She works half-time as a family physician and also holds a part-time position as Professor of Feminist Medical Research, University of Oslo, Norway. Her field of research deals with women's health, medical communication, and the theory of medicine, and her extensive list of publications includes articles reporting empirical research as well as methodological matters, book chapters, and an introductory book on qualitative methods in medical research.

HELEN E. McILVAIN, PhD, is Associate Professor, Department of Family Medicine, University of Nebraska Medical Center. Her research focus has been in the areas of smoking cessation and prevention, specifically looking at physician counseling behavior. She has contributed numerous articles and chapters on these topics. Since 1994, she has been a member of the Department of Family Medicine research division's qualitative analysis team, receiving on-the-job training in qualitative research. Recently, she adapted the genogram technique used in family systems therapy to the research division's current work in understanding the use of preventive services in family physicians' practices. The organizational genogram provides a clearer definition of the relational issues affecting the practice as well as potential avenues for change.

LYNN M. MEADOWS, PhD, is Assistant Professor and Alberta Heritage Foundation for Medical Research Population Health Investigator, Departments of Family Medicine and Community Health Sciences, University of Calgary. She has worked in the past as a research methodologist in the area of primary care. Her current research and writing foci are midlife women's experiences of health and health care utilization (the WHEALTH project) and case studies of seniors' experiences of acute health events. She is a qualified N4 instructor and is Adjunct Professor, International Institute for Qualitative Methodology and Department of Family Medicine, University of Alberta.

JESSICA H. MULLER, PhD, is a medical anthropologist and Assistant Professor, Department of Family and Community Medicine (DFCM) and Medical Anthropology Program, Department of Epidemiology and Biostatistics, University of California, San Francisco. She is currently Associate Director, DFCM Northern California Faculty Development Fellowship Program, as well as Associate Director, DFCM Medical Student Education Programs. Her research interests include professional socialization, death and dying, the culture of biomedicine, faculty development, and clinical teaching in medicine. She has published articles and book chapters in both the anthropological and medical literature that discuss the use of qualitative methods, including participant observation, stimulated recall using videotape, and in-depth interviewing.

KURT C. STANGE, MD, PhD, is Professor of Family Medicine, Epidemiology and Biostatistics, Oncology, and Sociology at Case Western Reserve University. A practicing family physician and epidemiologist, he is actively engaged in multimethod practice-based research designed to understand and improve primary care practice.

JANECKE THESEN, MD, is Research Fellow, Division for General Practice, University of Bergen, Norway, and has been a family doctor/ general practitioner for more than 20 years in a rural area in Norway. She is a specialist in Family Medicine and in Public Health. She is particularly interested in patient groups with serious or long-lasting illnesses that confine them to patient roles in major parts of their lives. Her writing and research interests spring from this, using both qualitative and quantitative methods.

HOWARD WAITZKIN, MD, PhD, is Professor and Director, Division of Community Medicine; Professor of Medicine; and Professor of Sociology, University of New Mexico. His work has focused on health policy in comparative international perspective and on psychosocial issues in primary care. He coauthored the proposal for a single-payer national health program that was published in the *New England Journal of Medicine* and later introduced in Congress. He has been involved in advocacy for improved health access and is currently conducting studies of Medicaid-managed care in New Mexico and the diffusion of managed care to Latin America, supported by the Agency for Health Care Policy and Research of the National Institutes of Health and by the World Health Organization. His work on patient-doctor communication and psychosocial issues in primary care is funded by the National Institute on Aging and the National Institute of Mental Health. He is the author of three books, including *The Politics of Medical Encounters: How Patients and Doctors Deal With Social Problems,* and more than 100 articles and chapters.

ROBERT L. WILLIAMS, MD, MPH, is Associate Professor, Department of Family Medicine, Case Western Reserve University. He is a Robert Wood Johnson Generalist Physician Faculty Scholar and a former Fulbright Senior Scholar. His professional work has centered on the delivery of health care to medically underserved populations, both domestic and international. He has conducted studies on methods for collecting and using qualitative data from communities in the planning and delivery of their health care.